Functional Disorders of the Gut

For Churchill Livingstone:

Senior Medical Editor: Rachael Stock
Project Supervisor: Mark Sanderson

Functional Disorders of the Gut

EDITED BY

Sidney F Phillips MD, FRCP, FACP
Professor of Medicine, Mayo Clinic and Mayo Medical School, Rochester, Minnesota, USA

David L Wingate DM, FRCP
Professor of Gastrointestinal Science, Royal London Hospital, London, UK

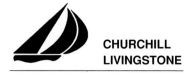

CHURCHILL LIVINGSTONE

LONDON EDINBURGH NEW YORK PHILADELPHIA SYDNEY TORONTO 1998

CHURCHILL LIVINGSTONE
is an imprint of Harcourt Brace and Company Limited

Harcourt Brace and Company Ltd 24–28 Oval Road
London NW1 7DX, UK

The Curtis Center
Independence Square West
Philadelphia, PA 19106-3399, USA

Harcourt Brace & Company
55 Horner Avenue
Toronto, Ontario M8Z 4X6, Canada

Harcourt Brace & Company, Australia
30–52 Smidmore Street
Marrickville, NSW 2204, Australia

Harcourt Brace & Company, Japan
Ichibancho Central Building, 22–1
Ichibancho, Chiyoda-ku,
Tokyo 102, Japan

A catalogue record for this book is available from the
British Library

ISBN 0–4430–5420–7

Typeset by Pure Tech India Limited, Pondicherry
Printed and bound in Hong Kong

Contents

SECTION 3
Functional disorders in context

Contributors

C Ainley, Newham General Hospital, London, UK

IJ Cook, Associate Professor of Medicine, University of New South Wales, St George Hospital, Kogarah, Australia

F Creed, Professor of Community Psychiatry, School of Psychiatry and Behavioural Sciences, Manchester Royal Infirmary, Manchester, UK

DF Evans, Reader in GI Science, St Bartholomew's and the Royal London School of Medicine & Dentistry, London, UK

W Gonsalkorale, Department of Medicine, University Hospital of South Manchester, Manchester, UK

WJ Hogan, Professor of Medicine, Medical College of Wisconsin, Milwaukee, USA

E Husebye, Consultant Physician, Department of Medicine, Ullevåal Hospital, Oslo, Norway

J-R Malagelada, a Professor of Digestive Diseases and Head Department of Digestive Diseases, Hospital General Vall'd' Hebron Autonomous, University of Barcelona, Spain

SF Phillips, Professor of Medicine, Department of Gastroenterology, Mayo Medical School and Clinic, Rochester, Minnesota, USA

CE Pope II, Division of Gastroenterology, University of Washington, Seattle, USA

RB Scott, Professor of Pediatrics, Alberta Children's Hospital, University of Calgary, Canada

AJPM Smout, Department of Gastroenterology, University Hospital Utrecht, The Netherlands

H Spiro, Professor of Medicine, Department of Internal Medicine, Yale University School of Medicine, New Haven, Connecticut, USA

DG Thompson, Professor of Gastroenterology, Hope Hospital, Salford, UK

WG Thompson, Professor of Medicine, Chief, Division of Gastroenterology, Ottawa Civic Hospital, Ottawa, Canada

RW Tobin, Division of Gastroenterology, University of Washington, Seattle, USA

PJ Whorwell, Consultant Physician Department of Medicine, University Hospital of South Manchester, Manchester, UK

DL Wingate, Professor of Gastrointestinal Science, GI Research Unit, University of London, London, UK

JD Wood, Professor of Physiology and Internal Medicine, Chairman, Department of Physiology, College of Medicine, Columbus, Ohio, USA

Preface

This book is an enterprise on which we embarked with some trepidation. The topic of functional disorders of the digestive tract is not characterised by a coherent corpus of solid scientific evidence, but rather by incomplete data and conflicting hypotheses. From an intellectually rigorous standpoint, there is a persuasive argument for a proper degree of reticence; rather than attempting to catalogue what might be regarded as scientific chaos, it would surely be better to wait until the dust of controversy has settled. This was our initial stance, but after protracted discussions with the publisher, we were persuaded by a compelling counter argument. This is the single undisputed fact in this field, which is that patients with functional disorders constitute the largest single cohort in gastroenterology clinics, and these ailments are a major cause of clinical, economic, and social morbidity. The patients are there now; neither they nor their physicians can indulge in the luxury of waiting for scientific certainty.

The structure of the book has been dictated by the complicated and incomplete contemporary scientific and clinical database. We cannot, at the time of writing, provide coherent accounts of the aetiology, pathophysiology, and management of specific disorders, while the identity of these problems is still obscure. The first section of the book deals with topics, including neurobiology, that we believe to be relevant to several, or even all, functional disorders of the gut. In the remainder of the book there are two parallel tracks through the successive regions of the digestive tract. The first summarises the present views on physiology and pathophysiology, while the second addresses the problems of clinical management. Finally, as a postscript to the book, an eminent contemporary who has seen it all before reminds us that there is nothing – or very little – new under the sun. This structure seemed to us to both logical and helpful to readers but, because of the nature of the topic, the boundaries between these compartments have defied precise delineation. Readers will find not only a degree of overlap between authors, but also occasional and perhaps inevitable discord. Rigorous editing could have produced a more discipline account, but such discipline would be arbitrary and artificial. As editors, we have no claim to superior knowledge, and no desire to indulge in scientific censorship.

We acknowledge that the science is not conclusive, and that the clinical strategies are sometimes arbitrary, but, nonetheless, we believe that physicians will find the information useful in helping them to understand the possible or even probable nature of these problems, and how they may be treated. Clinicians too often tend to dismiss functional disorders as trivial, or psychoneurotic, or the consequence of 'stress', but, in addition to being simplistic or even plain wrong, such judgements offer little comfort. It is our hope that the material in this book will enable doctors to provide insights for patients that will help them to cope with the chronic miseries of disturbed gut function.

Contributing to medical texts has to be regarded as a labour of love, as the material rewards are derisory; for this reason, we are all the more grateful to our contributors, all experts in their fields, for finding the time and energy to write chapters. They have made it possible, perhaps for the first time, to include, in a single volume, all the important information that is relevant to functional bowel disorders. We also acknowledge a debt of gratitude to Sheila Khullar who cajoled us into starting and persisting with this project. We hope that our readers will feel that it has all been worthwhile.

Sidney Phillips
David Wingate

Rochester, Minnesota, USA, & London, England

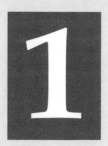

Biology of functional disorders

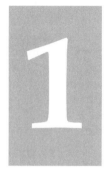

Functional anatomy and physiology

DL Wingate, SF Phillips

INTRODUCTION

The term 'functional disorders' implies, strictly speaking, a disorder of normal function, no less and no more. By convention, its usage in medicine is restricted to disorders in which the pathology and pathophysiology have yet to be identified. The emphasis on disordered motor activity in the discussion of functional gastrointestinal disorders might seem, at first sight, to be excessive, given that motility is only one of the functions of the digestive system. There is, however, a considerable surplus capacity of the other major functions – digestion, secretion and absorption – which allows compensation for major deficits in the tissues that subserve these functions. For example, the loss of more than half the exocrine pancreas or the entire production of gastric acid will still leave sufficient digestive capacity to enable the complete assimilation of food and if the jejunum is removed or excluded, the ileum is capable of increasing its absorptive capacity to compensate for the loss.

In this context, motility is the 'Achilles heel' of gut function; even modest alterations in the pattern of flow along the digestive tube can lead to significant derangement of the digestive process. Symptoms likely to be provoked by altered patterns of flow are integral to disorders of function; such symptoms include dysphagia, nausea, vomiting, bloating, abdominal pain, constipation and diarrhea. It must not be forgotten, however, that although the presence of such symptoms implies altered function, this relationship cannot be assumed.

WHAT IS MOTILITY?

Motility is a term that has been used for many years to denote an area of research interest but lacks precise definition and cannot be quantified; it refers to the propulsive nature of the digestive tube without distinguishing between the movement of material along the gut and the contractile mechanisms that govern flow. For many years, the smooth muscle of the gut was the focus of interest for research into motility but more recently, with the progress of research in the neurobiology of the enteric nervous system, attention has moved towards the systems that control movement and, in particular, to the innervation of the gut. As with the locomotor system, disordered gut motility has proved to be more commonly due to disorders of control rather than defective function of the smooth muscle itself. It is important to remember that the external operations of the gut – ingestion and excretion – are behavioral patterns that are governed by social constraints. The need to eat only two or three meals in a day and to defecate only once enables humans to devote much of their waking time to other activities. It is the property of motility that links the sporadic and voluntary acts of ingestion and excretion with the continuous physicochemical process of assimilation of nutrient and water and the separation of waste. When motility is disordered, it is projected into consciousness as difficulties with eating or defecation.

THE TRANSIT OF THE GUT

Because the mouth is higher than the anus, there is a tendency to assume that gravity is, at least to some degree, a factor in the propulsion of material through the digestive tube. In fact, gravity plays little part; it is the smooth muscle that mediates propulsion. The great difference in speed of transit through the different regions of the gut (Fig. 1.1) reflects the complexity of the movements of the gut wall and the close relation between structure and function. Each end of the gut has a reservoir capacity; the stomach retains a complete meal for slow and continuous delivery to the digestive zone of the small intestine, while the distal colon and rectum retain feces until expulsion is socially convenient. Transit time is a misleading concept except in the esophagus, where contents introduced at one end are rapidly propelled to the other by a sterotypic sequence of peristaltic movement; it is the only segment of the gut where there is no physicochemical modification of the contents. With a meal, the stomach is rapidly filled but emptying is a slow and prolonged process; the gastric transit of one fraction of the meal may be only a matter of minutes while for another, it may be a matter of hours. Marker studies have shown that small bowel transit is relatively constant but it must be remembered that most of the material that enters the

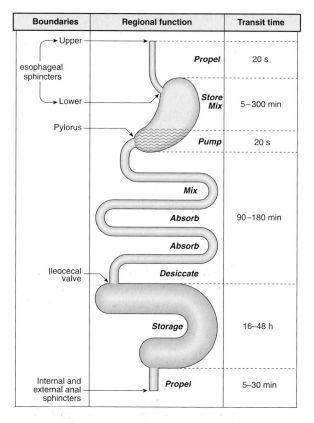

Boundaries	Regional function	Transit time
Upper esophageal sphincters	Propel	20 s
Lower	Store Mix	5–300 min
Pylorus	Pump	20 s
	Mix	
	Absorb	90–180 min
	Absorb	
Ileocecal valve	Desiccate	
	Storage	16–48 h
Internal and external anal sphincters	Propel	5–30 min

Fig. 1.1 Functional organization of the digestive tract. The different speeds at which luminal contents travel through the digestive tube (right) are related to the main functions of the region of the gut (center) and the residence time reflects the time required for material to be processed. The function of the sphincters within the gut (left) appears to be to prevent the retrograde transit of material; only the oropharynx and the anus, both partially under conscious control, act as barriers to onward flow.

duodenum will be absorbed before reaching the distal ileum. Colonic transit is again an unreal concept since colonic filling is gradual but emptying is abrupt, infrequent and incomplete.

The luminal continuity of the gut can be interrupted by *sphincters* (Fig. 1.1), specialized muscle zones that mark the boundaries of different segments. Physiologically, these serve to prevent retrograde flow rather than regulate forward flow, as the luminal contents of one segment may be destructive in the preceding segment: gastric acid damages the esophageal mucosa, pancreatobiliary secretions damage the gastric mucosa and colonic reflux into the ileum can lead to bacterial overgrowth of the small bowel. The sphincter arrangement at each end of the digestive tube is similar, with a sphincter under voluntary control on the outside and a smooth muscle sphincter on the inside; the difference is that proximally the interposition of the chest cavity between the pharynx and stomach requires the sphincter zones to be connected by a propulsive tube, whereas distally the sphincters are adjacent.

PERISTALSIS: THE UNIT OF PROPULSION

The 'building block' with which complex patterns of movement in the gut are constructed is peristalsis. This is discussed in more detail in the next chapter but it can be summarized by the statement that the presence of material in the digestive tube reflexly stimulates contraction orad to and relaxation aborad to the stimulus, thus propelling the bolus in an aboral direction to a new location where the same sequence is repeated. Stereotypic peristalsis that traverses an entire segment is only invariable in the esophagus, accounting for the rapid transit; in the rest of the gut, the incidence and spread of peristalsis is regulated by complex patterns of inhibition. In the stomach and small intestine, smooth muscle is governed by a cyclical and propagated pattern of excitation – the electrical slow wave or basic electrical rhythm – whose frequency is specific to the location (Fig. 1.2). Originally thought to be a property of the smooth muscle syncytium itself, it is now thought that the electrical rhythmicity is conferred by the interstitial cells of Cajal (ICCs), which act as an interface between smooth muscle and motor neurons; there is a close correlation between the density of ICCs and the dominance of rhythmicity.

Where the electrical rhythm is dominant, each wave of depolarization provides an opportunity for muscle contraction or the initiation of peristalsis, analogous to the electrical pacing of the myocardium. In the myocardium, however, the relation between depolarization and contraction is obligate whereas in the gut, it is the neural control networks that determine whether or not contraction will occur. It is this flexibility that allows complex patterns of contraction to occur. In 1921, in describing electrical rhythmicity for the first time, Walter Alvarez remarked that it reminded him of the engine of a car running, with motion not occurring until the clutch was engaged. Perhaps a more useful analogy is an octave on the keyboard of a piano. If all 10 fingers are used to strike notes on the beat, the resulting noise is monotonous, but by inhibiting most or all of the fingers on each beat according to a predetermined composition, different tunes can be played.

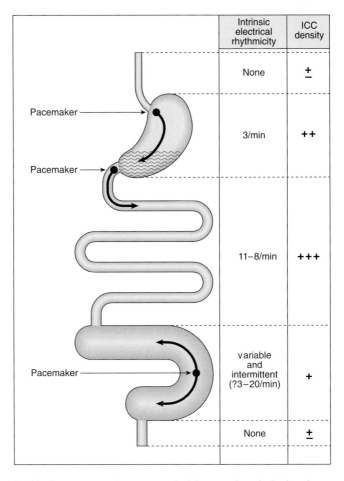

	Intrinsic electrical rhythmicity	ICC density
	None	±
Pacemaker	3/min	++
Pacemaker		
	11–8/min	+++
Pacemaker	variable and intermittent (?3–20/min)	+
	None	±

Fig. 1.2   Much controversy has surrounded the question of whether the regulation of gut function is 'myogenic' or 'neurogenic'. The key elements of the smooth muscle system are the pacemakers that confer rhythmicity; the pacemaking properties appear to be a function of the interstitial cells of Cajal (ICCs) and these cellular elements are found in the greatest numbers (right) where pacemaking and rhythmicity are prominent.

THE NEUROCHEMICAL CONTROL OF THE GUT

In the preceding section, complex control systems of gut function are postulated but it is only relatively recently that a coherent picture of these systems has begun to emerge. The neural components of this control system are the central nervous system (CNS), the enteric nervous system (ENS) and the two divisions of the autonomic nervous system (ANS), parasympathetic and sympathetic, that link ENS and CNS. In addition to neural control,

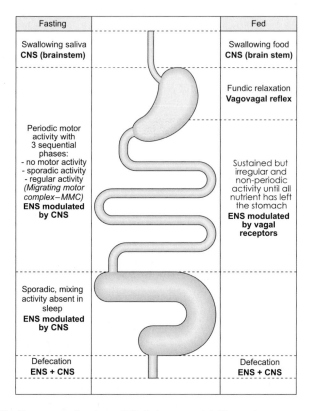

Fasting		Fed
Swallowing saliva **CNS (brainstem)**		Swallowing food **CNS (brain stem)**
		Fundic relaxation **Vagovagal reflex**
Periodic motor activity with 3 sequential phases: - no motor activity - sporadic activity - regular activity *(Migrating motor complex–MMC)* **ENS modulated by CNS**		Sustained but irregular and non-periodic activity until all nutrient has left the stomach **ENS modulated by vagal receptors**
Sporadic, mixing activity absent in sleep **ENS modulated by CNS**		
Defecation **ENS + CNS**		Defecation **ENS + CNS**

Fig. 1.3 Programmed motor activity is 'neurogenic'. The motor programs of the gut are resident in the enteric nervous system (ENS), but they can be modulated by the central nervous system (CNS). The entry and exit of material into and from the digestive tract is under CNS control (eating, drinking, defecation), but is coordinated with specialized local motor activities (esophageal peristalsis, internal anal sphincter relaxation).

some measure of regulation is provided by changing plasma levels of peptides ('hormones') released from the gut wall.

It has already been pointed out that entry to and exit from the gut (eating, drinking and defecation) are behavioral patterns under voluntary control. Except for swallowing, the programs of functional activity that determine the operations of the digestive tube on its contents appear to be largely within the domain of the ENS, but these programs are modulated by the activity of the CNS (Fig. 1.3).

Enteric nervous system (ENS)

The enteric nervous system consists not only of the intrinsic nerve plexuses of the gut wall, mainly the myenteric (Auerbach) and submucosal (Meissner) plexuses, but also the prevertebral ganglia. The nature and function of the ENS are considered in more detail in the following chapter but the main features are:

1. *The ENS provides the motor neurons to gut smooth muscle and mucosa.* It is important to appreciate that the gut structures are *not* directly innervated by sympathetic and parasympathetic fibers that synapse with ENS ganglia, but by the postganglionic fibers of the ENS.
2. *The ENS includes sensory afferents from mucosa and muscle to the ganglionic network.* These are only a proportion of gut afferents (see below), probably subserving touch (from the mucosa) and tension (from the muscle), but they are essential components of the peristaltic reflex.
3. *The neural circuitry of the ENS contains 'hard-wired' programs that determine gut function.* The program that has been most clearly identified is the fasting motor activity program marked by the recurrence of migrating motor complexes (MMCs), described in more detail in Chapter 12. The value of studying a phenomenon that is only present in the fasting state – and therefore of dubious physiological significance – has been questioned. The clinical relevance of the MMC is that (a) it has been clearly established in transplantation studies that the MMC program resides within the ENS and (b) it is the only validated index of ENS integrated activity that can be monitored in vivo. The circuitry that generates the MMC remains to be identified because MMC activity does not occur in ex vivo preparations of gut.

The prevertebral ganglia

The prevertebral (celiac, superior mesenteric, inferior mesenteric) ganglia are structures through which extrinsic nerve fibers run between the gut and the spinal cord; some terminate on the cell bodies of the prevertebral ganglia while others, such as small fibers mediating pain, pass through the ganglia without forming synapses. The ganglia not only form synapses between gut and spinal cord but also allow synapses between nerve fibers from the gut and cell bodies that project back to the gut directly or through intermesenteric nerves to other prevertebral ganglia (Fig. 1.4). Thus they form relay stations in a pathway of rapid communication between distant parts of the gut. These pathways serve *enteroenteric inhibitory reflexes* in which distension of one part of the gut will inhibit contractile activity in a remote area. It has been

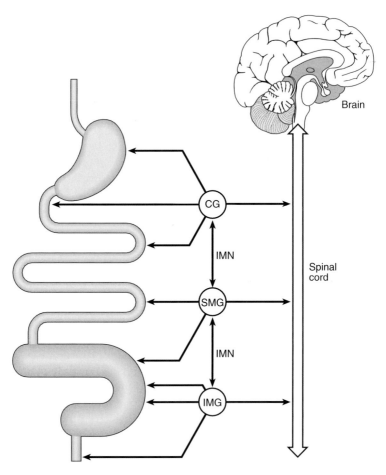

Fig. 1.4 The prevertebral ganglia (CG, celiac ganglion; SMG, superior mesenteric ganglion; IMG, inferior mesenteric ganglion) not only provide pathways between the spinal cord and the gut but also, via the intermesenteric nerves (IMN), enable information to be rapidly transmitted over long distances of the digestive tube. They provide pathways for enteroenteric reflexes, in which stimulation of one part of the gut affects function at a remote location.

shown, for example, that painless distension of the rectum will inhibit food-stimulated contractile activity in the proximal small bowel. They are also the probable route of the reflex response known as the *gastrocolonic response*, which is the stimulation of colonic motor activity by the arrival of a meal in the stomach.

The autonomic nervous system (ANS)

Before the recognition of the controlling function of the ENS, the parasympathetic and sympathetic pathways between brain and

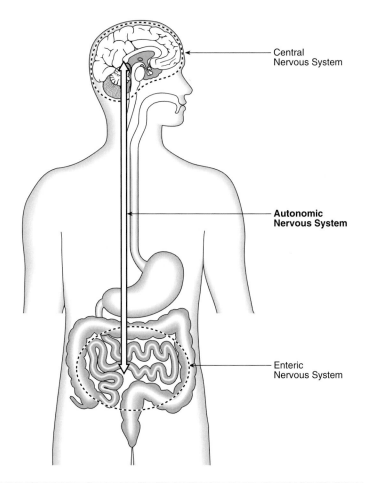

Central
Nervous System

**Autonomic
Nervous System**

Enteric
Nervous System

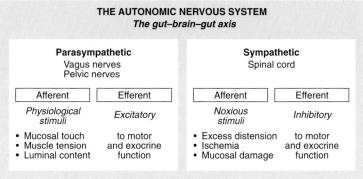

THE AUTONOMIC NERVOUS SYSTEM
The gut–brain–gut axis

Parasympathetic Vagus nerves Pelvic nerves		**Sympathetic** Spinal cord	
Afferent	Efferent	Afferent	Efferent
Physiological stimuli	*Excitatory*	*Noxious stimuli*	*Inhibitory*
• Mucosal touch • Muscle tension • Luminal content	to motor and exocrine function	• Excess distension • Ischemia • Mucosal damage	to motor and exocrine function

Fig. 1.5 The principal function of the two divisions of the autonomic nervous system that innervate the gut is the transmission of information between the enteric nervous system and the central nervous system.

gut were considered to be no more than the efferent pathways that allowed the CNS to control motor and secretory function in the gut. It is now recognized that these pathways have an important *afferent* function in the transmission of information from the gut to the brain. The parasympathetic (vagus and pelvic) nerves probably relay information on muscle movement and gut content, while the sympathetic (spinal) afferents are the route for the transmission of nociceptive (distension, inflammation) stimuli (Fig. 1.5). It has been estimated that 75–90% of vagal fibres are sensory afferents; the proportion of sensory afferents in the spinal innervation is not known but is likely to be similar. Autonomic motor efferents synapse on the ganglia of the ENS; in general, the parasympathetic fibers utilizing acetylcholine as a transmitter are excitatory while sympathetic fibers, with noradrenaline (norepinephrine) as transmitter, are inhibitory.

The sensory afferent activity of the autonomic nervous system is probably an important factor in the pathogenesis of functional disorders. Animal studies have shown that information on the activity and contents of the digestive tube is continuously relayed to the CNS, but human experience shows that this is not normally projected into consciousness. It has recently been shown, using non-invasive techniques in humans, that this information may reach the cerebral cortex even though it is not consciously perceived. Symptoms of gut dysfunction, which can be evoked by distension of the gut, appear to be marked by an increase in the traffic of information arriving in the brain. Normally, the amplification of afferent information is produced by increased stimulation within the gut, but if such amplification occurs within the brain, it would explain the genesis of symptoms in the absence of significant gut dysfunction (Fig. 1.6).

The vagovagal reflex arc

Vagovagal reflexes are a major pathway for initiating and maintaining the secretory and motor response of the gut to food. The chemosensitive receptors of the stomach and proximal small bowel, and also some of the touch and tension receptors of the gut wall, are vagal and they are the main system for the detection of the arrival and transit of a meal. Thus, the activity of the ENS in organizing the secretory and motor response to a meal is dependent on information that is transmitted along afferent fibers to the dorsal vagal complex in the brainstem and thence by descending vagal fibres to the ENS ganglia (Fig. 1.7). Disruption of this reflex arc by, for example, truncal vagotomy results in an

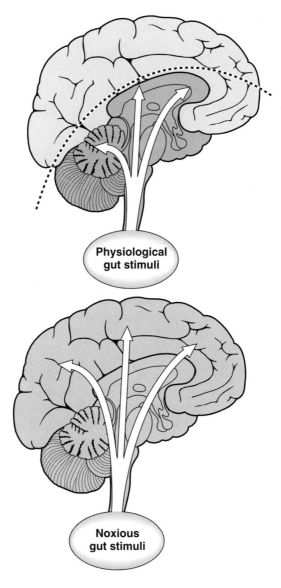

Physiological gut stimuli

Noxious gut stimuli

Fig. 1.6 Physiological stimulation of the gut results in the transmission of information to the brain (above) but there appears to be a functional barrier that prevents this information being projected to the cortex and thus into consciousness. For noxious stimuli (below) this barrier is removed so that, for example, excessive distension of the gut results in consciously perceived visceral pain. It is possible that some functional disorders occur because normal physiological changes (such as a full stomach) penetrate the functional brain barrier and, being projected into consciousness, are interpreted as noxious stimuli. It is also possible that sensitization of sensory receptors in the gut leads to a phsyiological change being recorded as noxious rather than normal.

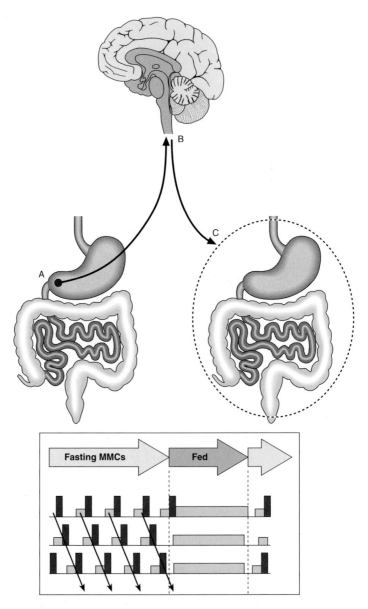

Fig. 1.7 The vagovagal pathway is utilized in the gut motor response to the presence of food. Vagal sensory receptors in the duodenum (A) convey the information about the arrival of food via the afferent vagus and the dorsal vagal complex (B) to the enteric nervous system (C); this information is distributed along the nervous systems via the prevertebral ganglia (see Fig. 1.4) so that the enteric nervous system alters activity not only in the stomach but also throughout the small and large bowel. The major change (lower panel) is the abolition of the fasting MMC pattern, which persists until all nutrient has left the stomach.

impaired and abbreviated response to food. This has been used therapeutically to blunt the gastric secretory response to food but the impaired motor response that is an inevitable accompaniment is responsible for the motor dysfunctions induced by feeding following vagotomy.

The central nervous system (CNS)

It is accepted without question that the activities that govern the filling of the digestive tube (eating, drinking and swallowing) are CNS functions, as is the act of defecation, since it is evident that these are conscious decisions. It is now also clear that CNS activity exerts a continuous modulatory activity on gut function. The motor activity of the small bowel and the colon is normally greatly altered during the diminished CNS arousal state of sleep. It has also been demonstrated that enhanced CNS arousal induced by stress also alters gut function; two such effects are a reduced rate of gastric emptying and an enhanced gastrocolonic motor response following a meal. Extensive studies on rats have shown that this is probably due to the release of corticotrophin-releasing factor (CRF) but, as yet, it remains to be confirmed that CRF release is an important mechanism in the modulation of gut activity by stress in humans.

Chemical (hormonal) control

Before the development of biochemical techniques for identifying molecules, hormones could only be detected by bioassay and the first hormone to be demonstrated in this way was secretin, by Bayliss and Starling in 1905. The existence of gastrin was proposed shortly afterwards by Edkins. Subsequently, cholecystokinin (CCK) and pancreozymin (PZ) were similarly identified as separate substances, until advances in chemistry showed them to be the same molecule. For the next few decades, it was generally accepted that there were three gastrointestinal hormones – gastrin, secretin and CCK-PZ – which were together responsible for the exocrine secretory response to a meal.

This coherent but limited concept of hormonal control of gut function was shattered during the two decades from 1970 by the discovery of numerous other peptides released from the gut into the circulation; many of these peptides had close structural affinities with gastrin and CCK or with secretin. From these discoveries a new view of gut endocrinology evolved, in which it was proposed that changes in humoral levels of these 'gut hormones' are the major controlling factors of gut secretory and motor function. Complex theories of hormonal control were elaborated, including not only endocrine actions (influence on remote target cells) but also paracrine actions (influence on adjacent cells).

The 'new dawn' in gut endocrinology has, however, not been sustained. At first it seemed likely that the new 'gut hormones', like gastrin, CCK and secretin, were released from specialized endocrine cells within the gut mucosa and this release was initiated by mucosal contact with different types of nutrient molecules. It then became clear that most, if not all, of these peptides were present in the neurons of the enteric nervous system and subsequently, that many were also present in the brain. It also became clear that many of the experiments in animal and human subjects from which 'hormonal' control of gut function was derived involved parenteral administration of peptides that were pharmacological but not physiological. It now seems likely that changes in the humoral levels of many of the plasma peptides signal rather than operate changes in function.

There does appear to be a measure of agreement on some functions of some of the 'regulatory peptides', as 'gut hormones' are now known.

- *Gastrin* is a true hormone. Released from the gastric antrum by mucosal stimulation into the bloodstream, it stimulates the parietal cells of the fundus to secrete hydrochloric acid.
- *Somatostatin* is a locally acting peptide that modulates the response of gastric parietal cells to gastrin and to cholinergic stimulation.
- Larger molecular forms of *cholecystokinin* (CCK-17 and CCK-34) may mediate gall bladder contraction and pancreatobiliary secretion but this may be complementary to neural control; *cholecystokinin octapeptide* (CCK-8) is probably a neurotransmitter in both gut and brain.
- *Pancreatic polypeptide* (PP) is a marker of vagal stimulation of the pancreas.
- *Substance P* is an important neurotransmitter in the ENS.
- *Motilin* is a marker of phase III of the MMC in the stomach and duodenum and motilin release may be a factor in the genesis of the contractile pattern of phase III. It is also unique among gut peptides in not being also a CNS peptide.
- *Vasoactive intestinal peptide* (VIP) is an important neuromodulator or neurotransmitter in the gut;

Hirschsprung's disease and achalasia of the cardia are marked by localized deficiencies of neurons containing VIP.
- *Neuropeptide Y* is a brain–gut regulatory peptide that may be important in the regulation of appetite and satiety.
- *Serotonin (5-hydroxytryptamine)* (5-HT) is an important neurotransmitter and/or neuromodulator in the ENS.

Scientists who are engaged in the study of the regulatory peptides of the gut may argue that the preceding list of peptide functions is incomplete, but many of their peers who are less involved and thus better placed to take a more detached view of the published evidence would argue that proofs of physiological actions that have been claimed are missing. For example, there are many reports of experiments in which gut peptides have been injected into the cerebral ventricles of laboratory animals and have induced changes in gut function, leading to claims that specific peptides 'play a role in the control of' specific gut functions, but the evidence that such effects occur in humans is lacking.

As for functional disorders, the only peptide that has been implicated in functional disorders is CCK; some evidence suggests that increased sensitivity to circulating CCK and/or increased release into the circulation may be part of the pathophysiology of the irritable bowel syndrome, but, again, conclusive evidence is lacking.

The brain–gut axis

In recent years, there has been much scientific and popular interest in the concept of the 'brain–gut axis'; for scientists because it is a fruitful area for the study of neural control systems and for the layman, because the effect of mood and thought on gut function is part of everyday experience. There is, for the man in the street, nothing new in the idea that the brain communicates with the gut.

What is important for the physician to appreciate is that this axis is a pathway for the bidirectional transmission of information between two nervous systems that are largely autonomous. The enteric nervous system can regulate gut function without central intervention; the effect of central nervous system activity is to perturb rather than enhance gut function. Functional disorders that depend upon the brain–gut axis are marked by the fact that dysfunction only occurs during the waking state. The irritable bowel syndrome (IBS) is a prime example of this; in contrast to diseases that are due to organic damage of the gut such as inflammatory bowel disease, IBS patients spend undisturbed nights.

We are thus left to consider the novel possibility that some functional disorders are due to disturbance of the normal interaction between brain and gut and for the dysfunction to be expressed, both systems must be operational (Fig. 1.5). Two consequences follow from this; first, the targets for specific therapy might be either at gut level or in the brain or both and, secondly, that if patients are aware of this, they will be better placed to understand why lifestyle changes may be an important limb of therapy.

SUMMARY

The digestive tract has, as discussed above, multiple controls, that are linked so as to ensure the assimilation of nutrient and the storage and rejection of waste. Functional disorders may be the consequence of no more than faulty interaction of the different elements that regulate transit; organ or system failure is not a required condition of dysfunction. Familiarity with computer technology has taught us that apparently trivial defects may disable complex programs and this may explain why the search for pathology in functional disorders has, so far, been largely in vain. The interdependence of the different elements of normal function also serves to illustrate why apparently similar dysfunctions may have diverse origins.

Enteric neuropathobiology

JD Wood

INTRODUCTION

The nervous system of the digestive tract controls contraction of the musculature, secretion and absorption by the mucosa and blood flow. Thus, the musculature, epithelium, blood and lymphatic vasculatures are effector systems of the gut (Cooke et al 1993, Wood 1993). Neural release of excitatory neurotransmitters evokes contractions of the muscles, whereas inhibitory transmitters suppress contractility. Malfunctions of these mechanisms are increasingly recognized as factors underlying the functional bowel disorders. The enteric nervous system is a 'minibrain', within which is stored a library of programs for different patterns of gut behavior. A specific program determines behavior in the postprandial state and another establishes the behavior characteristic for the fasting state. Upon intake of a meal, the program for the fasting state is switched off and the postprandial program is ordered into action. Emesis is another program which directs propulsion in the upper small intestine to be reversed for rapid movement of the contents toward the stomach. This program can be called from the library either by commands from the brain or by local sensory detection of noxious substances in the lumen (Lang & Sarna 1989). These and the other concepts explored here expand upon the overview of Chapter 1.

INNERVATION OF THE DIGESTIVE TRACT: PHYSIOLOGICAL PRINCIPLES

The digestive system is innervated by the autonomic nervous system; the sympathetic, parasympathetic and enteric divisions of the autonomic nervous system, together with sensory nerves from the spinal cord and brainstem, innervate the gut. Sensory nerves share some of the same projection pathways, as do the efferent autonomic nerves. *Sympathetic* and *parasympathetic* pathways transmit signals from the central nervous system to the gut. *Neurons of the enteric division* make up the local control circuits within the wall of the gut. The functional innervation includes interconnections between the brain, spinal cord and enteric nervous system.

The enteric nervous system

The enteric nervous system is populated by as many neurons as the spinal cord. This number of neurons required for the fine control of digestive processes would be excessive if inserted directly in the central nervous system. Rather, vertebrates have evolved systems in which most circuits for automatic control of gut function are placed close to the digestive effector systems.

Cell bodies of the neurons that make up the control circuits of the enteric nervous system are in ganglia inside the walls of the gut. The ganglia, together with interganglionic connections, form

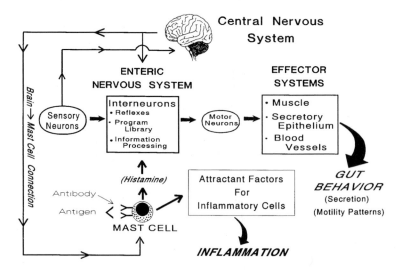

Fig. 2.1 The enteric nervous system behaves as an independent integrative nervous system, with functions like a 'minibrain'. It processes information derived from sensory neurons and inflammatory immune cells. Interneuronal processing involves reflex microcircuits and a library of programs responsible for stereotypic behaviors of the digestive tract. These include effects on systems that modulate motor, secretory and circulatory function. Mast cells detect threatening antigens and release several paracrine mediators simultaneously. Some mediators alert the enteric nervous system while others act as attractants for the inflammatory response. The central nervous system signals the enteric nervous system by direct neural pathways and through brain–mast cell connections.

a system that integrates and processes information like the brain and spinal cord. This underlies reference to the enteric nervous system as the 'brain in the gut'.

The enteric nervous system is organized as an independent integrative system, with information processing, reflex circuits and a library of motor programs placed in the wall of the bowel. Figure 2.1 is a conceptual diagram illustrating this.

Sensory neurons

The cell bodies of sensory neurons are in the nodose ganglia of the vagal nerves, the dorsal root ganglia and the enteric nervous system. Sensory afferent fibers of the nodose and dorsal root ganglia transmit information from the gastrointestinal tract to the central nervous system for processing; indeed, most fibers in the vagal nerves are sensory. Sensory neurons send a steady stream of information to the local processing circuits in the gut (mini-brain) and carry signals to prevertebral sympathetic ganglia and the central nervous system. The gut has mechano-, chemo- and thermoreceptors. Mechanoreceptors supply both the enteric minibrain and the central nervous system with information on the degree of stretch in the wall and on the movement of luminal contents as they brush the mucosal surface. Chemoreceptors generate information on the concentration of nutrients, osmolarity and pH in the luminal contents. Thermoreceptors supply the brain with deep-body temperature information used in-regulation.

Whether the sensory cell bodies for muscle stretch receptors belong to dorsal root ganglia, enteric ganglia or both is uncertain (Wood 1994, Furness et al 1995). Stretch-sensitive mechanoreceptors have pathophysiologic importance because a consistent finding in patients diagnosed with the irritable bowel syndrome is abnormally high sensitivity to stretch that translates into pain (Whitehead et al 1990, Lembo et al 1994). Heightened sensitivity to distension and conscious awareness of the GI tract, experienced by IBS patients, is a generalized phenomenon throughout the gut, including the esophagus (Richter et al 1986). The mechanism is unclear. However, three general explanations are apparent:

1. hypersignals from sensitized mechanoreceptors may be accurately decoded by the brain as hyperdistension;
2. a malfunctioning brain may be misinterpreting accurate information;

3. combined malfunctions of sensing and central processing could be occurring.

Hyposensory perception, particularly in the rectosigmoid region, is the opposite gastrointestinal sensory abnormality. Sensory suppression in this region of the gut, either in the pathway for rectoanal stretch reflexes or in the transmission pathway from the rectosigmoid to conscious perception of distension, can be an underlying factor in the pathogenesis of chronic constipation (Loening-Baucke & Yamada 1995).

Transduction of mucosal mechanoreception differs from the mechanism of transduction for muscle mechanoreceptors. Brushing the intestinal mucosa releases 5-hydroxytryptamine from enterochromaffin cells in proportion to the strength of the stimulus. The change in spike frequency in the enteric neuron becomes a transform of the stimulus strength that can be decoded by the enteric processing circuitry. This mechanism, first proposed by Bulbring & Lin (1959), is supported by evidence from recent research (Kirchgessner et al 1992, Sidhu & Cooke 1995).

Sensory transduction of chemosensitive information on nutrient concentrations in the small bowel utilizes cholecystokinin and the mechanism mimics sensory function in a taste bud (Fujita 1991). Mucosal enteroendocrine cells 'taste' the lumen and release cholecystokinin in direct proportion to the concentration of products of protein digestion and lipids. The vagal sensory fibers branch in the wall of the stomach and upper small bowel for simultaneous transmission to both the big brain and the enteric minibrain (Berthoud & Powley 1992). The spike frequency transmitted by each sensory neuron thereby becomes a transform of the stimulus strength for simultaneous decoding in the brain and enteric processing circuitry. The neuronal receptors for cholecystokinin belong to the CCK-A subtype (Smith et al 1985, Davison & Clarke 1988).

In vitro, receptors for both cholecystokinin and 5-hydroxytryptamine initiate spike discharge in vagal sensory nerve terminals. The 5-hydroxytryptamine receptors belong to the 5-HT_3 subtype. Identification of these receptors is relevant to the antiemetic efficacy of 5-HT_3 receptor antagonists. Vagal sensory mechanisms involving cholecystokinin are implicated in the complex nervous functions involved in the sensations of satiety and control of food intake (Smith et al 1985).

Interneurons

Interneurons are interposed between sensory and motor neuronal pools. Millions of synaptic connections between interneurons form the information-processing circuitry of the enteric nervous system. Synapses are made between axons and cell bodies, between axons and dendrites and from axon to axon. As in the central nervous system, the internuncial microcircuits account for the emergent functions responsible for the organized behavior of the effector systems.

Motor neurons

Motor neurons innervate the effector systems. The motor neuron pool includes both excitatory and inhibitory neurons. Excitatory motor neurons release neurotransmitters that stimulate the effector cells, whereas inhibitory motor transmitters suppress activity in the effector cells.

Enteric reflexes

Reflex responses reflect behaviors of the effector systems evoked by activation of sensory neurons. In a reflex circuit, sensory neurons connect with interneurons and interneurons connect to motor neurons. The pattern of effector behavior in a reflex response is stereotyped. It is always the same because the connections in the reflex circuit are 'hard-wired'. For example, brushing the intestinal mucosa initiates a motility ('peristaltic') reflex consisting of contraction of the circular muscle coat above the site and reflex inhibition of the circular muscle below the stimulus site. This pattern is reproduced each time the mucosal mechanosensors are activated.

Motor programs

Synaptic connections between interneurons form circuits responsible for programmed behavior of the effector systems. These are pattern-generating circuits with a repertoire of stored motor programs. The programs drive the motor neurons for control of repetitive cyclic behaviors, such as the cyclic patterns of intestinal motility observed after a meal. They determine the sequence of events in stereotyped repetitions of motor outflow to the effector systems. Programmed motor behavior, unlike reflex responses, is not initiated by sensory input and feedback from sensory neurons is not needed for the sequencing of the steps in the program. For repetitive behaviors generated by programmed motor circuits (e.g. walking, chewing, swimming), the motor program may be started by input signals from neurons called command neurons or by overlaying the circuit with a chemical neuromodulatory substance of neurocrine, endocrine or paracrine origin.

NEURONAL MOTOR PHYSIOLOGY

Enteric motor neurons are the final common pathways to the gastric, intestinal and esophageal effector systems (i.e. musculature, mucosa and blood vasculature). The effectors may be innervated by excitatory or inhibitory motor neurons or by both. Enteric excitatory motor neurons innervate mucosal secretory glands and stimulate secretion when they release their neurotransmitters at the neuroepithelial junctions. Motor neurons to the musculature are generally found in the myenteric plexus; those to the intestinal crypts and submucous vasculature are in the submucous plexus.

Motor neurons and peristaltic propulsion

Coordinated activation of both inhibitory and excitatory motor neurons to the musculature is an important component of basic peristaltic propulsion. Peristaltic propulsion is a neurally mediated pattern of intestinal motor behavior consisting of a propulsive and receiving segment (Fig. 2.2; Wood 1993, 1994). Propagated propulsion over extended distances occurs as receiving segments convert to propulsive segments while the next segment downstream becomes a receiving segment. This fundamental behavior is programmed in the internuncial circuits. It behaves like a polysynaptic spinal-motor reflex in response to gut distension or brushing the mucosa. The program simultaneously activates inhibitory motor neurons in the receiving segment and inactivates inhibition in the propulsive segment. At the same time, the program activates excitatory motor neurons to the longitudinal muscle of the receiving segment and inactivates excitatory input to the longitudinal muscle in the propulsive segment. The effect of one cycle of the program in a segment of intestine or along the esophagus is to relax the circular muscle while contracting the longitudinal muscle in the receiving segment. This expands the lumen and facilitates filling of the receiving segment with incoming material from the propulsive segment. Mounting evidence suggests that the neural program for peristalsis includes stimulation of mucosal secretion of mucus, water and electrolytes

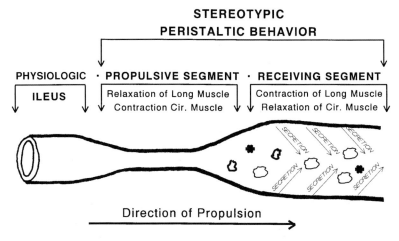

STEREOTYPIC
PERISTALTIC BEHAVIOR

PHYSIOLOGIC · **PROPULSIVE SEGMENT** · **RECEIVING SEGMENT**

ILEUS

Relaxation of Long Muscle
Contraction Cir. Muscle

Contraction of Long Muscle
Relaxation of Cir. Muscle

Direction of Propulsion

Fig. 2.2 Peristaltic propulsion is a stereotypic pattern (reflex) of muscle behavior. The receiving segment is formed by contraction of the longitudinal muscle and relaxation of the circular muscle. In the propulsive segment, the longitudinal muscle is relaxed while the circular muscle contracts. Secretomotor neurons are also activated, evoking secretion of electrolytes, water and mucus during formation of the receiving segment. The propulsive segment returns to a state of physiologic ileus (absence of activity) when peristaltic propulsion propagates to the next intestinal segment.

into the lumen of the receiving segment as the myomotor component of the program expands the segment.

Inhibitory motor innervation

Inhibitory motor neurons to the musculature are uniaxonal neurons with characteristic morphology. Nitric oxide (NO) and vasoactive intestinal polypeptide (VIP) are identified as the inhibitory neurotransmitters (Sanders & Ward 1992, Makhlouf & Grider 1993. However, an inhibitory role for purine nucleotides cannot be ruled out.

Binding of the inhibitory neurotransmitter to its receptors on the muscles leads to *hyperpolarization* of the membrane potential. Inhibitory junction potentials hyperpolarize the muscle membranes away from the threshold for action potentials and thereby prevent contractions.

Inhibitory neural control of the intestinal circular muscle differs from sphincteric circular muscle. A subset of inhibitory motor neurons for the circular muscle are continuously active; responses of the muscle occur when the inhibitory neurons are switched off by input from interneurons in the control circuits. In sphincters, the inhibitory neurons are normally off and are turned on with timing appropriate for coordination of sphincter opening with physiological events in adjacent regions.

Motor diseases characterized by 'disinhibition'

Malfunction of inhibitory motor neurons is the pathophysiologic basis of disinhibitory motor disease. It underlies several forms of chronic intestinal pseudoobstruction and sphincteric achalasia. The congenital absence of inhibitory motor neurons in Hirschsprung's disease is the cause of the constricted-hyperactive circular muscle in the terminal large bowel segment of the afflicted individual (Wood 1973, Wood et al 1986). Without inhibitory control, contractions of the autogenic musculature are continuous and disorganized. Inhibitory neuronal dysplasia also explains the findings of achalasia in the internal anal sphincter in Hirschsprung patients. Achalasia of the lower esophageal sphincter is likewise associated with loss of enteric inhibitory neurons (Csendes et al 1992). Some forms of biliary dyskinesia can be related to loss of inhibitory motor neurons and failure of relaxation of contractile tone in the sphincter of Oddi (Dodds et al 1988). Loss of inhibition and the resulting myogenic hyperactivity also underlie infantile hypertrophic pyloric stenosis (Vanderwinden et al 1992), analogous to the muscular hypertrophy found in unresolved Hirschsprung's disease.

Pseudoobstruction occurs in part because contractile behavior of the circular muscle is hyperactive and disorganized in the denervated regions. The hyperactive and disorganized contractile behavior reflects the absence of inhibitory nervous control of the muscles that are self-excitable (autogenic) when released from the braking action imposed by the inhibitory motor neurons.

The association of enteric neuronal loss and symptoms of pseudoobstruction in Chagas disease reflects autoimmune attack on the neurons. *Trypanosoma cruzi*, the bloodborne parasite that causes Chagas disease, has antigenic epitopes similar to antigens of enteric neurons (Wood et al 1982). This activates the immune system to assault the gut neurons coincident with the attack on the parasite.

Enteric secretomotor neurons

Secretomotor neurons are excitatory motor neurons that innervate the intestinal crypts of Lieberkuhn (Fig. 2.3). Acetylcholine and vasoactive intestinal polypeptide are identified as the neurotransmitters (Cooke & Reddix 1994). The postjunctional receptors

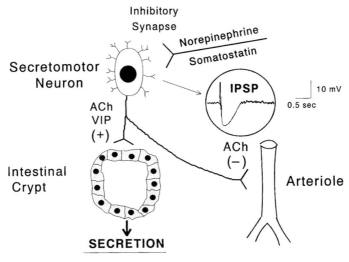

Fig. 2.3 Intestinal crypts of Lieberkuhn are innervated by secretomotor neurons which are stimulated by the release of vasoactive intestinal peptide (VIP) and acetylcholine. Simultaneously, axon collaterals to blood vessels dilate submucosal arterioles and increase mucosal blood flow. Secretomotor neurons receive inhibitory synaptic inputs from sympathetic postganglionic neurons (e.g. norepinephrine) and from other neurons in the enteric microcircuits (e.g. somatostatin). Activation of the inhibitory synaptic inputs evokes inhibitory postsynaptic potentials (IPSP) in secretomotor neurons.

for acetylcholine on the enterocytes are muscarinic. Collateral fibers from secretomotor axons innervate submucous arterioles and thereby link secretomotor activity in the crypts to submucous blood flow. When the secretomotor neurons fire, acetylcholine is released simultaneously at neuroepithelial and neurovascular junctions (Adriantsitohaina & Surprenant 1992, Evans et al 1994). Acetylcholine releases nitric oxide from the vascular endothelium which in turn dilates the blood vessels and increases blood flow for support of stimulated secretory activity in the crypts.

Secretomotor neurons receive inhibitory synaptic input. Activation of these inputs hyperpolarizes the neurons and decreases the probability of spike discharge. These hyperpolariz-ing potentials are *inhibitory postsynaptic potentials*. The physiologic effect of their activation is to suppress mucosal secretion. Norepinephrine released from postganglionic sympathetic axons acts at α_2 adrenergic receptors to hyperpolarize the secreto-motor neurons (North & Suprenant 1985). Opioid peptides and somatostatin are neurotransmitters that, like norepinephrine, hyperpolarize and suppress excitability in intestinal secretomotor neurons. Sympathetic inhibition of secretomotor neurons occurs in parallel with diversion of blood flow from the gut and is undoubtedly a component of sympathetic shutdown of function during demands on the body to maintain homeostasis when stressed by exercise, fear and other factors.

Generally, hyperactivity is associated with neurogenic secretory diarrhea; hypoactivity is associated with decreased secretion and dry stools. Neural linkage of secretion to motility may result in secretomotor hypoactivity being indirectly expressed as suppressed motility. Some of the neurotransmitters/modulators that inhibit secretomotor neurons also block synaptic transmission in the circuit linkages involving motility.

Synaptic inhibition in secretomotor neurons of the small and large intestine is fundamental to understanding the mechanism of action of some antidiarrheal drugs. Activation of α-adrenergic, opioid or somatostatin receptors on secretomotor neurons inhibits firing. This reduces the release of excitatory neurotransmitters at the junctions of secretomotor axons with epithelial cells in the crypts. The neuropharmacology of synaptic inhibition in secretomotor neurons helps explain the mechanism of antidiarrheal action of some drugs and the constipating action of others. Clonidine, an α_2 agonist and effective antidiarrheal drug, inhibits firing of secretomotor neurons (Morita & North 1981) and thereby reduces neuronal secretory drive to the crypts. Octreotide, a stable somatostatin analog, acts in similar manner, as does the opioid loperamide. Much of the well-known constipating action of morphine and other narcotics is undoubtedly related to the inhibitory effects of these agents on secretomotor neurons. In animals addicted to morphine, application of naloxone blocks the inhibitory action and dramatically increases the firing rate of the neurons (North & Tonini 1977).

Enhanced firing of the secretomotor neurons may be a normal functional event or may result from a variety of insults such as inflammation, sensitizing antigens and enterotoxins. Increased release of acetylcholine and/or vasoactive intestinal polypeptide at the crypt epithelium and consequent stimulation of secretion result from enhanced firing. *Vibrio cholerae*, a classic inducer of secretory diarrhea, has a neuronal secretomotor component that enhances firing (Jiang et al 1993).

INTERNUNCIAL CIRCUITS

Enteric internuncial microcircuits (Fig. 2.1) are integrated circuits formed by synaptic interconnections in pools of interneurons. They are involved in several functions characteristically found in integrative neural networks. In the digestive tract, they are responsible for:

1. processing of sensory information;
2. interpretation of signals from the brain and spinal cord;
3. storage of a variety of gut behavioral programs;
4. interpretation of signals from the immune system;
5. control of outflow in motor neurons to gut effector systems.

Significant synaptic events are:

1. fast excitatory postsynaptic potentials (fast EPSPs);
2. presynaptic inhibition;
3. presynaptic facilitation;
4. slow excitatory postsynaptic potentials (slow EPSPs);
5. inhibitory postsynaptic potentials;
6. neuromodulation.

Fast excitatory postsynaptic potentials

Fast EPSPs occur in the millisecond time range. They are the mode of rapid transmission of information from neuron to neuron as the circuits operate to process information or generate programmed outputs (Wood 1994). Acetylcholine acting at nicotinic receptors is the transmission mechanism for the majority of fast EPSPs found at all levels of the digestive tract, including the esophagus, stomach and small and large intestine. This holds for the internuncial circuitry, much of the excitatory synaptic input to motor neurons and the fast excitatory transmission occurring at the vagal and sacral parasympathetic interfaces with the enteric nervous system.

Presynaptic inhibition

Presynaptic inhibition is an important function at fast nicotinic synapses, at slow excitatory synapses and at sympathetic inhibitory synapses in the internuncial microcircuits and on motor neurons. It is a specialized form of neurocrine transmission whereby neurotransmitter released from one axon acts at receptors on a second axon to prevent the release of neurotransmitter from the second axon. Presynaptic inhibition resulting from actions of paracrine or endocrine mediators on receptors at presynaptic release sites is an alternative mechanism for modulation of synaptic transmission. Presynaptic inhibition in the enteric nervous system is mediated by multiple messengers and their receptors with variable combinations of the receptors working at each release site. The list of putative presynaptic inhibitory mediators, together with receptor subtypes, is shown in Table 2.1.

Table 2.1 Presynaptic inhibitory mediators

Mediator	Receptor subtype	Mechanism
Norepinephrine	α_2	Neurocrine
Histamine	H_3	Paracrine
Acetylcholine	Muscarinic	Neurocrine
Serotonin	$5\text{-HT}_{1A/4}$	Neurocrine
Adenosine	A_1	Neurocrine/paracrine
Pancreatic polypeptide		Endocrine
Neuropeptide Y		Endocrine
Peptide YY		Endocrine
Opioid peptides		Neurocrine
Tumor necrosis factor		Paracrine
Interleukin 1β & 6		Paracrine

Presynaptic inhibition mediated by paracrine or endocrine release of mediators is significant in pathophysiologic states such as inflammation. Release of histamine from mast cells in response to sensitizing antigens is an important example of paracrine-mediated presynaptic suppression in the enteric microcircuits (Frieling et al 1992, Wood 1993). Histamine acting at H_2 receptors produces a state of hyperexcitability like slow synaptic excitation in the cell bodies of a subset of interneurons. The outflow of spike discharge from these neurons activates neighboring neurons and eventually drives the activity of motor neurons to the effector systems. Presynaptic inhibitory action of histamine acts as a brake within the circuits to prevent runaway epileptic-like discharge from occurring across the synapses (Wood 1993).

Functional significance of presynaptic inhibition

Presynaptic inhibition operates normally in three important ways. First, it is a mechanism for selective shutdown or de-energization of a microcircuit. Prevention of transmission among the neural elements of a circuit inactivates the circuit. For example, a major component of shutdown of gut function by the sympathetic nervous system involves the presynaptic inhibitory action of norepinephrine on α_2 adrenoceptors at fast nicotinic synapses. This coincides with the inhibition of secretomotor function discussed earlier.

Presynaptic inhibition underlies gating functions in the microcircuits and this is a second aspect of its functional importance. Gating in this context involves the control of distance of spread of a behavioral event such as peristaltic propulsion along a length of intestine. Some events, such as mixing movements, occur over short lengths of intestine whereas others, such as power propulsion, occur over long reaches of bowel. Most, but not all, enteric neurons do not project for more than 3 cm up or down the bowel. Therefore, propagation distance of a behavioral event can be effectively controlled ('gated') by determining when information is permitted to pass through synapses connecting serial segments along the length of bowel.

The third important function of presynaptic inhibition in the enteric nervous system is autoinhibition. Autoinhibition occurs when transmitter released from an enteric neuron accumulates in the vicinity of the release site and activates presynaptic receptors to reduce further release. It functions in this respect as a negative feedback mechanism that automatically regulates the concentration of neurotransmitter within the synaptic space. Presynaptic muscarinic receptors mediate presynaptic autoinhibition at fast nicotinic synapses at many, but not all, specialized regions of the gut (Wood 1994).

Presynaptic inhibition is believed to be part of the programming for both physiological and paralytic (adynamic) ileus. Physiological ileus is interpreted as a state in which inhibition of transmission at synapses within motor control circuits prevents programming of contractile behavior (Wood 1994, Wood et al 1995b). Phase I of the migrating motor complex is an example of physiological ileus. In this circumstance, the 'gates' within the motor control circuits are in the closed state. Paralytic ileus is an exaggeration of physiological ileus brought on by conditions such as manipulation of the bowel during laparotomy or peritonitis. Unknown perturbations appear to sustain the synaptic gates in a closed configuration with unremitting activity of inhibitory motor neurons clamping the bowel musculature in an inactive state for extended periods of time. It is reminiscent of the paralysis of synaptic transmission seen in the spinal cord subsequent to injury and during the period of spinal shock.

Synaptic facilitation

Synaptic facilitation is the converse of presynaptic inhibition. It is augmentation of synaptic transmission by the action of a physiologic mediator or xenosubstance at the presynaptic terminal. At nicotinic synapses in the enteric nervous system, release of acetylcholine from the presynaptic terminal is enhanced, resulting in

EPSPs of larger amplitude. Identification of receptors for pre-synaptic facilitation in the gastric and intestinal microcircuits is incomplete; nevertheless, serotonergic receptors of the 5-HT$_4$ subtype appear to be involved (Pan & Galligan 1993).

Synaptic facilitation is the sole action of cholecystokinin in control of the guinea-pig gall bladder (Mawe 1991, Mawe et al 1994). A similar situation is found in pancreatic ganglia where cholecystokinin also acts to facilitate nicotinic neurotransmission (Ma & Szurszewski 1995). In both cases, release of acetylcholine from the vagal fibers evokes fast EPSPs that are below threshold and do not evoke spikes in the motor neurons. Cholecystokinin increases the EPSP amplitude to action potential threshold whereby firing of the motor neuron stimulates the effector.

Presynaptic facilitation takes on therapeutic importance as the mechanism of action of motility-enhancing drugs. Cisapride enhances the release of acetylcholine and augments fast EPSPs in the microcircuits of the gastric antrum and intestine (Tonini et al 1989, Tack et al 1991). These actions energize the circuits and thereby strengthen motor neuronal outflow to the effector systems.

Slow synaptic excitation

Slow synaptic excitation converts the neuronal cell body from hypoexcitability to a long-lasting hyperexcitable state. It is another of the mechanisms involved in energizing the internuncial microcircuits. Slow EPSPs occur in a population of internuncial neurons called AH/type 2 neurons. These are neurons with Dogiel type II morphology characterized by multipolar cell bodies with several long processes that project and branch extensively to release neurotransmitter at synapses with multiple neighboring neurons in the circuits. These neurons in the myenteric plexus of the guinea-pig have processes passing through the circular muscle coat into the mucosa where stimulation by 5-hydroxytryptamine released from mechanosensitive enterochromaffin cells can occur. Cell bodies of AH/type 2 neurons have low excitability when at rest and either do not fire action potentials or are capable of firing only a few action potentials before automatic mechanisms endogenous to the neuron lead to hyperpolarization and blockade of spike discharge (Wood 1994).

Functional significance of slow synaptic excitation

Slow synaptic excitation is evoked both by neurocrine release of neurotransmitters/modulators from presynaptic axons and by paracrine or endocrine release of chemical messengers from immune or endocrine cells in the gut wall. In the antigen-sensitized intestine, exposure to the sensitizing antigen (e.g. *Trichinella spiralis* protein or β-lactoglobulin) triggers release of histamine (Frieling et al 1994a, b). Once released, histamine acts as a paracrine messenger to mimic slow synaptic excitation in AH/type 2 neurons in the microcircuits of that region of intestine (Wood 1981, 1992, 1993, Frieling et al 1992). This action of histamine in the guinea-pig enteric nervous system is mediated by the histamine H_2 receptor subtype and persists without indications of tachyphylaxis as long as histamine is present (Tamura & Wood 1992).

Slow synaptic/paracrine excitation is mediated by multiple chemical messengers acting at a variety of different receptors. Different receptors, each of which mediates slow synaptic excitation, are found in variable combinations on individual neurons. A common mode of signal transduction, involving receptor activation of adenylate cyclase and second messenger function of cyclic 3',5'-adenosine monophosphate, links several different chemical messages to the behavior of a common set of ionic channels underlying generation of the slow excitatory response (Wood 1994). Putative messenger substances and specific receptor subtypes known to mimic slow synaptic excitation when applied experimentally to enteric neuron are given in Table 2.2.

Table 2.2 Messenger subtypes

Serotonin (5-HT_{1P})
Acetylcholine (muscarinic)
Motilin
Gastrin-releasing peptide
Calcitonin gene-related peptide (CGRP)
Tachykinins (NK3)
Cholecystokinin (CCK-A)
Histamine (H_2)
Vasoactive intestinal peptide (VIP)
Corticotrophin-releasing factor
Thyrotrophin-releasing factor
Adenosine (A2)
Pituitary adenylate cyclase-activating peptide

Inhibitory postsynaptic potentials

Slow IPSPs are the opposite of slow EPSPs. They act to hyperpolarize the membrane potential below the action potential threshold and decrease the probability of spike discharge. Part of their function, apart from inhibition of secretomotor neurons discussed above, may be to reverse the superexcitable condition of the slow EPSPs and return the membrane to the low excitability state.

Several putative neurocrine, paracrine and endocrine messenger substances evoke responses similar to IPSPs when applied experimentally to enteric neurons. Some of these substances are peptides, others are purine compounds and another is norepinephrine. Receptors for two or more of these substances may be localized to the cell body of the same neuron. Table 2.3 gives a list of the substances that may be found in enteroendocrine and inflammatory cells, as well as enteric neurons.

Table 2.3 Putative messenger substances

Acetylcholine	Purine nucleotides
Opioid peptides	Galanin
5-Hydroxytryptamine	Somatostatin
Norepinephrine	Neurotensin
Cholecystokinin	

Neuromodulation

Neuromodulation is defined as modification of neuronal excitability that is usually accomplished by chemically mediated synaptic, paracrine or endocrine signals. Excitability, in this context, is a qualitative reference to the probability of discharge of action potentials by the neuron within a specified time frame. Low excitability is none or a few spikes in a given time; as excitability increases, the frequency of spike discharge increases in direct proportion. Neuromodulation in enteric neurons can be long lasting and is related to the alterations in excitability associated with hyperpolarizing afterpotentials in AH/type 2 neurons and the prolonged increases or decreases in excitability during slow EPSP-like excitation or inhibitory synaptic events.

The significance of neuromodulation is threefold. First, it functions as a determinant of the frequency of spike discharge during any instant of time. Second, it alters the responsiveness (input–output relations) of the neuron to other synaptic inputs and to endocrine or paracrine messages. For example, fast nicotinic excitatory inputs are more likely to reach threshold for firing an action potential during a slow EPSP than during a slow IPSP. Third, it underlies the gating mechanism that regulates the spread of excitation between neurites at opposite corners of the multipolar Dogiel II neurons, as illustrated in Figure 2.4.

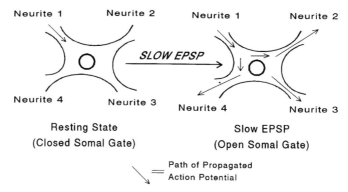

Fig. 2.4 Slow EPSPs (excitatory postsynapic potentials) underlie a gating mechanism by which the spread of spike information between neurites at opposite poles of the cell body is controlled. When the neuron is in the resting state, the excitability of the cell body is low and inbound spike information arriving at the soma in neurite 1 does not fire the cell body. In this state, the somal gate is closed and no information is relayed to the neurites at the opposite poles of the cell body. During the slow EPSP, the somal membrane is fired by inbound spikes in neurite 1; the somal gate is open and the inbound activity is transferred to neurites 2, 3 and 4 and relayed on to neighboring neurons.

ENTERIC NEUROIMMUNOPHYSIOLOGY

Observations in antigen-sensitized animal models suggest direct communication between the immune system and the enteric nervous system (Stead et al 1987, Castro 1989, Perdue et al 1990, Wang et al 1991, Wood 1991, 1992). The communication is meaningful and results in specialized adaptive behavior of the bowel in response to circumstances within the lumen that are threatening to the functional integrity of the whole animal. Communication is paracrine in nature and incorporates specialized sensing functions of the immune cells for specific antigens, together with the capacity of the enteric nervous system for intelligent interpretation of the signals. Immunoneural integration progresses sequentially, starting with immune detection – signal transfer to enteric microcircuits – neural interpretation – selection of a specific neural program of coordinated mucosal secretion and motor propulsion – effective clearance of the antigenic threat from the intestinal lumen (see Fig. 2.1).

A variety of cell types including polymorphonuclear leukocytes, lymphocytes, macrophages, dendrocytes and mast cells are present in varying numbers in the intestinal mucosa and/or lamina propria. These are often found in close histoanatomical association with the neuronal elements of the enteric nervous system (Stead et al 1987). The enteric immune system can be sensitized by foreign antigens in the form of foodstuffs, toxins or invading organisms. After sensitization, a second exposure to the same antigen triggers predictable integrated behavior of the intestinal effector systems (Harari et al 1987, Baird & Cutbert 1987). Neurally coordinated activity of the muscle, mucosa and blood vasculature results in organized behavior of the whole intestine that rapidly expels the antigenic threat. Recognition of an antigen by the sensitized immunoneural apparatus calls up a specialized propulsive motor program that is coordinated with copious secretion of water, electrolytes and mucus into the intestinal lumen (Baird & Cutbert 1987, Castro 1989, Cowles & Sarna 1991, Sarna et al 1991). Detection by the enteric immune system and signaling to the enteric minibrain initiates the adaptive behavior (see Fig. 2.1).

A frequently encountered pattern of muscle behavior in response to an offending antigen in the sensitized intestine is called power propulsion (Wood 1994). This specialized form of intestinal motility forcefully and rapidly propels any material in the lumen over long distances and effectively strips the lumen clean. Its occurrence is accompanied by abdominal distress and diarrhea (Sethi & Sarna 1991, Phillips 1995). Power propulsion is one of the neural programs contained in the library of programs stored in the enteric minibrain. Output of the program reproduces the same stereotyped motor behavior in response to radiation exposure, mucosal contact with noxious stimulants or antigenic detection by the sensitized enteric immune system (Sethi & Sarna 1991).

Immunoneural communication

Several cells in the lamina propria are putative sources of paracrine signals to the enteric minibrain. These include lymphocytes, macrophages, polymorphonuclear leukocytes and mast cells. Most is known about the signaling between mast cells and the neural microcircuits.

Intestinal mast cells proliferate during exposure to dangerous invaders such as *Trichinella spiralis*. Following an initial exposure to the nematode, immunoglobulin bound to receptors on the mast cells recognizes the sensitizing antigens. Crosslinking of a specific antigen with the bound antibody triggers degranulation of the mast cells. Degranulation releases a variety of paracrine messengers which may include serotonin, histamine, prostaglandins, leukotrienes, platelet-activating factor and cytokines.

Experimental application of histamine to simulate degranulation of mast cells in guinea-pig colon evokes cyclical bursts of chloride secretion coordinated with contraction of the musculature. The secretory behavior is activated for about 1 minute and then turned off for a few minutes prior to the next cycle (Wang & Cooke 1990, Frieling et al 1992). As the secretory cycle peaks, contraction of the muscularis externus occurs (Cooke et al 1993). Neural blockade with tetrodotoxin stops the secretory cycles. Drugs that selectively inhibit histamine H_2 receptors prevent the secretory cycles, whereas agonists selective for H_2 receptors mimic the cyclical behavior evoked by histamine. In guinea-pig colon several days after sensitization to either *Trichinella spiralis* or milk protein, exposure to the parasite or food antigen in Ussing chamber studies evokes a pattern of cyclical secretory behavior like that seen during exposure to histamine (Wang & Cooke 1990, Wang et al 1991).

Intracellular microelectrode recordings in neurons of the submucous plexus during histamine application show cyclical discharge of action potentials (Frieling et al 1992); antigen exposure in experimental preparations of sensitized intestine evokes similar excitatory responses in the neurons (Frieling et al 1994a,b). Both the action of histamine and the effects of antigen on neuronal behavior are mediated by histamine H_2 receptors.

Histamine signals in immunoneural communication

Immunophysiologic studies in the guinea-pig colon suggest that early stages of interpretation of histamine signals occur at H_2 receptors on the cell bodies of enteric interneurons and at presynaptic inhibitory receptors on axons at the sites of neurotransmitter release. Binding at the histamine H_2 receptors evokes a dramatic increase in neuronal excitability that mimics slow synaptic excitation (Frieling et al 1992, Tamura & Wood 1992, Nemeth et al 1984). This response is the same for several other slow EPSP mimetics that are putative neurotransmitters; nevertheless, histamine is not found in enteric neurons and is unlikely to be a neurotransmitter. Its signal functions appear to be related exclusively to mast cells and neuroimmune communication.

Presynaptic *inhibitory receptors* belong to the histamine H_3 subtype (Tamura et al 1987). These are inhibitory receptors that, when activated, suppress the release of acetylcholine at fast excitatory synapses in the internuncial microcircuits. This is a braking mechanism whereby the presynaptic inhibitory action of histamine prevents runaway excitation within the circuits as the H_2 excitatory receptors on the neuronal cell bodies are activated.

Brain–mast cell connection

Enteric mast cells appear to be involved in defense mechanisms apart from antigen sensing and local signaling to the enteric nervous system. An hypothesis that mast cells are relay nodes for transmission of selective information from the brain to the enteric nervous system is plausible and of sufficient importance to merit further attention (see Fig. 2.1). Evidence from ultrastructural and light microscopic studies suggests that enteric mast cells are innervated by projections from the central nervous system (Stead et al 1987, Williams et al 1995). Functional evidence supporting the brain to mast cell connection is found in reports of Pavlovian conditioning of mast cell degranulation in the gastrointestinal tract (MacQueen et al 1989).

PATHOPHYSIOLOGIC IMPLICATION OF THE BRAIN–MAST CELL CONNECTION

Functional bowel disorders

The brain–mast cell connection has clinical relevance for functional bowel disorders. It implies a mechanism linking central psychological status to irritable states of the digestive tract. An 'irritable state' of the bowel, known to result from degranulation of intestinal mast cells and release of signals to the enteric nervous system, is expected irrespective of the mode of stimulation of the mast cells (see Fig. 2.1). Degranulation and release of mediators evoked by neural input will have the same effect on motility and secretory behavior as does degranulation triggered by antigen detection.

Intestinal inflammation

Communication between the brain and mast cells may also be relevant in inflammation, including inflammatory bowel disease, because the enteric vascular system and circulating leukocytes are influenced by mast cell degranulation coincident with the delivery of the mast cell signal to the enteric nervous system. Degranulation releases mediators that are chemoattractant for circulating polymorphonuclear leukocytes known to be involved in the acute phase of an inflammatory response. This suggests that brain–gut interactions via mast cells can initiate an early phase of the mucosal inflammatory cascade coincident with calling up of the program for hypersecretion and power propulsion from the library of programs stored in the enteric nervous system. Associations between environmental stress and the initiation and progression of colitis in the cotton-top tamarin is thought to reflect this interaction (Wood et al 1995b).

CONCLUSION

The evidence from experimental enteric neurobiology leads to the inescapable conclusion that the moment-to-moment behavior of the gut, whether it be normal or pathological, is determined largely by integrative functions of the enteric nervous system. Input processed by the enteric minibrain is derived from local sensory receptors, immune cells (mast cells) and the brain. Mast cells utilize the immune system to detect new antigens and long-term memory permits recognition of the antigen if it ever reappears in the lumen. If it does, mast cells signal its presence to the enteric minibrain which then calls up from its program library the secretory and propulsive motor behavior that is organized for quick eradication of the threat. Operation of the program protects the integrity of the bowel, but at the expense of the side-effects of abdominal distress and diarrhea. The same sequence is to be expected from activation of neural pathways that link psychologic states to mast cells in the gut. These immunoneuro-physiology pathways are attractive putative mechanisms that could result in symptoms resembling the irritable bowel syndrome.

REFERENCES

Andriantsitohaina R, Surprenant A 1992 Acetylcholine released from guinea-pig submucosal neurones dilates arterioles by releasing nitric oxide from endothelium. Journal of Physiology (London) 453: 493–502

Baird WW, Cutbert AW 1987 Neuronal involvement in type 1 hypersensitivity reactions in gut epithelia. British Journal of Pharmacology 92: 47–655

Berthoud HR, Powley TL 1992 Vagal afferent innervation of the rat fundic stomach – morphological characterization of the gastric tension receptor. Journal of Comparative Neurology 319: 261–276

Bulbring E, Crema A 1959 The release of 5-hydroxytryptamine in relation to pressure exerted on the intestinal mucosa. Journal of Physiology (London) 146: 18–28

Castro GA 1989 Gut immunophysiology: regulatory pathways within a common mucosal immune system. News in Physiological Sciences 4: 59–64

Cooke HJ, Reddix RA 1994 Neural regulation of intestinal electrolyte transport. In: Johnson LR (ed.) Physiology of the gastrointestinal tract, 3rd edn. Raven, New York, pp. 2083–2132

Cooke HJ, Wang YZ, Rogers R 1993 Coordination of Cl-secretion and contraction by a histamine H(2)-receptor agonist in guinea pig distal colon. American Journal of Physiology 265: G973–G978

Cowles VE, Sarna SK 1991 *Trichinella spiralis* infection alters small bowel motor activity in the fed state. Gastroenterology 101: 664–669

Csendes A, Smok G, Braghetto I et al 1992 Histological studies of Auerbach's plexuses of the oesophagus, stomach, jejunum, and colon in patients with achalasia of the oesophagus – correlation with gastric acid secretion, presence of parietal cells and gastric emptying of solids. Gut 33: 150–154

Davison JS, Clarke GD 1988 Mechanical properties and sensitivity to CCK of vagal gastric slowly adapting mechanoreceptors. American Journal of Physiology, Gastrointestinal and Liver Physiology 255: G55–G61

Dodds WJ, Hogan WJ, Geenan JE 1988 Perspectives about function of the sphincter of oddi. Viewpoints on Digestive Diseases 20: 9–12

Evans RJ, Jiang MM, Surprenant A 1994 Morphological properties and projections of electrophysiologically characterized neurons in the guinea-pig submucosal plexus. Neuroscience 59: 1093–1110

Frieling T, Cooke HJ, Wood JD 1992 Histamine receptors on submucous neurons in the guinea-pig colon. American Journal of Physiology, Gastrointestinal and Liver Physiology 264: G74–G80

Frieling T, Cooke HJ, Wood JD 1994a Neuroimmune communication in the submucous plexus of guinea-pig colon after sensitization to milk antigen. American Journal of Physiology, Gastrointestinal and Liver Physiology 267: G1087–G1093

Frieling T, Palmer JM, Cooke HJ, Wood JD 1994b Neuroimmune communication in the submucous plexus of guinea pig colon after infection with *Trichinella spiralis*. Gastroenterology 107: 1602–1609

Fujita T 1991 Taste cells in the gut and on the tongue. Their common, paraneuronal features. Physiology and Behavior 49: 883–885

Furness JB, Johnson PJ, Pompolo S, Bornstein JC 1995 Evidence that enteric motility reflexes can be initiated through entirely intrinsic mechanisms in the guinea-pig small intestine. Neurogastroenterology and Motility 7: 89–96

Harari Y, Russell DA, Castro GA 1987 Anaphylaxis mediated epithelial Cl-secretion and parasite rejection in rat intestine. Journal of Immunology 128: 1250–1255

Jiang MM, Kirchgessner A, Gershon MD, Surprenant A 1993 Cholera toxin-sensitive neurons in guinea-pig submucosal plexus. American Journal of Physiology, Gastrointestinal and Liver Physiology 27: G86–G94

Kirchgessner AL, Tamir H, Gershon MD 1992 Identification and stimulation by serotonin of intrinsic sensory neurons of the submucosal plexus of the guinea pig gut – activity-induced expression of fos immunoreactivity. Journal of Neuroscience 12: 235–248

Lang IM, Sarna SK 1989 Motor and myoelectric activity associated with vomiting, regurgitation and nausea. In: Wood JD (ed.) Handbook of physiology, section 6, the gastrointestinal system, vol 1 motility and circulation. American Physiological Society, Bethesda, pp. 1179–1198

Lembo T, Munakata J, Mertz H et al, 1994 Evidence for the hypersensitivity of lumbar splanchnic afferents in irritable bowel syndrome. Gastroenterology 107: 1686–1696

Loening-Baucke V, Yamada T 1995 Is the afferent pathway from the rectum impaired in children with chronic constipation and encopresis? Gastroenterology 109: 397–403

Ma RC, Szurszewski JH 1995 Facilitating effect of cholecystokinin on nicotinic neurotransmission in cat pancreatic ganglion. American Journal of Physiology, Gastrointestinal and Liver Physiology (in press)

MacQueen G, Marchall J, Perdue M, Siegel S, Bienenstock J 1989 Pavlovian conditioning of rat mucosal mast cells to secrete rat mast cell protease II. Science 243: 83–84

Makhlouf GM, Grider JR 1993 Nonadrenergic noncholinergic inhibitory transmitters of the gut. News in Physiological Science 8: 195–199

Mawe GM 1991 The role of cholecystokinin in ganglionic transmission in the guinea-pig gall-bladder. Journal of Physiology (London) 439: 89–102

Mawe GM, Gokin AP, Wells DG 1994 Actions of cholecystokinin and norepinephrine on vagal inputs to ganglion cells in guinea pig gallbladder. American Journal of Physiology 30: G1146–G1151

Morita K, North RA 1981 Clonidine activates membrane potassium conductance in myenteric neurones. British Journal of Pharmacology 74: 419–428

Nemeth PR, Ort CA, Wood JD 1984 Intracellular study of effects of histamine on electrical behavior of myenteric neurons in guinea-pig small intestine. Journal of Physiology (London) 355: 411–425

North RA, Surprenant A 1985 Inhibitory synaptic potentials resulting from alpha 2 adrenoceptor activation in guinea-pig submucous plexus neurones. Journal of Physiology (London) 358: 17–33

North RA, Tonini M 1977 The mechanism of action of narcotic analgesics in the guinea-pig ileum. British Journal of Pharmacology 61: 541–549

Pan H, Galligan JJ 1993 5-HT4-mediated facilitation of fast synaptic transmission in the myenteric plexus of guinea pig ileum. Gastroenterology 104: A562

Perdue MH, Marshall J, Masson S 1990 Ion transport abnormalities in inflamed rat jejunum: involvement of mast cells and nerves. Gastroenterology 98: 561–567

Phillips SF 1995 Motility disorders of the colon. In: Yamada T (ed.) Textbook of gastroenterology, 2nd edn. JB Lippincott, Philadelphia, pp. 1856–1875

Richter JE, Barish CF, Castell DO 1986 Abnormal sensory perception in patients with esophageal chest pain. Gastroenterology 91: 845–862

Sanders KM, Ward SM 1992 Nitric oxide as a mediator of nonadrenergic noncholinergic neurotransmission. American Journal of Physiology, Gastrointestinal and Liver Physiology 25: G379–G392

Sarna SK, Otterson MF, Cowles VE, Sethi AK, Telford GL 1991 In vivo motor response to gut inflammation. In: Collins SM, Snape WJ (eds) Effects of immune cells and inflammation on smooth muscle and enteric nerves. CRC Press, Boca Raton, pp. 181–195

Sethi AK, Sarna SK 1991 Colonic motor activity in acute colitis in conscious dogs. Gastroenterology 100: 954–963

Sidhu M, Cooke HJ 1995 Role for 5-HT and ACh in submucosal reflexes mediating colonic secretion. American Journal of Physiology, Gastrointestinal and Liver Physiology 32: G346–G351

Smith GP, Jerome C, Norgren R 1985 Afferent axons in abdominal vagus mediate satiety effect of cholecystokinin in rats. American Journal of Physiology, Gastrointestinal and Liver Physiology 249: R638–R641

Stead RH, Tomioka M, Quinonez G, Simon GT, Felten SY, Bienenstock J 1987 Intestinal mucosal mast cells in normal and nematode-infected rat intestines are in intimate contact with peptidergic nerves. Proceedings of the National Academy of Sciences USA 84: 2975–2979

Tack JF, Janssens W, Janssens J, Vantrappen G, Wood JD 1991 Effect of cisapride on myenteric neurons in the guinea-pig gastric antrum. Journal of Gastrointestinal Motility 3: A203

Tamura K, Wood JD 1992 Effects of prolonged exposure to histamine. Digestive Diseases and Sciences 37: 1084–1088

Tamura K, Palmer JM, Wood JD 1987 Presynaptic inhibition produced by histamine at nicotinic synapses in enteric ganglia. Neuroscience 25: 171–179

Tonini M, Galligan JJ, North RA 1989 Effects of cisapride on cholinergic neurotransmission and propulsive motility in the guinea pig ileum. Gastroenterology 96: 1257–1264

Vanderwinden JM, Mailleux P, Schiffmann SN, Vanderhaeghen JJ, Delaet MH 1992 Nitric oxide synthase activity in infantile hypertrophic pyloric stenosis. New England Journal of Medicine 327: 511–515

Wang YZ, Cooke HJ 1990 H2 receptors mediate cyclical chloride secretion in guinea pig distal colon. American Journal of Physiology, Gastrointestinal and Liver Physiology 258: G887–G893

Wang YZ, Palmer JM, Cooke HJ 1991 Neuro-immune regulation of colonic secretion in guinea pigs. American Journal of Physiology, Gastrointestinal and Liver Physiology 260: G307–G314

Whitehead WE, Holtkotter B, Enck P et al 1990 Tolerance for rectosigmoid distension in irritable bowel syndrome. Gastroenterology 98: 1187–1192

Williams RM, Berthoud HR, Stead RH 1995 Association between vagal afferent nerve fibers and mast cell in rat jejunal mucosa. Gastroenterology 108: A941

Wood JD 1973 Electrical activity of the intestine of mice with hereditary megacolon and absence of myenteric ganglion cells. American Journal of Digestive Diseases 18: 477–488

Wood JD 1991 Communication between minibrain in gut and enteric immune system. News in Physiological Science 6: 64–69

Wood JD 1993 Neuro-immunophysiology of colon function. Pharmacology 47 (suppl. 1): 7–13

Wood JD 1994 Physiology of the enteric nervous system. In: Johnson LR (ed.) Physiology of the gastrointestinal tract, 3rd edn. Raven, New York, pp. 423–482

Wood JD, Brann LR, Vermillion DL 1986 Electrical and contractile behavior of the large intestine musculature of the piebald mouse model for Hirschsprung's Disease. Digestive Disease and Science 31: 638–650

Wood JD, Zafirov DH, Xia Y 1995a Daiichi DQ-2511 facilitates excitatory processes and suppresses inhibitory neuro-transmission in the enteric nervous system of guinea-pig small intestine. Gastroenterology 108: A711

Wood JD, Peck OC, Sharma HM et al 1995b Environmental stress as a factor in the etiology of colitis in the cotton-top tamarin. Gastroenterology 108: A943

Wood JN, Hudson L, Jessel TM, Yamamoto M 1982 A monoclonal antibody defining antigenic determinants on subpopulations of mammalian neurones and *Trypanosoma cruzi* parasites. Nature (London) 296: 34–37

Clinical pharmacology

DG Thompson

INTRODUCTION

This chapter aims to provide a general overview of the drug therapies which are currently available and those which may soon be available for the treatment of functional disorders of the gut. It is not intended to be an exhaustive review of pharmacology, either basic or clinical, nor is it designed to represent a systematic review of the randomized controlled trials of drug therapies for these disorders. Indeed, it has been claimed that few, if any, of the clinical trials of the great majority of therapies proposed for functional bowel disease are of satisfactory quality to justify their alleged efficacy. Nevertheless, many pharmacological approaches to the therapy of patients with functional bowel disorders currently exist and the temptation to prescribe them in response to patient pressure is great. This chapter therefore is constructed to provide a simple and practical guide to the therapy of patients' symptoms in functional disorders.

GENERAL PRINCIPLES OF DRUG THERAPY

In the absence of any clear understanding of the pathophysiology of functional bowel disorders (FBD), it is perhaps not surprising that the pharmacology and the therapeutic approaches to the various syndromes comprising FBD remain uncertain. Despite this fundamental ignorance, a number of classes of drugs have been proposed as possible therapeutic agents. While some of the drugs are rationally based on knowledge about the pharmacology of the enteric nervous system and the extrinsic neuronal control of the gut (see Chapter 1), most others are empirically based symptomatic remedies which, despite the lack of randomized controlled trial data to support their use, seem to have stood the test of time.

DRUGS USED IN THE TREATMENT OF FUNCTIONAL BOWEL DISEASE

Drugs which mimic neuropeptides in the enteric nervous system

A number of pharmacological agents, some of which have been available for many years, are now known to have an effect on gastrointestinal motility via an action which mimics the activity of naturally occurring neuropeptide transmitters. These include erythromycin (a motilin agonist), loxiglumide (a CCK-A receptor antagonist) and loperamide (an opiate receptor agonist).

Erythromycin and the macrolides

It is now over 10 years since the first observations that parenterally administered erythromycin was able to stimulate upper gastrointestinal motility in both animals and humans and to induce the production of phase 3 activity of the MMC. Before this, it was recognized that intravenous erythromycin in high doses induced cramping abdominal pains as one of its side-effects. Since these empiric observations were made, the relationship between macrolide antibiotics and the naturally occuring neuropeptide motilin has been recognized. Erythromycin and other macrolides act independently of their action as antibiotics and exert a direct stimulating effect on motilin receptors located on both smooth muscle and myenteric plexus neurons, in the stomach and duodenum. The ability of erythromycin to increase gastric tone and stimulate propagating contractile activity in the stomach has led to a series of studies into its therapeutic potential in a number of clinical problems. So far, the best developed application of erythromycin has been for the treatment of diabetic gastroparesis. Intravenous erythromycin and even oral erythromycin given to patients with severe gastric emptying delay and poor diabetic control are now known to be able to reduce the magnitude of the gastric emptying delay and as a consequence to improve diabetic control. Unfortunately, experience with non-diabetic gastroparetic syndromes appears to be rather less encouraging. The major limitations to the use of the drug relate to the need to provide a critical blood level before effective stimulation occurs. A further understandable concern about the long-term use of erythromycin is the possibility that resistant organisms will be encouraged; there is also a suspicion that the benefit of the drug tends to fall with repeated dosage.

Other macrolide-derived agents without antibiotic effects and improved bioavailability are being actively developed by several pharmaceutical companies. However, their exact role in the management of functional bowel diseases, in particular functional dyspepsia, remains to be determined.

Opiate agonists

As indicated in Chapter 1, the enteric nervous system of the gut contains many opiodergic neurons. It is also well recognized that morphine and other extrinsically administered opiates have profound effects on gastrointestinal motility, including delayed gastric emptying and colonic transit and induction of phase 3-like motor activity in the small intestine. Indeed, the traditional role for opiates as a therapy for diarrhea is based on these transit-delaying effects as well as their antisecretory actions. At present the only opiate agent currently in widespread use for functional disorders is loperamide, a synthetic agonist which mimics the action of endogenous opiates on gastrointestinal opiate receptors of enteric neurons. Loperamide differs from morphine in exerting its action almost exclusively on peripheral receptors without recognizable effects on the central nervous system. Despite its use in clinical practice for almost two decades, the pharmacokinetics of the drug remain somewhat mysterious and peripheral blood levels seem to bear little relationship to pharmacological effects. The most plausible explanation for its undoubted biological activity and its lack of CNS side-effects seems to be that it is functionally sequestered in the gut by recycling in the enterohepatic circulation and therefore does not reach the peripheral blood. This may also explain how it maintains its action for some time after ingestion without elevating peripheral blood levels or entering the central nervous system.

Cholecystokinin antagonists

There is much current interest in the possibility that synthetic antagonists of the cholecystokinin (CCK)-A receptor might prove to be clinically useful in functional bowel diseases. So far, no drugs have been given product licences but at least one is currently in advanced clinical trial development. Since CCK is a direct stimulant of gastric and colonic smooth muscle and also modifies gastric function via vagal neural stimulation, CCK antagonists might be expected to reverse nutrient-induced delay in gastric emptying and inhibit the gastrocolic excitatory reflex.

CCK receptor antagonists are currently undergoing clinical trials in irritable bowel syndrome, the rationale for their use being that the gastrocolic reflex is mediated at least in part by CCK and that CCK antagonists reduce the intensity of the response. If, as has been assumed, the pain in relation to meals in patients with irritable bowel syndrome is the result of either an excessive gastrocolic reflex or increased 'sensitivity' to a normal gastrocolic reflex, then CCK antagonists might be expected to relieve symptoms. Time will tell, however, whether the drug deserves a role in the treatment of irritable bowel syndrome (IBS) and whether any effects on symptom relief are indeed related to their role in modifying motility. A potentially undesirable side-effect of CCK-A antagonists, however, is a reduction of gall bladder emptying, since CCK is the major physiological stimulus for stimulation of gall bladder contraction.

Drugs which antagonize 5-hydroxytryptamine (5-HT) in the GI tract

As will be seen in Chapter 2, the mucosa and submucosa of the gastrointestinal tract are richly supplied with cells containing 5-HT and 5-HT receptors are present on many neurons in the enteric nervous system and extrinsic nerves. This has led to the exploration of potential use of 5-HT receptor antagonists, of which a large variety are now available as potential modifiers of gut function and sensation. Whilst the rationale for trials of such agents seems reasonable, unfortunately, despite much investigation their benefit in patients with painful functional bowel syndromes remains to be established.

In animal studies the induction of inflammation or mucosal damage clearly modifies sensation, reducing the pain threshold so that otherwise non-noxious stimuli become painful. When 5-HT receptor antagonists are administered to animals with experimentally inflamed mucosa, pain responses are reduced, implying a modulating role of 5-HT in the sensitization process.

There is a leap of faith required, however, to move from this information to the conclusion that the increased reporting of abdominal pain by patients with functional bowel diseases is also related to increased 5-HT mediated responses to inflammation. It is therefore perhaps not surprising that so far no clinical trial has clearly shown a benefit of 5-HT receptor antagonists in irritable bowel syndrome.

Drugs which influence cholinergic nerve pathways

Muscarinic antagonists

Acetylcholine plays a fundamental role in both myenteric and extrinsic neural control of the gut and it is well recognized that cholinergic muscarinic antagonists, e.g. atropine, modify gut function. The use of atropine, however, is not common in clinical practice, because of the unacceptability of extraintestinal side-effects In addition, quaternary anticholinergics such as hyoscine butylbromide (Buscopan) given orally are pharmacologically inactive yet continue to be prescribed as 'antispasmodics'. Their value beyond placebo therapy has yet to be established.

Cisapride

Cisapride is a drug with reproducible actions on human gastro-intestinal motor activity which appears to act at least partially via an enhancement of cholinergic neuronal activity. In healthy volunteers, the drug accelerates gastric emptying, increases esophageal peristalsis, accelerates transit and promotes colonic propulsion. Clinical trials have now also established its benefit in a number of clinical conditions, including mild reflux esophagitis, symptoms associated with delayed gastric emptying and in the milder forms of constipation. Unfortunately, however, most patients with the most severe gastroparesis or constipation are not greatly helped by the drug. Perhaps it is not surprising that drugs such as cisapride work best in patients with mild enteric neurological disease since its therapeutic benefit seems to derive from improving the function of neural activity rather than replacing it.

Drugs which act on the efferent sympathetic neurons to the gut

The gastrointestinal tract is innervated by sympathetic neurons from the spinal cord which exert an inhibitory influence on motility. Sympathetic neuronal discharge is a major factor in the induction of ileus postsurgery but there is also a tonic of sympathetic neuronal inhibition of normal gut function which can be uncovered by adrenergic neural blockade. However, although beta blockers such as propranolol accelerate transit through the gut they have yet to find a role in the treatment of functional bowel disorders.

Drugs which modify stool consistency

Given the above rather gloomy view that there is currently little therapeutic value in many of the therapies for functional disorders, most clinicians attempt symptomatic relief on an empirical basis. In the treatment of chronic constipation, where colonic contents become hardened and impacted, a simple but effective practical approach is often to render the colonic contents semiliquid to aid expulsion. Agents which soften the stool range from plant fiber substitutes, e.g. psyllium, to fermentable carbohydrates, e.g. lactulose, and osmotic laxatives, e.g. polyethylene glycol (Kleen-Prep).

Whilst none of these agents has any direct pharmacological effect on the colon they are undoubtedly of benefit in chronically constipated patients, working via transit enhancement.

Drugs which act via nitric oxide production

Gastrointestinal smooth muscle, like cardiovascular smooth muscle, is inhibited by nitric oxide so that agents which increased the nitric oxide availability at the gut smooth muscle reduce their contraction has led to the exploration of using GTN (glyceryl trinitrate) for gut symptoms which are thought to relate to increased contractility. The best example of GTN use is in the management of chest pain and dysphagia related to diffuse esophageal spasm and in dysphagia resulting from mild degrees of achalasia of the cardia. In both of these situations judicious use of sublingual GTN can modify symptoms.

Drugs which modify mood

In most patients with severe and chronic irritable bowel syndrome, there is a clear association between the severity of the symptoms and psychological state. In severe IBS a high degree of anxiety/depression symptoms can be identified, their severity correlating closely with the degree of gastrointestinal distress experienced by the patient. Because of these observations there is increasing interest in the employment of mood-modifying drugs to treat symptoms in IBS. The most frequently tested group of agents are the tricyclic antidepressants, e.g. amitriptyline or nortriptyline, and evidence from randomized trials exists to justify their use. The widespread adoption of such drugs in IBS, however, has been limited by their side-effects, particularly dry mouth and sedation. These difficulties have now led to interest in the newer SRI class antidepressants which are associated with fewer untoward effects. A number of large-scale trials are currently being conducted into their benefit in patients with IBS symptoms. Until the results of these trials are evaluated, however, their widespread use in IBS is not recommended unless there are clear depressive symptoms which would justify their use independently of the gut symptoms.

In addition to modification of mood by drug therapy, other approaches using psychotherapy or hypnosis are currently being employed. While such approaches are reported to provide benefit their use is restricted by the need to provide highly trained personnel to deliver the therapy and by the intense doctor–patient interaction required.

Drugs which act directly on intestinal smooth muscle

It is well known that many of the calcium channel antagonists which are employed in cardiovascular disease to reduce blood vessel tone also affect colonic function, which has led to interest in the drugs as possible agents for the therapy of IBS. Whilst drugs such as verapamil, for example, can reduce the degree of diarrhea in patients with predominant diarrhea IBS, in such patients the non-GI side-effects, e.g. headache, tend to limit their use.

Drugs which stimulate colonic neural activity

A number of naturally occurring products are capable of inducing colonic contractile activity via an effect on the colonic myenteric plexus. These traditionally used laxatives, e.g. anthroquinones, have an effect which is restricted to the colon because they need to be 'activated' by bacterial enzymes.

There seems to be little to choose between the many varieties of stimulant laxatives available, the choice of drug prescribed being determined by cost and convenience. There is a widespread view that the excessive use of non-specific neural stimulants in patients with severe constipation can damage the myenteric plexus and that their use must therefore be avoided if at all possible. In patients with severe constipation, however, where neuromuscular function is already impaired, the benefits of their use clearly outweigh any theoretical neurotoxic effect and their judicious use in conjunction with stool softeners improves quality of life and either delays or avoids colectomy.

A PRACTICAL APPROACH TO THE TREATMENT OF SYMPTOMS IN FUNCTIONAL GASTROINTESTINAL DISORDERS

Because the pathophysiology of functional GI disorders remains so unclear and because enteric neural pharmacology is still in its infancy, it is perhaps not surprising to discover that there is no single class of drugs capable of modifying functional bowel symptoms under all circumstances. The approach to the management of patients with such disorders therefore has to be an empiric one with therapy being designed to relieve specific symptoms rather than induce a specific neuromuscular effect.

What, then, can the practicing clinician do to help the patient with functional bowel disease? Whilst it is not the remit of this chapter to discuss in detail the care of patients with functional bowel disease, the following short summary provides a guide to the therapeutic approaches which are commonly adopted for symptom relief.

Symptomatic management of esophageal disorders

Once the diagnosis of an esophageal motility disorder such as diffuse esophageal spasm or achalasia has been established in a patient with dysphagia and chest pain, then smooth muscle relaxants, either verapamil or glyceryl trinitrate, can be employed.

A novel approach to the management of achalasia which is currently being explored is the use of botulinum toxin injected directly into the lower sphincter. Botulinum toxin provides an inhibition of cholinergic stimulatory nerves and reduces sphincter tone for up to 6 months in most instances.

Symptomatic management of functional dyspepsia

There is still no satisfactory drug therapy for most patients with severe functional dyspeptic symptoms despite the evidence of delayed gastric emptying in up to 40% of the patients. Dietary modification remains the most satisfactory approach with empiric clinical trials of erythromycin or cisapride being attempted in those in whom delayed emptying is suspected. It is important to note that adverse effects of cisapride have been recently reported when administered together with erythromycin so that simultaneous administration of the two is not recommended.

Symptomatic management of irritable bowel syndrome

There is no clear drug therapeutic regime for patients with irritable bowel syndrome and an empiric patient centered approach is required. The above therapies, either singly or in combination, are usually used to modify stool consistency together with attempts to elevate mood in depressed patients.

FURTHER READING

Camilleri M, Choi M-G 1997. Irritable bowel syndrome. Alimentary Pharmacology and Therapeutics 11: 3–15

Guthrie E, Creed F, Dawson D, Tomenson B 1991. A controlled trial of psychological treatment for the irritable bowel syndrome. Gastroenterology 100: 450–457

Janssens J, Peeters TL, Vantrappen G 1990. Improvement of gastric emptying in diabetic gastroparesis by erythromycin. New England Journal of Medicine 322: 1028–1031

Klein KB 1988. Controlled treatment trials in the irritable bowel syndrome. Gastroenterology 95: 232–241

Epidemiology

4

WG Thompson

Functional gut symptoms are difficult to recognize and quantify. By definition, they have no pathophysiologic marker and therefore there is no diagnostic test. Indeed, we only know of their existence by the words of those who suffer from them. There is evidence that most gut complaints seen in general practice are functional. Certainly, most of those seen by gastroenterologists have no demonstrable pathology or pathophysiology. To understand them better, working teams have developed definitions and symptom criteria for the functional gastrointestinal disorders. This chapter will discuss these syndromes, their classification, epidemiology, prognosis and cost.

CLASSIFICATION OF THE FUNCTIONAL GASTROINTESTINAL DISORDERS

> The bowels are at one time constipated, at another lax, in the same person . . . How the disease has two such different symptoms I do not profess to explain . . .
>
> W. Cumming, *London Medical Gazette*, 1849

Functional gastrointestinal disorders have been known for over 150 years. Complicated classifications of dyspepsia were offered by Osler in 1892 and Hutchison in 1927. In 1962 Chaudhary & Truelove subdivided the irritable colon syndrome into spontaneous and postinfectious. The first classification of all the functional gastrointestinal disorders was in my book *The Irritable Gut*, published in 1979. Beginning in 1986, a series of working teams meeting in Rome developed definitions and eventually a classification of these disorders (Thompson 1989, Thompson et al 1992, Drossman et al 1990). These are brought together in a book, *The Functional Gastrointestinal Disorders* (Drossman et al 1994).

Example definitions and the 'Rome' classification are shown in Tables 4.1 and 4.2. There is much to criticize in these working

Table 4.1 Some definitions

A functional gastrointestinal disorder
    A variable combination of unexplained, chronic or recurrent gastrointestinal symptoms not explained by structural or biochemical abnormalities. These may include symptoms attributable to the oropharynx, oesophagus, stomach, biliary tree, small or large intestine or anus.

A functional bowel disorder
    A functional gastrointestinal disorder with symptoms attributable to the mid or lower intestinal tract. The symptoms include abdominal pain, bloating or distension and various symptoms of disordered defecation.

The irritable bowel syndrome
    A functional bowel disorder in which abdominal pain is associated with defecation or a change in bowel habit, and with features of disordered defecation and with distension.

After Thompson et al 1992

Table 4.2 Functional gastrointestinal disorders – the Rome classification

A.   Functional esophageal disorders (41.6%)
    A1.   Globus (10.4%)
    A2.   Rumination syndrome (10.4%)
    A3.   Functional chest pain of presumed esophageal origin (12.5%)
    A4.   Functional heartburn (30.1%)
    A5.   Unspecified functional esophageal disorder (7.4%)

B.   Functional gastroduodenal disorders (26%)
    B1.   Functional dyspepsia (2.6%)
       B1a.   Ulcer-like dyspepsia (0.2%)
       B1b.   Dysmotility-like dyspepsia (1%)
       B1c.   Unspecified dyspepsia (1.5%)

C.   Functional bowel disorders (44.1%)
    C1.   Irritable bowel syndrome (11.2%)
    C2.   Functional abdominal bloating (30.7%)
    C3.   Functional constipation (3.6%)
    C4.   Functional diarrhea (1.7%)
    C5.   Unspecified functional bowel disorder

D.   Functional abdominal pain (2.2%)
    D1.   Functional abdominal pain syndrome
    D2.   Unspecified functional abdominal pain

E.   Biliary disorders
    E1.   Gall bladder dysfunction
    E2.   Sphincter of Oddi dysfunction (1.5%)

F.   Anorectal disorders (26.8%)
    F1.   Functional incontinence (7.8%)
    F2.   Functional anorectal pain (11.6%)
       F2a.   Levator ani syndrome (6.6%)
       F2b.   Proctalgia fugax (8%)
    F3.   Dyschezia (13.8%)
       F3a.   Pelvic floor dyssynergia
       F3b.   Internal anal sphincter dysfunction
    F4.   Unspecified anorectal disorder.

Those with any GI functional diagnoses (69.3%). see text

After Thompson et al 1992 and Drossman et al 1994

Table 4.3 The Rome criteria for irritable bowel syndrome

At least three months continuous or recurrent symptoms of:
1.   Abdominal pain or discomfort which is:
(a) relieved with defecation
(b) and/or associated with a change in frequency of stool
(c) and/or associated with a change in consistency of stools

AND

2. two or more of the following, at least a quarter of occasions or days:
(a) altered stool frequency*
(b) altered stool form (lumpy/hard or loose/watery stool)
(c) altered stool passage (straining, urgency or feeling of incomplete
    evacuation)
(d) passage of mucus
(e) bloating or feeling of abdominal distension
*For research purposes 'altered' may be defined as >3 bowel movements/day or
<3 bowel movements/week.

After Thompson et al 1992

Table 4.4 The Manning criteria for irritable bowel syndrome

Abdominal pain more than 6 times in the last year, plus two or more of:
1.   pain eased with defecation
2.   pain associated with a change in the frequency of defecation
3.   pain associated with a change in the consistency of defecation
4.   abdominal distension
5.   feeling of incomplete evacuation after defecation
6.   mucus in the stool.

After Manning et al 1978

team criteria. Subsequent work has found no scientific basis for the terms *ulcer-like* and *dysmotility-like* dyspepsia (Talley et al 1992a). Some of the anorectal disorders do have an 'organic cause'. The classification does not clearly delineate the 'gas' symptoms of bloating, aerophagia and passage of gas, which probably are distinct phenomena. It is not clear that chronic abdominal pain is a gut disorder at all. The Rome symptom criteria for the irritable bowel syndrome (IBS) are complex (Table 4.3). They exclude many patients with a clinical diagnosis of IBS and may not be an improvement on the simpler, more validated and still widely used 'Manning' criteria (Table 4.4). Nevertheless, like the *Diagnostic and Statistical Manual of Mental Disorders* (DSM) criteria employed by psychiatrists, the Rome classification is an important step (see below). While such a classification will require regular updating in the light of new knowledge, too frequent changes will promote confusion.

Why classify functional gastrointestinal disorders?

Some researchers are skeptical about these criteria (Read 1990). There is much evidence that there is both contemporary and sequential overlap of functional gut disorders with one another (Agreus et al 1995) and with dysfunction in other systems. Nevertheless, the criteria serve several important functions. The first is to bring some order into functional gut research. It is unlikely that the various functional gut disorders have identical causes, so it is very important that investigators accurately identify the subjects of physiological research. The elusive pathophysiologic markers that we seek require the most precise symptom definitions possible. It is less clear how important precise symptom criteria are to psychological research. The second important purpose of a proper nosology is to focus clinical trials on those who are most likely to benefit. Antisecretory drugs are unlikely to benefit those with IBS, while antispasmodic agents are likely to worsen those with functional heartburn. Drugs that speed up gut transit are unlikely to benefit an IBS patient with diarrhea. Klein (1988) and a working team (Talley et al 1994) have emphasized the importance of entry criteria and nomenclature in clinical trials of the IBS and other functional gut disorders.

Finally, and most importantly, identification of the various functional gut syndromes is very important in clinical medicine. The implied locus of the problem greatly influences the choice of investigations. While one might defend a sigmoidoscopy in the IBS or diarrhea, it makes little sense in heartburn or dyspepsia, where an upper endoscopy may prove more useful. Since there are many possible organic causes of chronic diarrhea, many tests must be done before it can be declared functional. While tests such as stool fat, laxative screen (Phillips et al 1995) or rectal biopsy may clarify persistent diarrhea, they are not indicated for typical IBS (McIntosh et al 1992). Similarly, an antidiarrheal agent will not benefit a patient with dyspepsia or IBS and a high fiber diet may worsen the symptoms of bloating and dyspepsia. Until we have reliable biological markers for functional gut disorders, we must strive for precise identification and quantification of the symptoms.

EPIDEMIOLOGY

Most epidemiological research has focused on IBS, dyspepsia and heartburn. A survey of over 8000 randomly selected householders (Drossman et al 1993) in the United States provides an estimate of those functional gut disorders strictly defined by the Rome criteria (Table 4.2. Prevalences of the various disorders are indicated in parentheses). However, the prevalences reported in this large survey must be interpreted with caution. The response was 66%. Householders are not a random sample of the US population, since the poor, the young, the elderly and non-whites are under-represented. The survey employed a self-completed questionnaire, without the guidance of an interviewer. The Rome criteria for IBS are very stringent. In dyspepsia, subgroups are no longer considered to be viable. Some of the definitions require updating and there is much overlap. Only 0.8% of the respondents who fulfilled any of the symptom criteria said they had a structural disorder. This is likely to be an underestimate. For example, it is not possible to determine how many with dyspepsia had an ulcer or how many with heartburn had esophagitis.

At face value, 69.3% of the householders had criteria for one or more of the functional gastrointestinal disorders. There was no overall difference between the sexes or with age. However, it is noteworthy that the IBS and constipation were twice as prevalent in females as males (7.7% and 2.4% versus 14.5% and 4.8%). Only 40% of those affluent people who had functional gastrointestinal disorders saw a doctor.

Irritable bowel syndrome

IBS is very common (Thompson 1986). We showed it to be present in 14% of British adults. Subsequent studies in the US (Drossman et al 1982, Longstreth & Wolde-Tsadik 1993), France (Bommelaer et al 1986), New Zealand (Welch & Pomare 1990), Denmark (Kay et al 1994) and even China (Bi-zhen & Qi-Ying 1988) and Nigeria (Olubide et al 1995) indicate that the prevalence of IBS is similar worldwide. Employing the Rome criteria, Drossman et al (1993) found the syndrome to be present in 11% of respondents in United States households. This study and one in Britain (Heaton et al 1992) indicate that IBS is twice as common in women as men. However, reports conflict as to whether the prevalence decreases with age or varies with culture (Kay et al 1994, Agreus et al 1994). Of course, these figures are sensitive to the definitions of IBS employed. In one instance, prevalences of 5–65% were found using different definitions (Kay et al 1994).

In one case, a population survey was repeated 1 year later (Talley et al 1992b). Thirty-eight percent of those who had IBS by Manning and Rome criteria (Tables 4.3 and 4.4) in the first survey did not on the second. Nine percent of those who did not have IBS initially had acquired it. The authors of this paper observed a similar turnover in chronic constipation, chronic diarrhea and dyspepsia. An even greater turnover occurs over

5 years, but only 5% of those who originally had IBS were free of symptoms (Kay et al 1994).

Epidemiological studies are hampered by their dependence on recall, which is notoriously flawed. For example, almost 40% of 961 adults with a previous fracture on their medical record had forgotten it when questioned 15 years later (Jonsson et al 1995). Most of several women who denied any gut symptoms reported abdominal pain during a 1-month period when they kept a diary. Thus the awareness and reporting of symptoms is less than their true occurrence. Most evidence suggests that IBS is a relapsing, chronic disorder that probably occurs in most adults during their lifetime. Since most of those who are aware of these symptoms do not consult a doctor, it may be important to know the factors that determine awareness and reporting of symptoms.

Most of those reporting IBS in population surveys have not sought medical help. Nevertheless, patients with IBS comprise about half of those seen in Western (Switz 1976) and Asian clinics (Kang et al 1994). Amongst Western clinic patients, women outnumber men by three or four to one (Harvey et al 1983, Thompson 1984). Curiously, in India and Sri Lanka, this ratio is reversed (Mathur et al 1966, Mendis et al 1982). If the two to one female to male ratio is true in Asia, there must be cultural or socioeconomic reasons why Asian men are more likely than women to consult a doctor for IBS.

Although most IBS sufferers in the community do not consult a physician for their symptoms, those that do present an important and costly health problem (Thompson 1986). Management strategy must be developed with these facts in mind. There are indications that IBS patients seen by specialists are a subgroup of the whole with psychosocial characteristics that are distinct from non-patients with the same symptoms (Drossman et al 1988, Whitehead et al 1988) and probably from those seen in primary care. A survey of 43 English general practitioners indicates that they refer only 14% of their IBS patients (Thompson et al 1997). This figure is similar to that actually found in general practice. About 14% of the population has IBS. If we accept that only 30% see doctors, then only 4% of all IBS sufferers see a specialist (Fig. 4.1). Even fewer may attend tertiary care centers where most of the IBS scientific literature originates. Therefore it is probably inappropriate to extrapolate physiological, psychological, pharmacological and clinical data gathered in academic centers to all IBS or, what is more important, to those treated in general practice.

Gastroenterologists have the impression that IBS is a major health problem, yet they see only those few difficult cases that fail

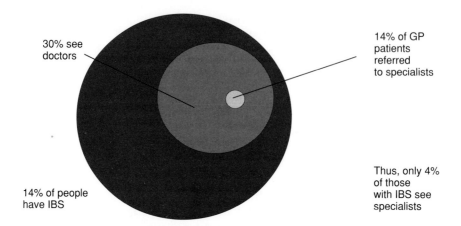

30% see
doctors

14% of GP
patients
referred
to specialists

14% of people
have IBS

Thus, only 4%
of those
with IBS see
specialists

Fig. 4.1 Venn diagram suggesting the prevalence and health care seeking of individuals with symptom criteria for IBS. Let's assume that only about 30% consult doctors. Eighty-five percent of these are cared for by their GP without referral so specialists may see as few as 4% of all individuals with IBS. This small group of individuals with IBS is not likely to be typical, so it may be inappropriate that they are the subjects of most physiological, psychological and therapeutic research into IBS.

to be satisfied by their GP. Overall, the GPs do not consider IBS a difficult problem (Thompson et al 1997). They rate backache and headache as more difficult problems in terms of diagnosis, patient satisfaction or time consumption. Their stated reasons for referral to specialists are patient dissatisfaction (56%) and uncertainty of diagnosis (35%). It seems that the small proportion of IBS patients that GPs send to specialists pose very different management problems from the remainder.

IBS has been associated with dysfunction in other systems. These include fibromyalgia, headache, dyspareunia, dysuria and backache (Whorwell et al 1986). Since most of the data supporting this view are reported from tertiary care centers, they may not apply to all IBS subjects. Similarly, the large amount of data indicating the association of depression, anxiety, stressful events and abuse with IBS applies to the patients of specialists, not necessarily to those seen in primary care. In the community, major depression, panic and agoraphobia are found more frequently in patients with unexplained gastrointestinal symptoms than in others (Walker et al 1993). However, unlike the tertiary care situation, the proportion of those with psychological disturbance was low. These may simply be the minority of functional gut patients in the community destined for tertiary care. Clearly future research in IBS must include those seen in primary care and those non-patients with IBS in the community.

Dyspepsia

It is difficult to determine the prevalence and incidence of peptic ulcer, even with its observable defect in the mucosa. It is much more difficult to acquire accurate figures for functional dyspepsia, given its lack of any physical marker! This task is doubly handicapped by lack of agreement on a definition of dyspepsia (George et al 1993). The disparate views of dyspepsia are illustrated in Table 4.5. Dyspepsia, like other functional disorders, may be recognized only by its symptoms. A 1980 estimate, that focused on epigastric pain or discomfort (that was not heartburn

Table 4.5 Some definitions of dyspepsia

1968 Rhind and Watson Epigastric discomfort after meals, a feeling of fullness so that tight clothing is loosened, eructation with temporary relief and regurgitation of sour fluid into the mouth and heartburn ('flatulent dyspepsia').

1982 Crean et al Any form of episodic or persistent abdominal discomfort or other symptom referable to the alimentary tract, except jaundice or bleeding.

1984 Thompson Chronic, recurrent, often meal-related epigastric discomfort initially suspected to be a peptic ulcer.

1984 Lagarde & Spiro Intermittent upper abdominal discomfort.

1985 Talley & Piper Pain, discomfort or nausea referable to the upper alimentary tract which is intermittent or continuous, has been present for a month or more, is not precipitated by exertion nor relieved by rest and is not associated with jaundice, bleeding or dysphagia.

1987 Nyren et al Epigastric pain or discomfort a key symptom, in absence of irritable bowel symptoms and organic disease ('epigastric distress syndrome').

1988 Talley & Phillips Chronic or recurrent (>3 months) upper abdominal pain or nausea which may or may not be related to meals.

1988 Colin-Jones et al Upper abdominal or retrosternal pain, discomfort, heartburn, nausea, vomiting or other symptom considered to be referable to the proximal portion of the digestive tract.

1989 Barbara et al Episodic or persistent abdominal symptoms, often related to feeding, which patients or physicians believe to be due to disorders of the proximal portion of the digestive tract.

1991 Heading Episodic or persistent abdominal symptoms, which include abdominal pain or discomfort. The term dyspepsia is not applied to patients whose symptoms are thought to be arising from outside the proximal gastrointestinal tract.

1991 Talley et al (Rome) Persistent or recurrent abdominal pain or abdominal discomfort centered in the upper abdomen.

1993 Klauser et al Complaints thought to emanate from the upper gastrointestinal tract, i.e. upper abdominal pain or discomfort, retrosternal pain or discomfort not related to physical activity, heartburn and nausea and vomiting.

1995 Thompson Chronic or recurrent (>3 months) epigastric pain or discomfort that suggests peptic ulcer disease; not GERD, IBS, angina, biliary colic, pancreatic or skeletal pain.

Updated from George et al 1993

or IBS), found a prevalence of about 6% (Thompson & Heaton 1980b).

A large survey of British general practice lists found a prevalence of about 30% (Jones et al 1990). However, this figure included people with heartburn, a common and totally different symptom from dyspepsia. The distinction is important since dyspepsia and heartburn pose different investigational and therapeutic challenges. In a Japan–Holland study of workers having regular health checks, the prevalence of dyspepsia in both countries was 13% (Schlemper et al 1993). Using the very restrictive Rome criteria, dyspepsia was found in only 2.7% of American householders (Drossman et al 1993) (66% of these relatively affluent people responded to the questionnaire). Therefore, at least 6 million Americans have dyspepsia and the true figure is probably much higher. All these population studies include patients with and without peptic ulcers since there is no way of determining which dyspeptics have ulcers. Among dyspeptic *patients* referred to specialist endoscopy clinics, roughly half have an ulcer (Table 4.6).

Table 4.6 Percentage of dyspeptic patients without ulcer by endoscopy

Study	n	No ulcer*
Williams et al 1988 (UK)	686	336 (49%)
Mansi et al 1990 (Italy)	2086	1293 (62%)
Hallisey et al 1990 (Ireland)	2659	851 (32%)
Bytzer et al 1992 (Denmark)	878	257 (64%)
Klauser et al 1993 (Germany)	220	55 (25%)
Hu et al 1995 (China)	1006	503 (50%)
Totals	7971	3857 (48%)

*or other gross lesion by endoscopy

Gastroesophageal reflux disease (GERD)

Determination of the prevalence and incidence of gastroesophageal reflux also presents problems. Heartburn is the most identifiable manifestation of GERD and therefore may give some idea of its occurrence. However, physiologists have demonstrated that most people reflux from time to time, usually with no complaint. On the other hand, esophagitis and its complications are relatively uncommon and may even occur without heartburn. Since the mechanism by which gastroesophageal reflux causes heartburn without esophagitis is unknown, simple heartburn is considered to be a functional disorder.

Table 4.7   Prevalence of heartburn

Study	n	At least one/year	At least one/month	Daily
Nebel et al 1976[a]	282		36%	7% M=F
Thompson & Heaton 1982[b]	330	33.6% M=33.6% F=33.5%	21.3%	4% (all female)
Drossman et al 1993[c]	543 0	30.1% M=30.5% F=29.7%		

[a] Hospital staff
[b] Unselected subjects with no hospital connection
[c] 66% of a random sample of US householders

Studies in Western countries indicate that one third of adults have heartburn at least once a year. About 3% have daily heartburn (Nebel et al 1976, Thompson & Heaton 1982, Drossman et al 1993). These figures hold for adults of both sexes and all ages (Table 4.7).

Population studies of esophagitis do not exist. The prevalences of esophagitis and its complications seen by doctors seem to increase with age. One complication, Barrett's esophagus, may be a precancerous condition, so determination of those at risk is an important subject for research.

Other functional gut disorders

Estimates of the prevalences of the functional gastrointestinal disorders as strictly defined by the Rome criteria are shown in Table 4.2. This work is a result of the canvasing of 8000 American householders (Drossman et al 1993) with 66% compliance and the limitations of the data that were discussed earlier. Nonetheless, the results provide a ballpark idea of the very great prevalences of these disorders.

A few more data are available. Proctalgia fugax occurred in 14% of 301 non-patients (Thompson & Heaton 1980a). Contrary to previous belief, it is not an affliction of young males and it is not uniquely experienced after sexual activity. In fact, it is commoner in young women and apparently unrelated to constipation or IBS. Eight percent of householders said they had the symptom.

Globus is very common. Described as a lump in the throat, it was found in 45% of young people (Thompson & Heaton 1982), but much less in the householders. Although related to strong emotion, it is not deserving of the epithet 'hystericus' that described it for many years.

PROGNOSIS

IBS (Table 4.8)

In terms of life expectancy, the prognosis of patients with IBS is excellent. The symptoms are themselves benign and there is no evidence that they predispose to any other disorder. A cohort of 112 IBS patients seen from 1961 to 1963 was followed for a median of 29 years and only three patients were 'misdiagnosed' (Owens et al 1995). Furthermore, their observed survival was similar to that expected in the population. Indeed, among 498 patients summarized in Table 4.8 in whom the outcome is known, only 10 (2.5%) had a subsequent change in diagnosis and most were new diagnoses. Therefore, the diagnosis of IBS is a safe one, both in terms of reliability and of life expectancy. In terms of cure of symptoms, the outlook is not so good. Many studies confirm that, despite a variety of treatments, most of those originally diagnosed as having IBS still had symptoms when interviewed 1–10 years later (Table 4.8). Given the fickleness of human memory, it is unlikely that many achieve a complete cure. Closer follow-up would likely show that most IBS patients continue to suffer symptoms periodically. In one survey, only 5% of IBS subjects interviewed at 5 years were completely free of symptoms (Kay et al 1994).

Data presented earlier suggest that there is an annual turnover of those reporting IBS criteria and memory of important symptoms can be faulty. The emerging picture is of a very common set of symptoms that seem to come in and out of awareness over a lifetime. For whatever reason, most can expect to be troubled

Table 4.8 Prognosis in the irritable bowel syndrome

Study	Patients	Years follow-up	Percent still symptomatic	Comment
Chaudhary & Truelove 1962	126	1–10	63	–
Waller & Misciewicz 1969	50	1	88	–
Holmes & Salter 1982	77	6	57	Diagnosis change in 4
Svendsen et al 1985	112	2	–	Organic disease in 3
Harvey et al 1987	97	5–8	74	No change in diagnosis
Talley et al 1992	1021	1	62	–
Kay et al 1994	4581	5	95	–
Owens et al 1995	112	32	–	Misdiagnosis in 3, observed survival same as expected

periodically. Perhaps a coping strategy should be the most important objective of the management plan.

FUNCTIONAL DYSPEPSIA (Table 4.9)

Non-ulcer dyspepsia also has a chronic, recurrent course and over 2–7 years 70% of dyspeptics continue to have symptoms (Thompson 1989). Very few of these develop ulcers, probably no more than can be expected in the normal population.

Table 4.9 Prognosis in functional dyspepsia

Study	Patients	Years follow-up	Percent still dyspeptic	Percent that developed ulcer
Gregory et al 1972	102	6	24	3
Talley et al 1987	110	2	70	3*
Sloth & Jorgensen 1988	37	5–7	80	0*

*endoscopically controlled

While there is a strong association of *Helicobacter pylori*-induced gastritis and non-NSAID peptic ulcers, there is no convincing evidence that this is so for non-ulcer (functional) dyspepsia (Thompson 1995). Older studies indicate a lack of relationship between chronic gastritis and symptoms. It is tempting to treat *H. pylori* in non-ulcer dyspeptics, but the evidence so far indicates that the treatment will fail to eliminate the dyspepsia. Indiscriminate use of antimicrobials to eradicate the organism may generate side-effects and bacterial resistance to antibiotics.

IMPLICATIONS OF FUNCTIONAL GUT DISORDERS

Functional gut problems are so common that it is likely that most adults experience some of them at some time. Nevertheless, the important syndromes are very troublesome and account for absenteeism and impaired quality of life (Drossman et al 1993). For example, among patients presenting to endoscopy for abdominal pain, those with functional dyspepsia had more interruption of their daily activities than those who were discovered to have structural disease, mainly peptic ulcer or esophagitis (Talley et al 1995b). They also scored more poorly than ulcer patients in mental health, social functioning and health perception. When people with functional gut disorders consult doctors for their symptoms, they may have many tests, referrals and treatments. These are costly and may contribute little to a person's wellness. Tests should be just sufficient to establish a confident diagnosis.

Patients with IBS symptoms should provoke a graded response from their doctors (Drossman & Thompson 1992). That is, treatments should be appropriate to the severity and confounding features of the disease. Cancer fear, depression, panic, abuse and other psychosocial problems will be greatest in patients seeing specialists. Few primary care patients fit the models developed in academic centers. Many primary care patients will be satisfied with a diagnosis and reassurance that there is no structural disease, especially cancer.

Health care seeking in IBS, particularly to tertiary care centers, may be as much due to a person's cultural and psychosocial state as the IBS symptoms themselves. How else can one explain why women are more likely than men to take their IBS symptoms to a gastroenterology clinic in Western cultures, while the opposite is true in India? Why do only a minority of those with IBS seek medical attention? Does the concurrence of threatening life events or psychosocial distress partially explain these phenomena?

Research should continue to inquire how symptoms are generated, what investigations are appropriate and what treatments are effective. However, it is equally important to understand why most individuals cope with such symptoms without tests, treatments or even consultation with a doctor. It seems likely that the small minority who cannot cope account for most of the suffering and cost.

COSTS

The costs generated by functional gastrointestinal disorders have been little studied. These common conditions are said to be the second most frequent cause of work absenteeism. In the US householders study (Drossman et al 1993), 7.3% of those with the criteria were unable to work or go to school compared to 4.2% of those with criteria for none of these conditions. Those with functional disorders missed 8.7 days of work or school in the previous year compared to 4.9 days in the others. Work loss was especially likely with IBS, constipation, dyspepsia and anorectal disorders.

Most available cost data apply to the IBS. Owens and colleagues (1995) undertook a study of a random sample of the white population of Olmsted County, Minnesota, where a comprehensive health and cost record is in place. Those with known organic disease were excluded from the calculations. They found that those subjects with IBS (abdominal pain +

two Manning criteria) accumulated $742 in health costs in 1942, compared to $429 by those with no functional gut symptoms. Those with gut symptoms that were insufficient to diagnose IBS generated $614. The excess charges for IBS alone amounted to $4 million annually which, when extrapolated to the whole US white population, becomes $8 billion. This astounding figure excludes non-whites and the costs of work loss and outpatient prescription and non-prescription drugs.

There are other indicators of the great costs of IBS and related disorders. Seventy-five percent of American office-based physicians (Longstreth 1995) and 100% of English GPs (Thompson et al 1996) prescribe medication for this benign, long-term disorder, despite lack of proven efficacy. The annual cost of over-the-counter laxatives in American chain drug stores is $348 million. IBS patients are more likely than others to have unnecessary surgery (Fielding 1988) or referral to gynecologists for pelvic pain (Prior et al 1989).

The costs of other gastrointestinal disorders must also be great. In the Minnesota study, patients with functional bowel disease but not IBS cost $185 more than controls, generating a few more billion dollars in national health costs. Dyspeptics are often mistakenly treated by inappropriate ulcer drugs. The annual cost for the management of a new dyspeptic is estimated to be about $1200, whether or not an initial endoscopy is performed (Silverstein et al 1993). In Sweden, Nyren et al (1992) estimated the annual cost of dyspepsia in 1981 to be $113, 630 per 1000 population in 1991 US dollars. In the United States these figures would generate costs of over $28 billion. Further, if one third of adult Americans suffer heartburn, one can imagine the costs if even 40% see a doctor.

Gastroenterologists should not ignore functional gut diseases. These disorders constitute half of our work and, without them, many of us would be out of a job. Costs are driven by worried patients, insecure physicians, free medical care, fee for service management, medicolegal concerns, cancer prevention programs and an increasing public belief that for every discomfort an explanation and cure are fundamental rights. The notion that these disorders are diagnoses of exclusion is costly and intellectually flawed. It generates needless and repeated investigations and tests, increases disability and impairs quality of life. The tendency to seek a quick pharmaceutical fix for these complex dysfunctions instead of more laborious counseling and follow-up is counterproductive.

SUMMARY AND CONCLUSIONS

Functional gastrointestinal disorders are very common. The absence of an anatomical or physiological marker makes their identification difficult. We are only aware of their existence because patients report their symptoms. To bring order to the field, a series of working teams has developed a classification and diagnostic criteria. While these are imperfect, they can guide physicians in clinical diagnosis and provide recognizable entry criteria for clinical research and therapeutic trials.

IBS is the prototype functional gastrointestinal disease, since it is the most common and the most studied. It occurs in 1–20% of most adult populations and appears to be more common in women. Most IBS sufferers do not consult a doctor for their complaint and only a small minority is referred to gastroenterologists, even less to research centers. Yet it is in these academic centers that most studies of the physiology, psychology and treatment of IBS occur. Therefore, the results may not be applicable to the whole IBS population.

The prevalence of dyspepsia is problematic, since there are many definitions and some of them include heartburn. Using the strict Rome criteria in US householders, the prevalence is about 6%. The proportion of dyspeptics that have a peptic ulcer is unknown, but half of those coming to endoscopy are so afflicted. Peptic ulcers can be cured, but people with functional dyspepsia usually continue to have symptoms.

Heartburn occurs in a third of adults and is a daily phenomenon in 3%. It is a marker of GERD, but physiological studies indicate that most people reflux from time to time. There are few data on the prevalence of esophagitis.

These common disorders generate billions of dollars in costs. Were it not for them, half of our gastroenterologists would be unemployed, along with many surgeons, gynecologists, radiologists and other specialists. Much is made of the great costs of medical care, but few realize the economic impact of these benign disorders. They divert funds from the care of more serious disease.

REFERENCES

Agreus L, Svardsudd K, Nyren O, Tibblin G 1994 The epidemiology of abdominal symptoms: prevalence and demographic characteristics in a Swedish adult population A report from the abdominal symptom study. Scandinavian Journal of Gastroenterology 29: 102–109

Agreus L, Svardsudd K, Nyren O, Tibblin G 1995 Irritable bowel syndrome and dyspepsia in the population: overlap and lack of stability over time. Gastroenterology 109: 671–680

Bi-zhen W, Qi-Ying P 1988 Functional bowel disorders in apparently healthy X-Chinese people. Chinese Journal of Epidemiology 9: 345–349

Blau JN 1992 Migraine: theories of pathogenesis. Lancet 339: 1202–1207

Bommelaer G, Rouch M, Dapoigny M et al 1986 Epidemiology of functional bowel disorders in apparently healthy people. Gastroenterology and Clinical Biology 10: 7–12

Bytzer P, Schaffalitzky de Muckadell OB 1992 Prediction of major pathologic conditions in dyspeptic patients referred for endoscopy. A prospective validation study of a scoring system. Scandinavian Journal of Gastroenterology 27: 987–992

Chaudhary NA, Truelove SC 1962 The irritable colon syndrome. Quarterly Journal of Medicine 31: 307–322

Cumming W 1849 Electro-galvanism in a peculiar affliction of the mucous membrane of the bowels. London Medical Gazette NS9: 969–973

Drossman DA, Thompson WG 1992 Irritable bowel syndrome: a graduated, multicomponent treatment approach. Annals of Internal Medicine 116: 1009–1016

Drossman DA, Sandler RS, McKee DC, Lovitz AJ 1982 Bowel patterns among subjects not seeking health care. Use of a questionnaire to identify a population with bowel dysfunction. Gastroenterology 83: 529–534

Drossman DA, McKee DC, Sandler RS et al 1988 Psychosocial factors in the irritable bowel syndrome. A multivariate study of patients and nonpatients with irritable bowel syndrome. Gastroenterology 95: 701–708

Drossman DA, Funch-Jensen P, Janssens J, Talley NJ, Thompson WG, Whitehead WE 1990 Identification of subgroups of functional bowel disorders. Gastroenterology International 3: 159–172

Drossman DA, Li Z, Andruzzi E et al 1993 U.S. householder survey of functional gastrointestinal disorders: prevalence, sociodemography and health impact. Digestive Diseases and Sciences

Drossman DA, Richter J, Talley N et al 1994 Functional gastrointestinal disorders. Little, Brown, Boston.

Fielding JF 1988 Surgery and the irritable bowel syndrome: the singer as well as the song. Journal of Irish Medicine 76: 33–34

George R, Hellier MD, Kennedy HJ, Smits BJ 1993 Definition and sub-typing of non-ulcer dyspepsia. Gastroenterology International 6: 93–99

Gregory DW, Davies GT, Evans KT, Rhodes J 1972 Natural history of patients with x-ray negative dyspepsia in general practice. British Medical Journal 4: 519–520

Hallisey MT, Allum WH, Jewkes AJ, Ellis DG, Fielding JWL 1990 Early detection of gastric cancer. British Medical Journal 301: 513–515

Harvey RF, Salih SY, Read AE 1983 Organic and functional disorders in 2000 gastroenterology outpatients. Lancet i: 632–634

Harvey RF, Mauad EC, Brown AM 1987 Prognosis in the irritable bowel syndrome: a five-year prospective study. Lancet 963–965

Heaton KW, O'Donnell LJD 1994 An office guide to whole gut transit time: patients' recollection of their stool form. Journal of Clinical Gastroenterology 19: 28–30

Heaton KW, O'Donnell LJD, Bradden FEM, Mountford RA, Hughes AO, Cripps PJ 1992 Symptoms of irritable bowel syndrome in a British urban community: consulters and nonconsulters. Gastroenterology 102: 1962–1967

Holmes KM, Salter RH 1982 Irritable bowel syndrome – a safe diagnosis. British Medical Journal 285: 1533–1534

Hu PJ, Li YY, Zhou MH et al 1995 Helicobacter pylori associated with high prevalence of duodenal ulcer disease and a low prevalence of gastric cancer in a developing country. Gut 36: 198–202

Hutchison R 1927 Lectures on dyspepsia, 2nd edn. Edward Arnold, London

Jones RH, Lydeard SE, Hobbs FDR et al 1990 Dyspepsia in England and Scotland. Gut 31: 401–405

Jonsson B, Gardsell P, Johnell O, Redlund-Johnell I, Sernbo I 1995 Remembering fractures: fracture registration and proband recall in southern Sweden. Journal of Epidemiology and Community Health 48: 489–490

Kang JY, Yap I, Gwee KA 1994 The pattern of functional and organic disorders in an Asian gastroenterology clinic. Journal of Gastroenterology and Hepatology 9: 124–127

Kay L, Jorgensen T, Jensen KH 1994 The epidemiology of irritable bowel syndrome in a random population: prevalence, incidence, natural history and risk factors. Journal of Internal Medicine 236: 23–30

Klauser AG, Voderholzer WA, Knesewitsch PA et al 1993 What is behind dyspepsia? Digestive Diseases and Sciences 38: 147–154

Klein KB 1988 Controlled treatment trials in the irritable bowel syndrome: a critique. Gastroenterology 95: 232–241

Longstreth GF 1995 Irritable bowel syndrome: a multibillion-dollar problem. Gastroenterology 109: 2029–2042

Longstreth GF, Wolde-Tsadik G 1993 Irritable bowel-type symptoms in HMO examinees: prevalence, demographics and clinical correlates. Digestive Diseases and Sciences 38: 1581–1589

Mansi C, Mela GS, Pasini D et al 1990 Patterns of dyspepsia in patients with no clinical evidence of organic diseases. Digestive Diseases and Sciences 35: 1452–1458

Mathur A., Tandon BN, Prakkash OM 1966 Irritable colon syndrome. Journal of the Indian Medical Association 46: 651–655

McIntosh D, Thompson WG, Patel D, Barr JR, Guindi M 1992 Is rectal biopsy necessary in irritable bowel syndrome? American Journal of Gastroenterology 87: 1407–1409

Mendis BLJ, Wijesiriwardena BC, Sheriff JHR, Dharmadasa K 1982 Irritable bowel syndrome. Ceylon Medical Journal 27: 171–181

Nash P, Gould SR, Barnardo DE 1986 Peppermint oil does not relieve the pain of irritable bowel syndrome. British Journal of Clinical Practice 40: 292–293

Nebel OT, Fornes MF, Castell DO 1976 Symptomatic gastroesophageal reflux: incidence and precipitating factors. American Journal of Digestive Diseases 21: 953–956

NIH Consensus Conference 1994 *Helicobacter pylori* in peptic ulcer disease. Journal of the American Medical Association 272: 65–68

Nyren O, Lindberg G, Lindstrom E, Marke L, Seensalu R 1992 Economic costs of functional dyspepsia. Pharmacoeconomics 1: 312–324

Olubide IO, Olawuya F, Fasanmade AA 1995 A study of irritable bowel syndrome in an African population. Digestive Diseases and Sciences 40: 983–985

Osler W 1892 Principles and practice of medicine. Pentland, Edinburgh

Owens DM, Nelson DK, Talley NJ 1995 The irritable bowel syndrome: long term prognosis and the patient–physician interaction. Annals of Internal Medicine 122: 107–112

Phillips S, Donaldson L, Geisler K, Pera A, Kochar R. Stool composition in factitial diarrhea: a 6-year experience with stool analysis. Annals of Internal Medicine 1995; 123: 97–100.

Prior A, Wilson K, Whorwell PJ, Faragher EB. Irritable bowel syndrome in the gynecological clinic. Digestive Diseases and Sciences 1989; 34: 1820–1824.

Read NW. Functional gastrointestinal disorders: building castles in the air. Gastroenterology International 1990; 3: 182–183.

Schlemper RM, van der Werf SD, Vandebrouke JP, Biemond I, Lamers CB. Peptic ulcer, non-ulcer dyspepsia and irritable bowel syndrome in The Netherlands and Japan. Scandinavian Journal of Gastroenterology Suppl 1993; 200: 33–41.

Silverstein MD, Petterson T, Talley NJ 1993 Initial endoscopy or empiric therapy for dyspepsia: a toss-up. Medical Decision Making 4: 398

Sloth H, Jorgensen LS 1988. Chronic non-organic upper abdominal pain:

diagnostic safety and prognosis of gastrointestinal and non-intestinal symptoms. A 5- to 7-year follow-up study. Scandinavian Journal of Gastroenterology 23: 1275–1280

Svendsen JH, Munck LK, Andersen JR 1985. Irritable bowel syndrome: prognosis and diagnostic safety. A 5-year follow up study. Scandinavian Journal of Gastroenterology 20: 415–418

Switz DM 1976 What the gastroenterologist does all day. A survey of a state society's practice. Gastroenterology 70: 1048–1050

Talley NJ, McNeil D, Hayden A, Colreavy C, Piper DW 1987 Prognosis of chronic unexplained dyspepsia. A prospective study of potential predictor variables in patients with endoscopically diagnosed nonulcer dyspepsia (published erratum appears in Gastroenterology 1987; 93 (1): 223). Gastroenterology 92: 1060–1066

Talley NJ, Zinsmeister AR, Schleck CD, Melton III LJ 1992a Dyspepsia and dyspepsia subgroups: a population-based study. Gastroenterology 102: 1259–1268

Talley NJ, Weaver AL, Zinsmeister AR, Melton III LJ 1992b Onset and disappearance of gastrointestinal symptoms and functional gastrointestinal disorders. American Journal of Epidemiology 136: 165–177

Talley NJ, Nyren O, Drossman DA et al 1994 The irritable bowel syndrome: toward optimal design of controlled treatment trials. Gastroenterology International 6: 189–211

Talley NJ, Gabriel SE, Harmsen WS, Zinsmeister AR, Evans RW 1995a Medical costs in community subjects with irritable bowel syndrome. Gastroenterology 109: 1736–1741

Talley NJ, Weaver AL, Zinsmeister AR 1995b Impact of functional dyspepsia on quality of life. Digestive Diseases and Sciences 40: 584–589

Thompson WG 1979 The irritable gut. University Park Press, Baltimore

Thompson WG 1984 Gastrointestinal symptoms in the irritable bowel compared with peptic ulcer and inflammatory bowel disease. Gut 25: 1089–1092

Thompson WG 1986 Irritable bowel syndrome: prevalence, prognosis and consequences. Canadian Medical Association Journal 134: 111–113

Thompson WG 1989 Gut reactions. Plenum, New York

Thompson WG 1995 Dyspepsia: is a trial of therapy appropriate? Canadian Medical Association Journal 153: 293–289

Thompson WG, Heaton KW 1980a Proctalgia fugax. Journal of Royal College of Physicians of London 14: 247–248

Thompson WG, Heaton KW 1980b Functional bowel disorders in apparently healthy people. Gastroenterology 79: 283–288

Thompson WG, Heaton KW 1982 Heartburn and globus in apparently healthy people. Canadian Medical Association Journal 126: 46–48

Thompson WG, Creed F, Drossman DA, Heaton KW, Mazzacca G 1992 Functional bowel disorders and functional abdominal pain. Gastroenterology International 5: 75–91

Thompson WG, Heaton KW, Smyth T, Smyth C 1996 Irritable bowel syndrome: the view from general practice. European Journal of Gastroenterology 1997: 9; 689–692

Walker EA, Katon WJ, Jemelka RP, Roy-Byrne PP 1993 Comorbidity of gastrointestinal complaints, depression, and anxiety in the epidemiological catchment area (ECA) study. American Journal of Medicine (suppl.) 1A92: 26–30

Waller SI, Misiewicz JJ 1969 Prognosis in the irritable bowel syndrome. Lancet ii: 753–756

Welch GW, Pomare EW 1990 Functional gastrointestinal symptoms in a Wellington community sample. New Zealand Medical Journal 103: 418–420

Whitehead WE, Bosmajian L, Zonderman AB, Costa PTJ, Schuster MM 1988 Symptoms of psychologic distress associated with irritable bowel syndrome.

Comparison of community and medical clinic samples. Gastroenterology 95: 709–714

Whorwell PJ, McCallum M, Creed FH, Roberts CT 1986 Non-colonic features of irritable bowel syndrome. Gut 27: 37–40

Williams B, Lucas M, Ellingham JHM, Dain A, Wicks ACB 1988 Do young patients with dyspepsia need investigation? Lancet ii: 1349–1351

Psychopathology of functional disorders of the gut

F Creed

INTRODUCTION

It has long been recognized that functional bowel disorders are associated with psychological symptoms. In their seminal work, Chaudhury & Truelove (1962) identified psychological factors which appeared to influence the onset or exacerbation of irritable colon syndrome in over 80% of their 130 cases. The list of psychological factors considered by Chaudhury & Truelove included three separate dimensions which would now be measured individually:

1. personality types – for example, lifelong worrier
2. psychiatric illness – for example, anxiety or depressive disorders
3. environmental stress – for example, business or family problems.

These dimensions will each be considered below, with the additional dimension of illness attitudes and beliefs. Modern research allows independent measurement of each of these dimensions.

Gastroenterologists need to be aware of recent findings and also of some of the methodological pitfalls in this area of research. This chapter will introduce the reader to relevant research and indicate how these empirical data lead to a model of clinical assessment that can be used in routine practice.

TERMINOLOGY

Figure 5.1 indicates the main areas of assessment and some of the measures used for this purpose.

Personality

The term 'personality' refers to habitual responses and coping mechanisms that are stable over time and that are considered to

SOCIAL STRESS		PERSONALITY	MENTAL STATE	
Childhood	Recent	Habitual response to stress/coping Attitudes to illness Independence/ Tendency to worry	Psycho- logical distress	Psych- iatric disorder
e.g. parental illness e.g. sexual abuse	e.g. death in family e.g. divorce			
* Childhood experience and childhood abuse	* Social stress and support interview * Life events and difficulties schedule	* MMPI * Eysenck personality inventory	* SCL-90 * STAXI	* GHQ * HADS * BDI * PSE * SCID

Fig. 5.1 Psychological assessment in functional bowel disorder.

arise from constitutional factors and early environmental experiences. The latter may include loss of a parent or exposure to abnormal parental attitudes. Important dimensions of personality include: self-reliance versus dependence on others, attitudes towards illness and health, characteristic responses to stress. Such attributes will be part of a person's personality prior to the development of any gut disorder.

Mental state

This refers to symptoms of anxiety (e.g. excessive worry and somatic symptoms of anxiety) and depression (depressed mood, crying, gloomy view of the future, etc.). This chapter will distinguish between individual symptoms of anxiety and depression ('psychological distress') and the recognizable clusters of symptoms (syndromes) of anxiety and depressive disorders. The latter are diagnosed when the symptoms are present in sufficient numbers and severity to merit a diagnosis (see below). Anxiety and depressive disorders are the two principal psychiatric disorders that the gastroenterologist needs to diagnose and manage in the clinic.

Social stress

This is considered in two forms. *Early environmental experiences* refer to major experiences during childhood (e.g. loss of a parent, sexual and childhood abuse) which may shape the personality, including characteristic response to stress and attitudes towards illness. *Recent life events* refer to bereavement, marital separation, accidents or illness in the family which may have occurred over recent weeks or months and determine a person's current mental state. They may also be important in precipitating functional gut disorders.

Illness attitudes determine a person's response to symptoms. Whereas one person may tend to deny symptoms (e.g. abdominal pain and diarrhea), another may be inclined to dwell on them and even appear to exaggerate them. Attitudes to illness may be shaped by current mental state, by personality and recent or early stresses. Thus depression, hypochondriacal traits in the personality and recent bereavement may all increase anxieties that normal abdominal sensations imply serious illness. Extreme attitudes and abnormal illness behaviors may amount to a psychiatric diagnosis of somatization or hypochondriacal disorder (see below).

ASSESSMENT AND DIAGNOSIS

This chapter will firstly review advances in measurement of psychiatric disorder and then discuss other psychosocial measures.

Unstandardized clinical assessments

Gomez & Dally (1977) performed clinical interviews on a series of patients presenting to a gastroenterology clinic who did not have an organic cause for their pain. They were all classified as abnormal: 12 drank excessively, 31 were diagnosed as depressed, 21 had chronic tension and 17 manifested 'hysterical symptoms and used their abdominal pain as communication or to obtain necessary narcissistic satisfaction'. This idiosyncratic classification suggests, firstly, that 100% of patients with functional bowel disorders are psychologically abnormal and, secondly, that the psychiatrists were prepared to diagnose psychiatric disorder simply on the presence of abdominal pain. Such a study does not advance our knowledge in a systematic way – it reflects the preconceived notions of the psychiatrists.

Use of psychiatric diagnostic criteria

The use of specific diagnostic criteria improves the reliability of diagnosis; the often quoted studies of Liss et al (1973) and Young et al (1976) used the recognized Feighner's diagnostic criteria. In the Liss study of 25 patients with irritable bowel syndrome eight had anxiety or depressive disorders, seven were diagnosed as hysteria, eight had mild (but non-specific) psychiatric diagnoses and only two did not have a diagnosis of psychiatric disorder. The diagnosis of hysteria would have been made on the basis of multiple bodily symptoms – the gastrointestinal symptoms would have contributed to this diagnosis. Recent research has confirmed that patients attending gastrointestinal clinics with irritable bowel syndrome may have many bodily symptoms (Whorwell et al 1986), but this does not necessarily imply that a psychiatric disorder – hysteria – is present. Thus standardized diagnostic criteria need to be used with care in certain medical clinic populations. This is done using standardized research interviews (see below).

THE PSYCHIATRIC DISORDERS

Anxiety and depressive disorders

The symptoms of anxiety and depressive disorders are well known to most doctors. The criteria for diagnosis are listed in Tables 5.1–3.

Table 5.1 Diagnostic criteria for major depressive disorder

Five (or more) of the following symptoms:

c must include either (1) or (2)
c present during the same 2-week period
c represents a change from previous functioning and causes clear distress &/or impairment in social, occupational functioning
c not due to general medical illness or drugs
c symptoms occur every day or nearly every day.

1. *Depressed mood* most of the day (e.g. feels sad or empty or observed to be tearful)
2. *Loss of interest or pleasure* in all or almost all activities most of the day
3. *Significant weight loss* or *weight gain* (e.g. 5% or more change of body weight in a month) or change in appetite
4. *Insomnia or hypersomnia*
5. Observable *psychomotor agitation* or *retardation*
6. *Fatigue* or *loss of energy* nearly every day
7. Feelings of *worthlessness* or excessive or inappropriate *guilt*
8. Diminished ability to *think or concentrate* or *indecisiveness*
9. Recurrent *thoughts of death* (not just fear of dying), recurrent *suicidal ideation* with or without a specific or a *suicide attempt*

Table 5.2 Diagnostic criteria for generalized anxiety disorder

A. Excessive anxiety and worry (apprehensive expectation), occurring more days than not for at least 6 months, about a number of events or activities (such as work or school performance)

B. The person finds it difficult to control the worry
C. The anxiety and worry are associated with three (or more) of the following six symptoms:
  1. restlessness or feeling keyed up or on edge
  2. being easily fatigued
  3. difficulty concentrating or mind going blank
  4. irritability
  5. muscle tension
  6. sleep disturbance (difficulty falling or staying asleep or restless unsatisfying sleep)
D. The anxiety, worry or physical symptoms cause clinically significant distress or impairment in social, occupational or other important areas of functioning
E. The disturbance is not due to the direct physiological effects of a substance (e.g. a drug of abuse, a medication) or a general medical condition (e.g. hyperthyroidism)

Table 5.3 Criteria for panic attacks

Note: A panic attack is not a diagnosable disorder. Such attacks occur in panic disorder and depressive disorders.

A discrete period of intense fear or discomfort, in which four (or more) of the following symptoms developed abruptly and reached a peak within 10 minutes.
  1. Palpitations, pounding heart or accelerated heart rate
  2. Sweating
  3. Trembling or shaking
  4. Sensations of shortness of breath or smothering
  5. Feeling of choking
  6. Chest pain or discomfort
  7. Nausea or abdominal distress
  8. Feeling dizzy, unsteady, lightheaded or faint
  9. Derealization (feelings of unreality) or depersonalization (being detached from oneself)
  10. Fear of losing control or going crazy
  11. Fear of dying
  12. Paresthesias (numbness or tingling sensations)
  13. Chills or hot flushes

Somatizing and factitious disorders

In addition to anxiety and depressive disorders, the gastroenterologist should be aware of a further diagnostic category – the somatoform disorders. This term refers to patients who have chronic symptoms in numerous bodily systems which are distressing, disabling but which cannot be explained on the basis of organic disease. The recent diagnostic schemes (ICD-10 and DSMIIIR) have grouped together the overlapping 'somatoform disorders', which are listed in Table 5.4. The somatoform disorders are characterized by a number of abnormal illness behaviors:

- disability disproportionate to detectable disease
- a relentless search for causes and cures

- adoption of lifestyle around the sick role, with a repertoire of passive – aggressive behaviors to sustain the sick role and avoidance of healthy roles due to lack of skills or fear of failure
- reinforcement of sick role by family, disability payments and, possibly, health care providers.

Table 5.4 Classification of somatoform and related disorders

Chronic somatizing disorders	
Somatization disorder	* 2 years of multiple/variable physical symptoms for which no adequate physical explanation can be found * Persistent refusal to accept reassurance from doctor * Impairment in social function as a result of the symptoms
Somatoform pain disorder	* Persistent pain unexplained by organic disorder or physiological process
Hypochondriacal disorder	* Persistent preoccupation with possibility of serious disease * Refusal to accept reassurance from doctor and normal investigation results
Simulated disorders	
Dissociative (conversion) disorders	* Acute onset of dramatic symptom(s) which mimic organic disease * Unconscious simulation
Malingering	* Feigned illness * Conscious motivation to avoid responsibility
Factitious disorders	* Self-induced symptoms and signs * Patient aware of the deception but has little insight into underlying motivation (unlike malingerer) * Includes Münchhausen syndrome (and 'by proxy')

There are a number of factors which lead to such behaviors. Firstly, the patient may have marked personality problems and there may also be current relationship difficulties. There may have been a history of prolonged illness during childhood (either in the patient themselves or their parent) and/or a history of lack of parental care during childhood (Craig et al 1993). There may also be current depressive illnesses, which exacerbates the somatizing syndrome.

The term 'factitious disorders' refers to patients who present with various physical symptoms and signs, which are eventually found to be self-induced. This includes surreptitious laxative abuse. In 'Munchausen's syndrome' simulated disease presents dramatically to A & E departments; abdominal pain is common. These people may have been neglected or unwanted as children and appear to gain reward by entering and maintaining the sick role (Ford 1983). They are well aware of the deception involved in these disorders but, unlike malingering, the disorders appear to confer no obvious advantage to the patient – they appear to be driven by underlying psychopathology. The patient has often had previous experience of organic disease (either in themselves or through working in the medical/nursing sphere) and a personality disorder with pronounced dependent, masochistic and hostile traits.

Standardized research interviews for psychiatric diagnosis

The specific diagnostic criteria for psychiatric diagnoses can best be applied, for research purposes, using a standardized research interview. Such interviews record each symptom, using severity and duration criteria to decide whether a symptom is present. For example, the actual loss of weight and number of panic attacks over the preceding month will be recorded – depressed mood and free-floating anxiety are rated on a four-point scale. The reliability and validity of such diagnoses, when used by a trained rater, are excellent. In addition, when used by an experienced clinician, such interviews can exclude symptoms directly attributable to functional bowel disorders to prevent (wrongly) making a psychiatric diagnosis solely on the presence of physical symptoms.

The results of such psychiatric interviews are remarkably consistent, demonstrating that 40–60% of patients attending GI clinics with functional bowel disorders have anxiety and depressive disorders (Table 5.5). There have not been adequate studies of somatoform disorders in gastroenterology clinics; much will depend on the type of clinic and the proportion of chronic attenders (Guthrie et al 1992).

Thus, to many psychiatrists, the term 'psychopathology' may indicate the presence of one or more of the above disorders. Modern training of psychiatrists allows them to state when there is no evidence of such disorders. This is why some patients referred by gastroenterologists to psychiatrists receive a reply indicating that no psychiatric disorder is present.

Psychological distress versus psychiatric disorder

In contrast to the above section regarding a formal psychiatric diagnosis, many patients with functional gut disorders may

Table 5.5 Prevalence of current psychiatric disorder in functional bowel disorder (FBD)/irritable bowel syndrome (IBS) using standardized research psychiatric interviews and a minimum of 30 subjects

Study	Number of subjects	Instrument for psychiatric disorder	Functional bowel disorder	Organic gastrointestinal disorder	Healthy controls
McDonald & Bouchier 1980	32 (FBD[1])	CIS[3]	53%	20%	–
Colgan et al 1988	37 (FBD)	CIS	57%	6%	–
Corney & Stanton 1990	48 (IBS)	CIS	48%	–	
Craig & Brown 1984	79 (FBD)	PSE[4]	42%	18%	–
Ford et al 1987	44 (IBS[2])	PSE	42%	6%	8%
Toner et al 1990a	44 (IBS)	DIS[5]	61%	–	14%
Blanchard et al 1990	68 (IBS)	DIS	56%	25%	18%

[1] FBD = Functional bowel disorder (i.e. consecutive non-organic gastrointestinal disorders in the clinic)
[2] IBS = Irritable bowel syndrome patients
[3] CIS = Clinical interview schedule
[4] PSE = Present state examination
[5] DIS = Diagnostic interview schedule

report symptoms of distress which do not amount to disorder, e.g. occasional crying or anxiety, without the other symptoms listed in Tables 5.1–3.

These symptoms can readily be recorded on self-administered questionnaires. Such questionnaires can be used to provide the clinician with an indication of the level of a patient's distress or, more usually, allow the researcher to compare the levels of distress between two groups of patients (e.g. functional bowel disorder patients with other groups). It is important to note that, for the clinician, the questionnaire cannot be a substitute for clinical assessment (Goldberg 1986).

Methodological aspects of psychosocial measurement in functional gut disorders

Numerous instruments have been used to measure psychosocial variables in functional gut patients; these are referred to in this section and in Table 5.6. However, none of these questionnaires has been designed and validated in a population of patients with functional gut disorders. The responses obtained may therefore need to be viewed with caution. There are two ways in which the results may be distorted.

1. *Bodily symptoms.* We have already seen that patients with functional gut disorders, who have many bodily symptoms, might wrongly be diagnosed as having psychiatric disorder partly on the basis of their bodily symptoms. For example, the frequently used GHQ (28-question version) includes the following items: 'Have you been feeling perfectly well and in good health?',

' . . . been feeling in need of a good tonic?', ' . . . been feeling run down and out of sorts?', ' . . . felt that you are ill?'. Such items are bound to be scored by FBD patients but would not necessarily indicate depression. The Beck Depression Inventory has items of weight loss, concerns about aches and pains, upset stomach, constipation and changes in appetite. It also has items about ability to work that may result directly from bowel disturbance rather than depression. On a questionnaire such symptoms might lead to a spuriously high score, suggesting psychiatric disorder.

2. *Response style*. Abnormal scores may also reflect a general response tendency, which is unrelated to current psychological status; irritable bowel syndrome patients have been noted to respond with socially desirable responses or in a particularly gloomy way (Gomborone et al 1992).

Bearing in mind these two caveats, the psychological measures used among patients with functional GI disorders can be categorized into the following specific domains:

1. personality traits
2. psychological distress
3. psychiatric symptoms
4. illness attitudes and beliefs.

Table 5.6 lists the commonly used instruments for these domains.

Table 5.6 Commonly used psychosocial measures

Dimension	Measure	Comment
Personality	MMPI Minnesota Multiphasic Personality Inventory	550 true/false items. Previously widely used but impractically long and results are contaminated by physical disease
	EPI Eysenck Personality Inventory	57 true–false items. Widely used, reliable and valid. Measures personality dimensions of neuroticism and introversion and extroversion
	STAXI Speilberger Trait Anxiety Inventory	20 items scored on Likert scale. Widely used trait anxiety measure – validity and reliability established
Psychological distress Crown Crisp (CCEI) Experiential Index	SCL-90 Hopkins Symptom Checklist	90 questions scored on Likert scale. Designed for medical and psychiatric patients. Used as screening and outcome measure. Scored on several scales including depression and anxiety

Table 5.6   (contd)

Psychiatric symptoms – self-administered questionnaires	GHQ General Health Questionnaire	12, 28, 30 and 60-item versions. Emphasis on recent change of symptoms. Validated in general population and medical patients (need to adjust 'cut-off' score in latter)
	BDI Beck Depression Inventory	A measure of severity of depression – 21-item scale, with graded statements. 14 + regarded as 'cut-off' but requires higher score in medically ill because it includes somatic items
	HADS Hospital Anxiety and Depression Scale	Designed for medical populations as it excludes somatic items – items each for anxiety and depression graded for severity. Has 'cut-off' scores for anxiety and depression each but not widely validated. Easy to use
	Zung Depression Scale	20 items – quantitative scale of severity of depression
Psychiatric disorder – structured interviews	PSE Present State Interview (now updated as SCAN – Schedules for Clinical Assessment Neuropsychiatry)	Long detailed interview requires trained mental health researcher. CATEGO computerized diagnostic system. Highly reliable in trained hands. Provides psychiatric diagnosis, not severity or change measure
	DIS Diagnostic Interview Schedule	Structured interview for psychiatric diagnosis. Lay interviewers can be trained to use it
	SCID Structured Clinical Interview for DSM-IIIR	Structured diagnostic interview – needs trained mental health researcher
	HRSD Hamilton Rating Scale of Depression	Structured interview for severity of depression – a suitable measure of change
Life stress – self-administered questionnaires	SRE Schedule of Recent Experience	Self-administered questionnaire
	SSRI Cairns and Clare	
Life stress – structured interview	PERI Psychiatric Epidemiology Research Interview LEDS Life Events and Difficulties Schedule	
Illness attitudes and beliefs	IBQ Illness Behaviour Questionnaire IAS Illness Attitude Scale	

Personality

The instruments used to measure personality in functional gut disorders include the MMPI and EPI. The former is not advised

as the results can be profoundly distorted by a disabling illness (Pincus et al 1986). The items such as inability to work and
sleep loss are interpreted as symptoms of depression when
they may equally be due to the disabling effect of a physical
illness.

A number of studies have demonstrated that irritable bowel
syndrome clinic patients are more neurotic and anxious in their
personality than people without health problems or a non-clinical
population with organic bowel disorders (for details, see
Drossman et al 1995a). Esler & Goulston (1973) found that IBS
clinic patients have higher scores in terms of neuroticism
than healthy controls but include some people who are as neurotic and anxious as patients under the care of psychiatrists and
others who are as free of neurosis as healthy controls.

Psychological distress

Scores on psychological distress scales (e.g. Speilberger State
Anxiety Inventory, Crown Crisp Experiential Index.) demonstrate higher scores amongst functional bowel disorder patients
in the clinic than healthy groups but these findings are not confined to this patient group; other medical patient groups show
elevated levels of depression, anxiety and somatization, which
may reflect the distress associated with many disorders (Palmer
et al 1974).

Psychiatric symptoms

These scales may be used as an overall score, which corresponds
to a measure of psychological distress. Alternatively, scores
above a predefined 'cut-off' score indicate probable psychiatric
disorder (usually anxiety or depression). The common scales
used in functional bowel disorders are listed in Table 5.6. The
GHQ provides a measure of psychiatric symptoms as a whole.
The Hospital Anxiety and Depression Scale (HADS) provides a
score for anxiety and depression separately; it may be particularly useful in this population as it specifically excludes items
concerning bodily symptoms – it was designed for use in medical
populations. The Beck Depression Inventory (BDI) is a measure
of severity of depression alone.

The generally accepted cut-off score for the GHQ (28-question
version) is 4/5. Using this cut-off, Whorwell et al (1984) noted
that 10% of the sample of IBS subjects in their hypnotherapy trial

were possible 'cases' of psychiatric disorder. By contrast, 60% of the sample treated by Lancaster-Smith et al (1982) were above the cut-off score; these were, therefore, very different samples of patients.

Heaton (1992) recorded a mean score of 11 for clinic patients with IBS on the anxiety scale of the Hospital and Anxiety Depression Scale (HADS) (Table 5.7); 50% of this sample had probable anxiety disorder. The mean score on the depression scale was 6–11% scored above the cut-off for probable depressive disorder. This sample of patients was very similar, in this respect, to that of Rumsey (1991) who entered into a treatment trial a group of IBS patients whose mean HAD anxiety score was also 11 and mean depression score 6.5. After psychological treatment the HAD score of the treatment group had fallen to 7 for anxiety and 3 for depression.

This illustrates two valid uses of such scales: they are very useful for comparing two populations and comparing change before and after treatment in two groups rather than as a measure of the prevalence of psychiatric disorder. Any tendency to bias should affect both populations similarly, making the comparison valid. The only reliable way to measure prevalence is to use research interviews (see above).

Abnormal illness attitudes and beliefs

The way that a person responds to their functional bowel symptoms, especially in relation to medical treatment seeking, is determined primarily by the patient's attitude towards their symptoms. It is well recognized that patients attending a pain clinic may show abnormal illness behaviors. Two scales have been developed in the pain clinic and used in other patient groups – the Illness Behavior Questionnaire (IBQ) (Pilowsky & Spence 1983) and Illness Attitude Scale (IAS) (Kellner 1983).

Examples of the items that make up the hypochondriacal beliefs, disease phobia and bodily preoccupation scales of the IAS are: 'Do you believe that you have a physical disease but the doctors have not diagnosed it correctly?', 'When your doctor tells you that you have no physical disease, do you refuse to believe him?', 'Are you afraid that you have cancer/another serious illness?', 'If you feel unwell and someone tells you that you are looking well, do you get annoyed?'.

Patients with irritable bowel syndrome have been shown to have abnormal scores on the IBQ especially general hypochondriasis and disease conviction scales. These abnormal scores may be accounted for by the subgroup of patients who have anxiety and depressive disorders (Colgan et al 1988). This is important because it indicates that patients who have anxiety/depressive disorders worry more about their illness, are more convinced that there is an organic cause and see it in somatic (rather than psychological) terms compared to patients who have organic GI disorders.

Studies using the IAS show different results (Gomborone et al 1995). These workers found that certain illness beliefs were more extreme in IBS subjects than in depressed patients under the care of a psychiatrist (Fig. 5.2). This study found highly significant differences between IBS patients and patients with organic gastrointestinal disorders on most scales. IBS patient scores were higher than depressed patients seeing a psychiatrist on the following scales: hypochondriacal beliefs, disease phobia and bodily preoccupation.

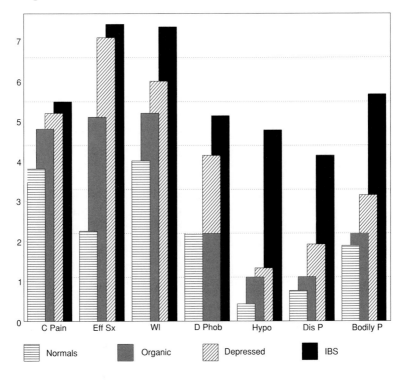

C Pain=   , Eff Sx = Effect of Symptoms, WI = Whitely Index, D Phob = Death Phobic, Hypo = Hypochondriacas beliefs, Disp = Disease Phobia, Bodily P = Bodily Perception

Fig. 5.2 IAS subscale scores (Gomborone et al 1995).

RELATIONSHIP OF FUNCTIONAL BOWEL SYMPTOMS AND PSYCHIATRIC SYMPTOMS

The relationship between bowel and psychiatric symptoms has been considered by Craig (1989), Walker et al (1990) and Creed (1994). One suggestion is that the psychiatric disorder is a consequence of, or a reaction to, the chronic stress of coping with gastrointestinal symptoms. For this to be the case, two conditions must be satisfied: first, functional bowel disorder must precede the psychiatric symptoms. Secondly, psychiatric symptoms must be as common in other (organic) gastrointestinal disorders as the stress of coping with gastrointestinal symptoms will be at least as severe in those with organic GI disorders. Table 5.5 demonstrates that the second condition is not met; psychiatric symptoms are 2–3 times more common in functional bowel disorders than organic disorders.

Only a few studies have paid close attention to the timing of onset of psychiatric and bowel symptoms (Walker et al 1990). Craig (1989) noted that 49% of patients with functional gut disorders had a psychiatric disorder; in 24% the psychiatric disorder occurred first and in 25% the onset of the psychiatric disorder coincided with the onset of the functional bowel disorder. Lydiard et al (1993) noted that 43% of their sample of IBS patients had psychiatric disorder prior to the onset of IBS and an additional 34% experienced the onset of IBS and psychiatric disorder at approximately the same time. Thus the evidence does not support the notion that psychiatric disorder is a consequence of the functional gut disorder.

The alternative explanation is that the functional gut disorder (FGD) is in some way related to the psychiatric disorder. The latter may cause the FGD or exacerbate preexisting subclinical FGD so that treatment is sought. For this relationship to be established, four conditions must be met:

1. psychiatric symptoms must be common in functional bowel disorder patients – we have already seen that this is so (Table 5.5)
2. psychological symptoms must precede or coincide with the onset of functional gut symptoms – this has been reported above
3. other characteristics of psychiatric disorder – childhood antecedents, previous episodes of depression and precipitating life events – should be present
4. response to psychological treatment should be similar to that expected from other psychiatric disorders.

Patients with functional gastrointestinal disorders have the characteristics of other patients with psychiatric disorders.

Childhood antecedents

McDonald & Bouchier (1980) reported that patients with non-organic gastrointestinal illness were significantly different from patients seen in the same clinic with organic GI illness in that they experienced more frequent separation from their parents when young and were more likely to have had an unhappy childhood. Creed (1985) also noted that patients with a normal appendix removed at appendicectomy more frequently had a family history of psychiatric disorder, more difficulties in their relationships with their parents and more disruptions of their parent relationships compared to patients with appendicitis. More recent research has demonstrated more frequent sexual abuse (see below).

Previous episodes of depression

McDonald & Bouchier (1980) reported that patients with non-organic gastrointestinal illness were significantly more likely than patients with organic GI conditions to report previous treatment for depression. Craig & Brown (1984) and Creed (1985) also noted that a greater percentage of patients with functional gut disorders had previous psychiatric disorder compared to patients with organic GI conditions.

Precipitating life events

Two thirds of IBS patients have experienced a severe social stress, such as bereavement, marital separation or major argument leading to a broken family relationship just before onset of the abdominal symptoms. This compares with approximately a quarter of patients with organic disease/healthy controls. The pattern of social stress before the onset of IBS is strikingly similar to that preceding depression and deliberate self-harm, where precipitating stress is well recognized (Creed et al 1988, Creed 1990).

Response to psychological treatment should be similar to that expected from other psychiatric disorders

Lydiard et al (1986) and Noyes et al (1990) showed significant improvement in bowel symptoms concurrent with improved anxiety when patients were treated with psychotropic medication. Greenbaum et al (1987) had found that reduction of depression was associated with improved diarrhea.

Studies using psychological treatments (Guthrie et al 1991, Rumsey 1991) have illustrated that improved anxiety and depression are highly correlated with improved bowel symptoms, suggesting that anxiety and depression are very closely linked to the bowel symptoms.

Are functional gut disorders really psychiatric disorders?

Walker et al (1990) described the irritable bowel syndrome as a 'forme fruste' of psychiatric illness. This is erroneous. Table 5.5 demonstrates that approximately 40% of patients with functional bowel disorders do not have psychiatric disorder. Similarly, studies using personality assessments have indicated that many patients with functional gut disorders fall well within the normal range (Esler & Goulston, 1973).

It is preferable to consider FGD and psychiatric disorders as frequently coexisting disorders; either can occur alone but when they occur together, they can exacerbate each other. Clinically, each must be evaluated in its own right.

PSYCHIATRIC DISORDER, ILLNESS BEHAVIOR AND TREATMENT SEEKING

Many authors have suggested that psychological symptoms are not an integral part of functional bowel disorders but are important concomitants, which lead to treatment seeking. In this model, tertiary referral clinics, which have been the focus of most research, have an overrepresentation of psychiatric diagnoses and abnormal illness behavior.

It is clear from community studies that psychiatric disorder and reported gastrointestinal symptoms are significantly associated (Walker et al 1992, Lydiard et al 1994). Self-reported gastrointestinal symptoms are not the same as a clinical diagnosis of IBS, however. Whitehead et al (1988) have shown that reported gastrointestinal symptoms are associated with psychological distress but this is not so for symptoms fulfilling restricted criteria for irritable bowel syndrome.

On the other hand, one community study which did attempt a clear definition of IBS showed that more severe IBS-type symptoms were clearly associated with higher depression and anxiety scores (Longstreth & Wolde-Tsadik 1993). These symptoms were also associated with more non-gastrointestinal symptoms and greater number of physician visits.

Two studies have found that clinic populations have both more severe gastrointestinal symptoms and more severe psychological symptoms than people in the community who report with IBS symptoms, but who are not consulting a doctor for them. Drossman et al (1988), using multivariate analysis, found that severity of bowel symptoms and psychological symptom score both independently contributed to clinic attendance. Heaton (1992) reported that there was a linear relationship between the number of bowel symptoms and the likelihood of consulting a physician. These authors also reported increased anxiety and depression scores in the clinic attenders (Fig. 5.3) (Table 5.7).

Sandler et al (1984) found that patients with bowel dysfunction who consulted a doctor were also more likely to consult for non-gastrointestinal symptoms. Others have reported that people

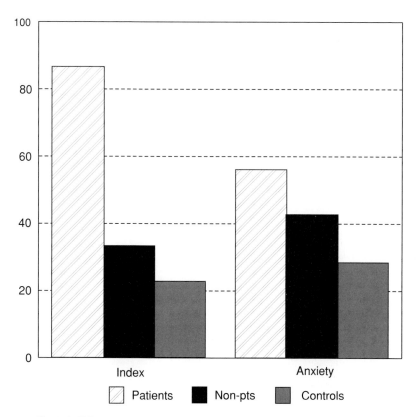

Fig. 5.3 IBS severity index and HAD anxiety scores (Heaton et al 1991).

Table 5.7 Results of anxiety and depression scores on the Hospital Anxiety and Depression Scale (HADS) (Heaton et al 1991) and on the Beck Depression Inventory (Greenbaum et al 1983). The table shows median scores for patients with IBS attending a gastroenterology clinic, those in the community who have IBS symptoms but do not seek medical treatment and healthy controls in the community

	HADS anxiety	HADS depression	BDI depression
Clinic patients	11	6	7
Non-clinic symptomatic	9	3	5
Healthy comparison subjects	5	3	2

who complain of symptoms of IBS are more likely to seek treatment frequently from doctors than those who have a peptic ulcer (Whitehead et al 1982). Thus illness behavior, particularly fear of serious illness, is an important determinant of treatment seeking (Lydiard & Jones 1989).

Drossman et al (1988) recorded IBQ scores for three groups of people: IBS patients in the clinic, people in the community with IBS symptoms but who were not seeking treatment, and healthy controls. The clinic patients had significantly higher scores than the other groups for abdominal pain, affective disorder, health worry and illness disruption scales of the IBQ (Fig. 5.4).

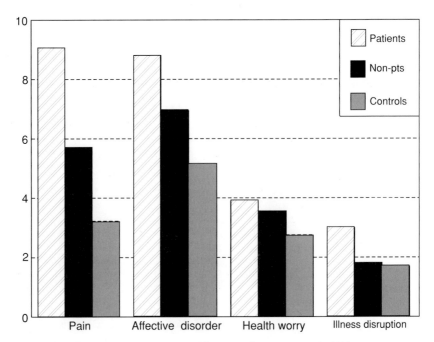

Fig. 5.4 Symptom reports and IBQ scores (Drossman et al 1988).

In summary, there may be several factors that distinguish clinic attenders from non-attenders: more severe more bowel symptoms, presence of anxiety/depression, illness behavior.

SEXUAL ABUSE

In tertiary referral clinics, sexual and physical abuse have been reported by a significant number of women and the proportion is generally higher in patients with functional GI diagnoses compared to those with organic diagnoses (Table 5.8). These results have been confirmed in two community studies. Longstreth & Wolde-Tsadik (1993) found that all forms of abuse were significantly more frequent in people reporting severe IBS-type symptoms compared to those reporting less severe IBS-symptoms and normal controls. Talley et al (1994) reported that the rate of sexual abuse was twice as high amongst those with IBS or functional dyspepsia compared to healthy subjects.

Such abuse is associated with a higher frequency of pelvic pain, multiple somatic symptoms and more lifetime surgery. Drossman et al (1996) found that women who reported a history of abuse experienced significantly more pain, more days in bed, more psychological distress, poorer daily function, more frequent physician visits and more lifetime surgery than those who had not been abused.

Mechanism of relationship with sexual abuse

It is recognized that patients with a prior history of sexual abuse are more likely to have depression and anxiety. In addition, abuse history is strongly associated with increased symptom reporting, including pelvic pain, headache, back pain and multiple somatic symptoms (Golding 1994). Physician attendance is also significantly higher in those who have been abused.

Table 5.8   Prevalence of reported sexual abuse in patients with functional GI disorders, organic GI disorders and healthy controls

Study	No. of subjects	% WITH HISTORY OF ABUSE		
		functional disorders	GI organic disorder	GI healthy controls
Drossman et al 1990	200	31	18	
Longstreth	1264	22.2	–	5.2
Talley et al 1994	919	43		19.4
Drossman et al 1996	239	33	20	

There may be a non-specific relationship between patients presenting with functional gut disorders and sexual abuse; abuse is associated with continuing psychological distress and the social conditions in which abuse has occurred may be those where the person has poor social support and ongoing stressful life events. There may also be several more direct ways to explain the relationship, including psychophysiological mechanisms, enhanced visceral sensitivity or lowered pain threshold (Scarinci et al 1994; Drossman et al 1996).

Interviews of women with irritable bowel syndrome and women with inflammatory bowel disease or duodenal ulceration have indicated a higher frequency of sexual problems in the former; these results hold even when present psychiatric disorder is controlled (Guthrie et al 1987). It is likely that part of the reason for such sexual problems is prior sexual abuse.

RATIONALE FOR A PSYCHOSOCIAL ASSESSMENT

Owens et al (1995) assessed the quality of the physician–patient interaction at the first appointment with functional bowel disorder using the following eight criteria:

1. documentation in the notes of the patient's psychosocial history
2. notation of reassurance about the diagnosis
3. reference to the patient's name within the physician's notes
4. use of pronouns and adjectives that suggest the collaboration of patient and physician
5. referral for psychiatric counseling only if evidence of a definite psychiatric diagnosis existed
6. no unnecessary invasive procedures ordered without firm indication
7. notation of a factor or factors that precipitated the patient seeking medical help
8. notation of discussion with the patient about test results and diagnosis.

The key variables which were related to number of return IBS visits were three: notation of the patient's psychosocial history, the precipitating factors causing the patient to seek medical help and discussion with the patient. The patients in whose notes these were recorded were less likely to make return visits.

Van Dulmen et al (1995) recorded changes reported by the patient after consultation with a gastroenterologist for functional bowel disorders. Following consultation there was a significant reduction in the patient's overall anxiety, fear of having cancer and preoccupation and helplessness in relation to the pain. Since these factors are related to outcome, the reduced anxiety, reduced fear of cancer and understanding of the relationship between stress and gut function could lead to a better outcome.

CLINICIAN'S ASSESSMENT OF PSYCHOSOCIAL DIMENSIONS

Whatever the theoretical relationship between psychological symptoms and functional gut disorders, the task facing the clinician is clear. In the gastrointestinal clinic, patients with functional gut disorders need to be assessed on the following dimensions:

c psychological distress, including the possible presence of an anxiety or depressive disorder
c personality dimensions – a possible lifelong tendency to worry, including longstanding excessive concerns about the significance of the gut and other bodily symptoms and habitual response to stress
c current difficult social situations and ineffective coping strategies
c abnormal illness attitudes and behaviors.

Each of these requires assessment in its own right as well as assessment of the bowel symptoms. The aim of the following section is to indicate how these assessments may be completed in a short period of time so that they can be applied routinely to all patients with functional gut disorders. They do not provide a way of distinguishing between functional and organic GI disorders – patients with duodenal ulcer or ulcerative colitis may have depressive disorder, neurotic personality and abnormal illness attitudes.

Detection of psychological problems

When gastroenterologists assess patients, they need to cover any psychological disorders or specific psychosocial problems which might accompany the gastrointestinal symptoms. There are two ways of doing this. The first is to use a screening questionnaire, the second is to use direct clinical interview. For research purposes, a screening questionnaire alone may suffice. In clinical practice a specific clinical interview is also required (Goldberg 1986).

The questions to ask

Specific questions that the gastroenterologist should ask include the following:

1. When did your symptoms start?
The doctor may also ask: 'When did you last feel quite well?'. This enables the patients to indicate the time course of the physical symptoms, which may be related to a stressful event, and indicate that the feeling of being unwell may have started with psychological symptoms prior to the current somatic symptom.

2. What do you think your symptoms are due to?
Further questioning enables fears of illness to be detected and explored.

3. Have you had difficulties sleeping?
This is followed by the questions in Table 5.9 to detect anxiety or depression.

4. Have there been any recent stresses in your life?
These questions will demonstrate to the patient that the gastroenterologist is interested in psychological and social aspects of the patient's disorder as well as the bowel symptomatology. They will also help the gastroenterologist to decide if referral to a psychologist or psychiatrist is required.

Table 5.9   An example of a brief mood scale is provided in Goldberg et al 1994

Anxiety	Depression
1. Have you felt keyed up and on edge?	1. Low energy?
2. Have you been worrying a lot?	2. Loss of interest?
3. Have you been irritable?	3. Loss of confidence in yourself?
4. Have you had difficulty relaxing?	4. Felt hopeless?
If 'yes' to any two of the above, go on to:	*If 'yes' to any one of above, go on to:*
5. Have you been sleeping poorly?	5. Unable to concentrate?
6. Have you had headaches or tightness in head or neck?	6. Lost weight (poor appetite)
7. Dizzy, trembling, sweating, diarrhea, frequency, tingling? (autonomic anxiety)	7. Early waking?
8. Been worried about your health?	8. Felt slowed up?
9. Difficulty falling asleep?	9. Felt worse in the morning?
1 point for each answer.	*1 point for each answer.*
Add A-score – anxiety states usually score 5+	*Add D-score – depression usually scores 3+*

Referral to a psychologist/psychiatrist

When to consider a referral

Referral to a psychiatrist may be appropriate when the gastroenterologist:

c believes that the patient has a psychiatric disorder which requires assessment and treatment

c discovers that the patient is seriously depressed and/or has suicidal ideas

c needs advice regarding the use of psychotropic drugs (e.g. antidepressants in chronic pain)

c finds serious impairment of social functioning that cannot be explained by the functional gut disorder

c believes the patient shows chronic somatization with multiple referrals to many different departments

c uncovers a history of sexual abuse or other major trauma which requires more specialized psychological treatment than the gastroenterologist and GP can offer.

How to make the referral

Many patients are loath to see a psychiatrist or psychologist. The suggestion may lead a patient to protest that (s)he is not mad or to accuse the doctor of considering that the pain is being imagined.

This most commonly occurs when the suggestion of seeing a psychiatrist is made at the end of the diagnostic search, which has included technological investigations to detect organic disease but without a parallel interest in the patient's psychosocial problems. An earlier explanation that the symptoms are often linked to stress and that exploration of stress is an important part of the assessment will overcome these difficulties in most cases. There are a few patients, however, in whom the mildest suggestion of seeing a psychiatrist or psychologist is greeted with the most vehement refusal coupled with clear annoyance at the doctor who suggested it – possibly apparent from the patient's accusation that the doctor does not believe his symptoms or is indicating that the symptoms are 'all in the mind'.

The patient with chronic abdominal pain

The patient with chronic abdominal pain provides the gastroenterologist with a special problem (Drossman & Thompson 1992). The form of assessment outlined above provides a framework for such patients. The gastroenterologist should assess whether the patient has a depressive disorder, which commonly accompanies chronic pain syndromes, acknowledge (repeatedly if necessary) the reality of the pain and assess abnormal illness behavior. In their descriptive paper, Drossman & Thompson indicate that this group of patients should be managed in a different way, resembling the management for chronic pain patients (see Chapter 6).

REFERENCES

Blanchard EB, Scharff L, Schwartz SP, Suls JN, Barlow DH 1990 The role of anxiety and depression in the irritable bowel syndrome. Behaviour Research Therapy 28: 401–405

Chaudhury NA, Truelove SC 1962 Irritable colon syndrome. A study of the clinical features, predisposing causes, and prognosis in 130 cases. Quarterly Journal of Medicine 31: 307–322

Colgan S, Creed FH, Klass H 1988 Symptom complaints, psychiatric disorder and abnormal illness behaviour in patients with upper abdominal pain. Psychological Medicine 18: 887–892

Corney RH, Stanton R 1990 Physical symptom severity, psychological and social dysfunction in a series of outpatients with irritable bowel syndrome. Journal of Psychosomatic Research 34: 483–491

Craig TK 1989 Abdominal pain. In: Brown G, Brown, TO (eds) Life events and illness. Guilford Press, New York

Craig TK, Brown GW 1984 Goal frustrating aspects of life events stress in the aetiology of gastrointestinal disorder. Journal of Psychosomatic Research 28: 411–421

Craig TK, Boardman AP, Mills K, Daly-Jones O, Drake H 1993 The south London somatisation study. I: Longitudinal course and the influence of early life experiences. British Journal of Psychiatry 163: 579–588

Creed FH 1985 Psychosocial variables and appendicectomy. MD Thesis, University of Cambridge

Creed FH 1990 Functional abdominal pain in somatization: physical symptoms and psychological illness. In: Bass C (ed.) Blackwell, Oxford

Creed F 1994 Controversies in management. Irritable bowel syndrome. Psychological treatment is essential for some. British Medical Journal 309: 1647–1648

Creed FH 1996 Conceptual issues in psychosomatics. Proceedings of the Royal College of Physicians of Edinburgh 26: 26–35

Creed FH, Guthrie E 1989 Psychological treatment of the irritable bowel syndrome: a review. Gut 30: 1601–1609

Creed FH, Craig T, Farmer R 1988 Functional abdominal pain, psychiatric illness and life events. Gut 29: 235–242

Drossman DA, Thompson WG 1992 The irritable bowel syndrome: review and a graduated, multicomponent treatment approach. Annals of Internal Medicine 116: 1009–1016

Drossman DA, McKee DC, Sandler RS et al 1988 Psychosocial factors in irritable bowel syndrome. A multi-variate study of patients and non-patients with IBS. Gastroenterology 91: 701–708

Drossman DA, Leserman J, Nachman G et al 1990 Sexual and physical abuse in women with functional or organic gastrointestinal disorders. Annals of Internal Medicine 113: 828–833

Drossman DA, Creed FH, Fava GA et al 1995a Psychosocial aspects of the functional gastrointestinal disorders. Gastroenterology International 8(2): 47–90

Drossman DA, Talley NJ, Leserman J, Olden KW, Barreiro MA 1995b Sexual and physical abuse and gastrointestinal illness. American College of Physicians 123: 782–794

Drossman DA, Zhiming L, Leserman J, Toomey TC, Yuming JB 1996 Health status by gastrointestinal diagnosis and abuse history. Gastroenterology 110: 999–1007

Esler MD, Goulston KH 1973 Levels of anxiety in colonic disorders. New England Journal of Medicine 288: 16–20

Ford CV 1983 The somatising disorder. Illness as a way of life. Elsevier, New York

Ford MJ, Miller PM, Eastwood J et al 1987 Life events, psychiatric illness and the irritable bowel syndrome. Gut 28: 160–165

Goldberg D 1986 Use of the General Health Questionnaire in clinical work. British Medical Journal 293: 1188–1189

Goldberg DP, Benjamin S, Creed F 1994 Psychiatry in medical practice, 2nd edn. Routledge, London

Golding JM 1994 Sexual assault history and physical health in randomly selected Los Angeles women. Health Psychology 13: 130–138

Gomborone JE, Dewsnap PA, Libby GW, Farthing MJG 1992 A specific illness-related schema in irritable bowel syndrome (IBS). Abstract British Society of Gastroenterology S23

Gomborone J, Dewsnap P, Libby G, Farthing M 1995 Abnormal illness attitudes in patients with irritable bowel syndrome. Journal of Psychosomatic Research 39: 227–230

Gomez J, Dally P 1977 Psychologically mediated abdominal pain in surgical and medical outpatient clinics. British Medical Journal i: 1451–1453

Greenbaum D, Abitz L, van Egeren L, Mayle J, Greenbaum R 1983 Irritable bowel symptoms prevalence, rectosigmoid motility and psychometrics in symptomatic subjects not seeing physicians. Gastroenterology 84: 1174

Greenbaum D, Mayle J, van Egeren L et al 1987 Effects of desipramine on irritable bowel syndrome compared with atropine and placebo. Digestive Diseases and Sciences 32: 257–266

Guthrie E, Creed FH, Whorwell P 1987 Severe sexual dysfunction in women with the irritable bowel syndrome: comparison with inflammatory bowel disease and duodenal ulceration. British Medical Journal 295: 577–578

Guthrie E, Creed FH, Dawson D, Tomenson B 1991 A controlled trial of psychological treatment for the irritable bowel syndrome. Gastroenterology 100: 450–457

Guthrie E, Creed FH, Whorwell PK 1992 Outpatients with irritable bowel syndrome: a comparison of first time and chronic attenders. Gut 33: 361–363

Heaton K 1992 What makes people with abdominal pain consult their doctor? In: Creed F, Mayon R, Hopkins A (eds) Medical symptoms not explained by organic disease. Royal College of Psychiatrists and Royal College of Physicians, London, pp 1–8

Heaton K, Ghosh S, Braddon FEM 1991 How bad are the symptoms and bowel dysfunction of patients with irritable bowel syndrome? A prospective, controlled study with special reference to stool form. Gut 32: 73–79

Kellner R 1983 Abridged manual of the Illness Attitude Scale. University of New Mexico, Albuquerque

Lancaster-Smith MJ, Prout BJ, Pinto T, Anderson JA, Schiff AA 1982 Influence of drug treatment on the irritable bowel syndrome and its interaction with psychoneurotic morbidity. Acta Psychiatrica Scandinavica 66: 33–41

Liss JL, Alpers D, Woodruff RA 1973 The irritable colon syndrome and psychiatric illness. Diseases of the Nervous System 34: 151–157

Longstreth GF, Wolde-Tsadik G 1993 Irritable bowel-type symptoms in HMO examinees. Prevalence, demographics and clinical correlates. Digestive Diseases and Sciences 38: 1581–1589

Lydiard RB, Laraia MT, Howell EF et al 1986 Can panic disorder present as irritable bowel syndrome? Journal of Clinical Psychiatry 57: 470–473

Lydiard RB, Fossey MD, Marsh W, Ballenger JC 1993 Prevalence of psychiatric disorders in patients with irritable bowel syndrome. Psychosomatics 34: 229–234

Lydiard RB, Greenwald S, Weissman MM, Johnson J, Drossman DA, Ballenger JC 1994 Panic disorder and gastrointestinal symptoms: findings from the NIMH Epidemiologic Catchment Area Project. American Journal of Psychiatry 151: 64–70

Lydiard S, Jones R 1989 Factors affecting the decision to consult with dyspepsia: comparison of consulters and non-consulters. Journal of the Royal College of General Practitioners 39: 495–498

McDonald AJ, Bouchier PAD 1980 Non-organic gastro-intestinal illness: a medical and psychiatric study. British Journal of Psychiatry 136: 1276–1283

Noyes R, Cook B, Garvey M et al 1990 Reduction of gastrointestinal symptoms with treatment for panic disorder. Psychosomatics 31: 75–79

Owens DM, Nelson DK, Talley NJ 1995 The irritable bowel syndrome: long-term prognosis and the physician–patient interaction. Annals of Internal Medicine 122: 107–112

Palmer RL, Stonehill E, Crisp AH, Waller SL, Misiewicz JJ 1974 Psychological characteristics of patients with the irritable bowel syndrome. Postgraduate Medical Journal 50: 416–419

Pilowsky I, Spence ND 1983 Manual for the Illness Behaviour Questionnaire (IBQ), 2nd edn. University of Adelaide, Australia

Pincus T, Callahan LF, Bradley LA, Vaughn WK, Wolfe F 1986 Elevated MMPI scores for hypochondriasis depression, and hysteria in patients with rheumatoid arthritis reflect disease rather than psychological status. Arthritis and Rheumatism 29: 1456–1466

Rumsey N 1991 Group stress management versus pharmacological treatment in the irritable bowel syndrome. In: Heaton K, Creed F, Goeting N (eds) Towards confident management of irritable bowel syndrome. Duphar Laboratories Ltd

Sandler RS, Drossman DA, Nathan HP, McKee DC 1984 Symptom complaints and health care seeking behaviour in subjects with bowel dysfunction. Gastroenterology 87: 314–318

Scarinci IC, McDonald-Haile J, Bradley LA, Richter JE 1994 Altered pain perception and psychosocial features among women with gastrointestinal disorders and history of abuse: a preliminary mode. American Journal of Medicine 97: 108–117

Talley NJ, Fett SL, Zinsmeister AR, Melton III LJ 1994 Gastrointestinal tract symptoms and self-reported abuse: a population-based study. Gastroenterology 107: 1040–1049

Thompson WG, Creed F, Drossman DA, Heaton KW, Mazzacca 1992 Functional bowel disease and functional abdominal pain. Working Team Report. Gastroenterology International 5: 75–91

Toner BB, Garfinkel PE, Jeejeebhoy KN 1990a Psychological factors in irritable bowel syndrome. Canadian Journal of Psychiatry 35: 161

Toner BB, Garfinkel PE, Jeejeebhoy KN et al 1990b Self-schema in irritable bowel syndrome and depression. Psychosomatic Medicine 52: 149–155

Van Dulmen AM, Fennis JFM, Mokkink HGA, van der Velden HGM, Bleijenberg G 1995 Doctor-dependent changes in complaint-related cognitions and anxiety during medical consultations in functional abdominal complaints. Psychological Medicine 25: 1011–1018

Walker EA, Roy-Burne PP, Katon WJ 1990 Irritable bowel syndrome and psychiatric illness. American Journal of Psychiatry 147: 565–572

Walker EA, Katon WJ, Jemelka RP, Roy-Byrne PP 1992 Comorbidity of gastrointestinal complaints, depression, and anxiety in the epidemiologic catchment area (EAC) study. American Journal of Medicine 92: 26–30

Whitehead WE, Winget C, Fedoravicius AS, Wooley S, Blackwell B 1982 Learned illness behaviour in patients with IBS and peptic ulcer. Digestive Diseases and Sciences 27: 202–208

Whitehead WE, Bosmajian L, Zonderman A, Costa P, Schuster MM 1988 Symptoms of psychological distress associated with irritable bowel syndrome: comparison of community and clinic samples. Gastroenterology 92: 709–714

Whorwell P, McCallum M, Creed FH, Roberts CT 1986 Non-colonic manifestations of irritable bowel syndrome. Gut 27: 37–40

Young SJ, Alpers DH, Norland CC et al 1976 Psychiatric illness and the irritable bowel syndrome. Gastroenterology 70: 162–166

Chronic abdominal pain

6

PJ Whorwell, W Gonsalkorale

Amongst the long list of causes of chronic abdominal pain found in any large textbook of medicine (Table 6.1) there is usually a category entitled 'functional'. This is the somewhat derisive term that is reserved for those patients in whom no obvious etiology for their problem can be established. These patients are the focus of this chapter and it is assumed that all the other possibilities listed in Table 6.1 have already been excluded.

It seems reasonable to suppose that the syndrome of chronic abdominal pain is a heterogeneous condition which will only become more clearly understood as we acquire a better knowledge of the neurophysiology of the gut/brain axis, particularly as it relates to the perception of pain (see Chapter 2). Most patients with this problem are referred to gastroenterologists but this does not necessarily mean that the pain is always gastrointestinal in origin. In women, the gynecological system has to be seriously considered particularly when the pain is below the umbilicus or confined to the pelvis. In some patients the anterior abdominal wall may be the origin of the pain whilst in others root pain has to be ruled out. The role of postoperative adhesions in the genesis of chronic pain remains highly controversial and in some cases the patient seems to actually wake up with pain after an operation, making adhesions implausible and raising the possibility of some form of 'neurogenic' pain. The nature of the pain (e.g. colicky or burning) and its duration (e.g. continuous) can sometimes be helpful in predicting responsiveness to treatment, with subjects complaining of unrelenting pain often appearing not to do quite so well.

When the pain is gastrointestinal in origin it can presumably arise from any anatomical site including the biliary tract. Some of the more severe cases turn out to have problems such as visceral neuropathy but the vast majority of patients appear to have irritable bowel syndrome in which, for some reason, pain is the overwhelmingly predominant symptom. Why pain should

Table 6.1 Some important causes of abdominal pain

Pain originating in the abdomen
  A. Parietal peritoneal inflammation
    1. Bacterial contamination, e.g. perforated appendix, pelvic inflammatory disease
    2. Chemical irritation, e.g. perforated ulcer, pancreatitis, mittelschmerz
  B. Mechanical obstruction of hollow viscera
    1. Obstruction of the small or large intestine
    2. Obstruction of the biliary tree
    3. Obstruction of the ureter
  C. Vascular disturbances
    1. Embolism or thrombosis
    2. Vascular rupture
    3. Pressure or torsional occlusion
    4. Sickle cell anaemia
  D. Abdominal wall
    1. Distortion or traction of mesentery
    2. Trauma or infection of muscles
  E. Distension of visceral surfaces, e.g. hepatic or renal capsules

Pain referred from extraabdominal sources
  A. Thorax, e.g. pneumonia, referred pain from coronary occlusion
  B. Spine, e.g. radiculitis from arthritis
  C. Genitalia, e.g. torsion of the testicle

Metabolic causes
  A. Exogenous
    1. Black widow spider bite
    2. Lead poisoning and others
  B. Endogenous
    1. Uraemia
    2. Diabetic ketoacidosis
    3. Porphyria
    4. Allergic factors (C1 esterase inhibitor deficiency)

Neurogenic causes
  A. Organic
    1. Tabes dorsalis
    2. Herpes zoster
    3. Causalgia and others
  B. Functional

Adapted from, Harrison's Principles of Internal Medicine

predominate so much in a particular patient is unknown but in some, certain factors such as psychological problems or previous physical or sexual abuse may be contributory. Table 6.2 gives a more exhaustive list of the many possible causes of 'functional' chronic abdominal pain including some syndromes of questionable significance.

Management of chronic abdominal pain

It is essential to try and give the patient a diagnosis but in some instances this is just an impossible goal. It is our practice to admit difficult patients to our investigation unit for a week where they are submitted to an in-depth evaluation. This includes clinical,

Table 6.2 Causes of chronic (functional) abdominal pain

Functional bowel disorders
  Irritable bowel syndrome
  Functional dyspepsia
  Biliary dyskinesia
Visceral myopathy/neuropathy
Chronic abdominal wall pain
  Myofascial pain
  Nerve entrapment
  Skeletal pain
  Spinal pain
  Hernias
  Rectus syndrome
Pelvic pain/pelvic congestion
Postoperative pain
  Incisional pain
  Nerve 'damage'
  Adhesions
Hyperventilation
Dietary allergy/intolerance
Disaccharide intolerance
Celiac artery compression syndrome
Celiac (solar) plexus syndrome

investigational, psychological, physiological and dietary assessments. They are also seen by the pain management team. All diagnostic possibilities are reviewed and where indicated, additional investigations that have not been previously undertaken may be contemplated to either exclude other organic diseases (Table 6.1) or to try and define the type of functional disorder further (Table 6.2). From the point of view of functional disorders these may include various scanning procedures, contrast radiology, endoscopic cholangiopancreatography and laparoscopy as well as hematological tests such as the measurement of gastrointestinal hormones. Physiological assessments vary from patient to patient but the most commonly performed tests are transit measurements and anorectal motility/sensitivity recordings as these can help with the more rational 'targeting' of therapeutic strategies. All patients are seen by a member of the hypnotherapy/counseling team and the pain management unit for an assessment regarding their suitability for either of these approaches to management. The dietitian decides whether some form of exclusion diet is worth trying as there is evidence that some patients benefit from avoidance of certain dietary constituents (Alun Jones et al 1982).

If a reasonable diagnostic label can be applied to a patient then all the standard pharmacological approaches suitable for that condition are tried alone or in combination before they are judged refractory. After all this we are then left with a group of patients with chronic abdominal pain in whom a diagnosis may or may not have been made. From then on we take the stance that pain control is the main priority rather than worrying too much about applying a specific diagnostic label to them.

Pain control

This can take three basic forms which can be broadly categorized under the headings pharmacological, physical and psychological.

Pharmacological approaches involve trying a variety of medications, altering their dose as necessary and establishing whether there is a response or not. Similar principles apply to physical methods. Psychological approaches are far more complex and in recent years have received a considerable amount of attention. Thus, proportionally much more space is devoted to the latter in this chapter, particularly as the practising gastroenterologist is less likely to be familiar with the techniques involved and the jargon used with these types of approach. Furthermore, a good understanding of the psychotherapeutic principles involved in pain control is undoubtedly useful even when delivering more traditional remedies for pain as even when these are effective, the patient often needs some form of support system.

PHARMACOLOGICAL APPROACHES

Antidepressants

Although many patients will have already tried this group of drugs they are still worthy of consideration. Traditionally, tricyclics are used and some appear to be more effective than others (Pace et al 1995). It is worth noting that a response can often be achieved at a relatively low dose (sub-antidepressant) which enables the drug to be better tolerated particularly if there has been intolerance before. It is important that the side-effects of these drugs are fully explained as initially patients can often feel worse before they feel better. Constipation can be a feature with this group of antidepressants which may be advantageous if there is coexistent diarrhea but undoubtedly constipated patients are often made worse. This can usually be overcome by the use of a laxative but can sometimes be so severe that discontinuation of treatment is necessary. Terminal care specialists sometimes use extremely high doses of tricyclic antidepressants to aid pain control and we sometimes try this approach especially if there is coexistent depression, although we often then encounter problems with the bowel habit. The more modern selective serotonin re-uptake inhibitors do not cause constipation but can induce nausea which is a common preexisting symptom in patients with chronic abdominal pain. In addition, the effect of this class of drugs on chronic pain syndromes has yet to be fully evaluated but obviously does not preclude their use in the meantime.

Narcotics

We are not afraid to introduce narcotics in this problem and are able to obtain reasonable pain control in a substantial proportion of patients. We usually use slow-release morphine preparations or diamorphine elixir, sometimes in combination with tricyclic antidepressants and always under the strict supervision of the pain management team with the use of pain charts, etc. Constipation can be a problem but this can often be overcome with a laxative although rather generous doses may be needed. An alternative which is not associated with so much bowel disturbance and has a longer duration of action is fentanyl in the form of transdermal patches. We feel that once the 'alarm' associated with the use of such drugs in a benign disorder has been overcome in both the patient and their medical attendants, they are an extremely useful adjunct in the management of this difficult condition.

Other drugs

If the pain appears to have a 'neurogenic' component, carbamazepine is worthy of trial and it has been suggested that gonadotrophin-releasing hormone analogs (Mathias et al 1994) might be effective in some patients with chronic abdominal pain. Homeopathic remedies are often tried by such patients and although we have no experience of this approach, we do not discourage patients from trying this form of treatment if they want to.

PHYSICAL APPROACHES

Transcutaneous electrical nerve stimulation (TENS)

Transcutaneous nerve stimulation (TNS) in various forms has been used for many years although the use of an electrical current as the stimulant (TENS) is a more recent innovation. It is an extremely simple technique using electrodes (often two) rather similar to those used for electrocardiographic monitoring and placing them on the surface of the skin overlying the pain (McMeeken & Stillman 1987). They are connected to a small battery-powered stimulation unit which can be worn unobtrusively and delivers a current which can be adjusted in terms of both frequency and intensity. The 'gate' theory of pain control is often suggested as the mechanism by which TENS exerts its benefit but a full understanding of how it works still eludes us (McMeeken & Stillman 1987). TENS is currently enjoying widespread popularity in fields as diverse as childbirth and cancer pain control. There is some evidence that it may have some application in abdominal pain syndromes (Sylvester et al 1986) and we find that it is undoubtedly helpful in a small but significant proportion of our patients. If it does help pain, it does not change any of the other features commonly observed in functional bowel disorders such as bowel habit, distension or noncolonic manifestations. It is certainly free of any side-effects other than occasional cutaneous reactions to adhesives or electrode gels.

Acupuncture

It is not within the scope of this chapter to discuss whether this technique is just another form of transcutaneous nerve stimulation or has other unique qualities that make it a separate entity. Although widely used in the field of pain control, there are surprisingly few data on its use in chronic abdominal pain. We have some experience with it for this indication and have found it rather disappointing but should emphasize that we have never attempted to assess its efficacy in a formal clinical trial.

Adhesiolysis

Adhesions can undoubtedly cause acute abdominal pain as a result of intestinal obstruction or strangulation. However, their role in the genesis of chronic abdominal pain is much less certain and an even more controversial issue is whether their surgical division is ever beneficial. It is probably fair to say that the majority view is that adhesions do not cause chronic symptoms (Alexander-Williams 1987) but it would not be surprising if there was the occasional exception to that rule. Thus, until recently, operations to divide adhesions were relatively rare, a trend that has been abruptly reversed by the current wave of enthusiasm for laparoscopic surgery. Unfortunately, the technique has an extremely powerful placebo effect, particularly when the patient is given a graphic videotape of the proceedings and great care will be needed in assessing the increasing claims for great success with this approach (Ikard 1992). It is to be hoped that carefully controlled trials will emerge on the subject as it is a procedure that does have complications.

Celiac plexus blockade (CPB)

This technique has been successfully used for many years to help with the management of pain associated with upper gastro-intestinal malignancies (Fugere & Lewis 1993). Its use in benign conditions has been inhibited by the somewhat invasive nature of the technique, the fact that the effect may not be long lasting and the potential for complications such as hematoma formation, hypotension, pneumothorax and very occasionally paraplegia. These issues should become much less of a problem as ultra-sound or CT scanning is used to improve accuracy and safety. Thus, it could be that CPB should be more formally evaluated in patients with severe chronic abdominal pain where quality of life is extremely poor and some degree of risk might be justifiable (Hastings & McKay 1991). There does not appear to be much information in the literature on the effect of CPB on the physio-logy of the bowel although there have been reports of diarrhea following the procedure. This could be an important point since so many patients with chronic abdominal pain complain of coexistent bowel dysfunction.

Papillotomy

Even when gall stones are present, it can often be quite difficult to decide whether the right hypochondriacal pain of which the patient complains is due to this problem. Thus, it is not surpris-ing that patients without gall stones or those who have already had a cholecystectomy pose even more of a management prob-lem. They are usually subjected to numerous scans and other imaging techniques all to no avail and are often then diagnosed as having biliary dyskinesia. There is some evidence that some of these patients may actually have a motility disturbance of the sphincter of Oddi and the possibility of endoscopic sphinctero-tomy for such subjects has been suggested (Choudhry et al 1993). Unfortunately, sphincter of Oddi manometry is not without risk of pancreatitis and papillotomy also has a definite morbidity, making this an extremely difficult decision area. We have encountered patients benefiting from papillotomy but good guidelines on how to approach this problem are badly needed.

PSYCHOLOGICAL APPROACHES

General considerations

Pain is not simply a physical sensation. It is a complex phenomenon, a multidimensional experience which involves many psychosocial factors, such as cognitive, emotional, perceptual, interpersonal and personality variables, all of which have the potential to contribute to the pain (Chaves 1993). Therefore, pain cannot be seen in isolation, particularly when it has developed into a chronic condition. Because of this, the psychology of pain control has grown greatly in the past two decades. A number of psychological techniques have been applied successfully to the regulation of both acute and chronic pain and are increasingly being used, either on their own or as part of a multimodal approach to pain management. Although much of the work has been carried out and published in relation to such conditions as low back pain and arthritis, these are generally applicable to chronic pain of any origin, including chronic abdominal pain, whether that pain is the only symptom the patient experiences or whether it is part of the IBS picture.

Psychological interventions aim to reduce pain perception where possible, to maximize the patient's ability to cope with pain and to enable a reasonable quality of life. Different approaches have been adopted in the management and treatment of chronic pain, which can be grouped as:

c dynamic or interpretive psychotherapy
c cognitive-behavioral therapy
c hypnosis/hypnotherapy.

Their uses will be described and discussed in relation to chronic pain in general and reference made specifically to chronic abdominal pain as applicable. The reader should bear in mind, however, that coverage of these different interventions is not extensive and inevitably some omissions will be made. We have intentionally included some psychological jargon in order to allow the interested reader to understand the literature in this area a little better. Jargon terms have been underlined and, in some instances, defined in a little more detail.

Dynamic psychotherapy

Treatment of chronic pain by dynamic psychotherapy is based on the assumption that the pain represents some underlying psychological conflict or trauma. The symptom is thus a metaphor for the underlying problem, a purposeful signal that needs to be listened to. It has been suggested that physical and sexual abuse, loss of a significant other (e.g. spouse or relative), severe life events or even an unexpressed emotion such as anger could be involved in chronic pain, including abdominal pain and IBS (Lakoff 1983, Jenkins 1991, Whitehead et al 1992). Recent reports suggest that past abuse, particularly when severe, is associated with greater symptom reporting and somatization disorders, including chronic abdominal or pelvic pain (Drossman et al 1990, Walker et al 1992).

This type of therapy can take various forms, all of which in some way involve exploration of and help the patient to deal with any psychological conflicts or trauma forming the basis for symptoms. Use of this approach has been reportedly rather sparse and success has been varied. For instance, in one study of chronic 'psychogenic' pain, amitriptyline was found to be more effective than dynamic psychotherapy in that while both treatments increased patient activity levels, pain intensity was reduced by amitriptyline but actually increased by psychotherapy (Pilowsky & Barrow 1990). Lakoff (1983) reported several cases in which dynamic psychotherapy was useful in treating pain within a multimodal approach combining other psychotherapeutic techniques such as behavioral modification, relaxation and physical therapies. Similarly, Guthrie and colleagues (1991) have used a psychodynamic approach combined with relaxation successfully to reduce the symptoms of IBS, including abdominal pain, although constant pain responded poorly.

Cognitive-behavioral therapy

Cognitive-behavioral methods comprise the mainstay of current chronic pain management programs (Weisenberg 1987, Pither & Nicholas 1991). These are based on cognitive and learning theories which recognize that particular patterns of behavior are set up in response to pain. These can become reinforced, according to operant conditioning paradigms (reward or punishment for displayed behavior), by significant others such as family members and by environmental factors. In addition, chronic pain itself is a stressor and therefore all the variables which are significant and important in dealing with any stress are relevant to pain. Maladaptive cognitions, coping strategies, beliefs about the pain and the ability to control this can maintain or exacerbate pain. So, too, can the presence of secondary gain which results when the pain serves underlying psychological needs or is useful

Table 6.3   Common cognitive-behavioral strategies for pain

Goal setting
Reinforcing 'well' behaviors
Discouraging pain behaviors
Time-contingent medication
Relaxation/autogenic training
Cognitive restructuring – self-statements
Imagery
Distraction

to the patient in some way. Anxiety, psychophysiological arousal and depression can accompany the pain and may be a consequence of the pain rather than vice versa (Main & Spanswick 1991). Cognitive-behavioral methods may be used alone or in combination with other forms of treatment in a multimodal treatment plan, which involves patient education about pain mechanisms, medication and physiotherapy.

Behavioral interventions focus on modifying behavioral patterns associated with pain, aiming to reduce pain behaviors and replace them with more appropriate 'well' behaviors. Cognitive methods, originally developed for use in depression and anxiety and incorporated into therapeutic approaches for pain, serve to modify maladaptive cognitions and teach more appropriate strategies both to cope with the pain and to reduce perception of pain (Fernandez 1987). Methods from both approaches are commonly used in various combinations and include those listed in Table 6.3 and described below.

Many patients become locked into certain ways of responding to pain, building up habitual patterns of behavior reflected, for example, in speech, facial expressions, postural changes, attention seeking, work refusal and avoidance behavior. When pain becomes chronic, these can become reinforced, often unintentionally, e.g. through attention from others, avoidance of unpleasant situations, such as work or a difficult relationship. These patterns need to be broken by encouraging the patient to do something different, otherwise progress can be difficult. Where a pattern of pain is identified, e.g. 'I always wake up with the pain', the expectation of pain can become a self-fulfilling prophesy, the mind building an association between external or internal cues and the experience of pain (as in Pavlovian classical conditioning).

Goal setting

This aims to instil new and more appropriate behaviors and to increase the patient's activity levels. It is also a way of orientating the patient to the future and the possibility of change. Specific goals and activities that are appropriate for and within the present capabilities of the patient are planned and gradually increased as progress is made. For example, a patient who spends much of the time in bed would be encouraged to spend less time in bed and to do other things. Such 'well' behavior can be reinforced by others giving appropriate praise and encouragement when these activities are carried out, while at the same time any pain behavior is ignored in order to discourage it. However, it is also important for patients to 'pace' themselves, allowing appropriate rest periods.

Time-contingent medication

Although it is usual clinical practice to prescribe medication for pain relief on a <u>pain-contingent</u> or 'as necessary' basis, this could be viewed as building an association between taking medication and pain relief in the form of a conditioned response. In order to prevent this happening, psychologists often advocate that medication should be taken at regular intervals (<u>time contingent</u>) and this approach is particularly appropriate if one has to resort to opiates.

Relaxation

Pain is often accompanied by general physiological arousal and increased muscular tension associated with changes in autonomic nervous activity. The patient is usually vigilant, expecting the pain to get worse or being unable to cope as it continues. <u>Progressive relaxation techniques</u> reduce sympathetic drive and increase parasympathetic activity and thus can help reduce perception of pain as well as giving the patient a coping strategy when in pain. Typically, patients are taught a progressive relaxation method to practice daily, possibly with the aid of an audiotape. <u>Autogenic training</u>, which is similar to relaxation, can be used and involves the use of self-statements to promote certain physiological changes such as warmth.

Cognitive restructuring

The way a person thinks about pain influences how it is felt. For instance, <u>catastrophic thinking</u> (such as 'This pain is awful', 'I can't stand this pain, it's killing me!') increases pain perception. A person's thoughts also give clues about the beliefs that person has regarding the pain, their ability to cope with or influence it and also about feelings of hopelessness and helplessness. Poor coping strategies are associated with increased levels of impairment, pain, anxiety and depression (Turner & Clancy 1986). Not surprisingly, those with a high <u>internal locus of control</u> (believing that they can influence their condition) do better using psychological interventions (Toomey et al 1991) than those with an <u>external locus of control</u> (relying on others to do something about it). Thus, the more control, self-esteem and problem-solving abilities a person perceives himself to have, the more able that person is to cope and live effectively despite any pain (Dolce 1987, Jacob et al 1993). This has implications for the treatment of IBS and pain, since a recent study examining cognitive and behavioral strategies among IBS patients attending an outpatient clinic showed that many had catastrophic cognitions and avoided at least one activity because of abdominal pain. In addition, the majority of patients expected the doctor to do something about the condition, in terms of advice or medication (Van Dulmen et al 1994).

Cognitive restructuring is an important intervention through which maladaptive cognitions can be changed. The role of 'negative' or maladaptive beliefs and thoughts in pain perception is explained to the patient. Such thoughts can be elicited by careful questioning or by asking patients to monitor and note them down over a period of time. More appropriate, 'positive' thoughts are then formulated which the patient would regularly practice as <u>coping self-statements</u>, especially when pain is noticed. For example, a patient who thinks 'This pain is killing me' could change this to 'This discomfort is unpleasant, but it won't kill me; I can meet the challenge'. <u>Reinterpretative self-statements</u> are also used to transform the pain sensation and to emphasize positive aspects of the experience. For example, the person could think of a burning pain as a 'radiating heat' which is more pleasurable and enjoyable. Some advocate that words such as 'pain' and 'hurt' are never used. In addition, asking patients about how comfortable they feel as opposed to how much pain they are in can introduce a subtle yet important shift in perceptual experience.

Distraction techniques

These are designed to engage conscious attention on something other than the pain, focusing either on the external environment or being involved in mental distraction such as reciting poems or pleasant imagery. Distraction techniques are probably only useful for pain of short duration and recent experimental evidence calls into question the efficacy of such attention-based coping strategies for chronic persistent pain (Eccleston 1995).

Imagery

This is not necessarily visual but can involve any or all of the senses, such as auditory, tactile and olfactory. It can be used to promote a number of pain-reducing or pain-coping strategies in different ways, such as:

c distraction, e.g. imagining a pleasant scene which is incompatible with pain,

c transformation – the pain is relabeled and imagined as other sensations such as tingling, throbbing, etc.

c metaphor/symbolic – the pain is imagined in symbolic form, such as a color, which is then changed in some way.

Evaluation of cognitive-behavioral strategies in chronic pain

Overall, cognitive-behavioral strategies in chronic pain have been rather poorly evaluated until fairly recently. Certainly, such an approach can produce significant improvement in symptoms, increasing the patient's activity levels and ability to cope, but because studies have used a different mix of methods it is uncertain which interventions may be the most useful (Malone & Strube 1988, Keefe et al 1992). The impression has been that cognitive-behavioral interventions are superior to those that use behavioral methods alone, although this is not clearcut (Vlaeyen et al 1995). Generally speaking, the particular methods used are probably best guided by the patient's individual needs, abilities and preferences.

The use of these methods in treating chronic abdominal pain as an isolated symptom has not been formally evaluated in the scientific literature. For pain as part of IBS, studies have reported the effectiveness of both behavioral and cognitive-behavioral interventions. Behavioral methods, which included bowel-retraining techniques as well as patient education, were as effective as medical treatment, although behaviorally treated patients also had less avoidance behavior in the long term (Corney et al 1991). Therapy consisting of progressive muscle relaxation, thermal biofeedback, cognitive coping strategies and a focus on patient education led to significant improvement in all symptoms, including pain, maintained at long-term follow-up (Schwarz et al 1990). In a later study, which included modification of cognitions and beliefs, challenging of beliefs and altering 'self-talk', significant improvement was produced in 80% of patients compared with 10% of non-treated controls (Greene & Blanchard 1994).

Hypnosis and hypnotherapy

The use of hypnosis for pain relief predates all the other psychological interventions described. Its most dramatic application has been for non-chemical anesthesia and analgesia during major surgery (Wain 1992) and hypnosis can therefore claim to have an important role to play in any painful condition.

To date, there is no adequate definition or explanation as to what hypnosis actually is, although it is useful to think of it as a form of influential communication and the hypnotic state as a natural state characterized by focused or selective attention (Yapko 1990). Hypnosis involves the intentional induction of 'hypnotic trance', which can be achieved by a variety of techniques including deep relaxation, imagery, ritualistic techniques and indirect methods. During this state, therapeutic interventions are used, which may take the form of suggestions by the therapist, which may be worded directly or indirectly, such as in the form of metaphors or analogies of the message the therapist wants to communicate. Therapy may be interactive whereby the patient communicates with the therapist and it may also incorporate approaches usually delivered in the fully orientated state, such as psychodynamic and cognitive-behavioral techniques. By definition, hypnotherapy is any therapy delivered in the hypnotic setting. Hypnosis is the tool used to bring about therapeutic change because the person can more readily accept and assimilate changes at the subconscious level since it is assumed that critical thought processes are less active, thus making rejection of new ideas less likely. In the context of treating pain, hypnotherapy can be used to:

c attain pain relief
c modify relevant psychological factors, such as negative cognitions and beliefs that maintain or exacerbate the pain
c explore and resolve possible causes, such as past trauma or psychological conflict.

Techniques for pain relief

A number of different strategies can be used in the hypnotic setting and these are outlined in Table 6.4 (Carasso et al 1988, Wain 1992). Techniques which will be successful for a particular individual depend, at least to some extent, on that person's

Table 6.4 Outline of specific hypnotic techniques for pain relief

Technique	Description
Relaxation	See cognitive-behavioral methods
Distraction	See cognitive-behavioral methods
Imagery	See cognitive-behavioral methods
Direct suggestion	Suggestions made that patient feels less/no pain
Indirect suggestion	Suggestions made that patient feels comfortable, etc.
Transformation	Changing pain into another sensation, e.g. tingling, itching, warmth
Displacement	Pain is moved to another part of body where it will be less troublesome
Anesthesia/analgesia	Numbness produced in affected part or in hand and transferring this to painful area by direct suggestion or imagery
Dissociation	Imagining self removed from direct experience, e.g. watching from distance, or dissociating painful part from body
Time distortion	Changing perception of time so that periods of pain seem very short and times of comfort very long
Amnesia	Patient forgets previous pain experiences
Age regression	Regression to time before onset of pain

'natural ability'. While <u>high hypnotizables</u> are generally considered more able to achieve greater levels of pain reduction than those with 'low' susceptibility, and hypnotic ability has been considered a rather stable individual trait, it is now more consistently viewed as a skill which can be enhanced with practice (Golden et al 1987, Chaves 1993). Most patients are not capable of total abrogation of pain but many advocate that this is not desirable except in special circumstances such as surgical anesthesia and phantom limb pain, in case the pain is serving protective or subconscious purposes. However, it is not necessary for a person to achieve a 'deep' level of trance to benefit from pain relief techniques, but it probably determines which methods of intervention would be most useful and successful, based on the individual's skills and preferences. For instance, a patient would probably need to have good hypnotic ability to achieve amnesia for pain or to acquire pain relief through direct suggestion. For chronic or severe intractable pain, hypnosis can be most effective when carried out at frequent intervals, i.e. two or three times a day, in the early stages of treatment. More recently, Crasilneck (1995) has suggested that using five or six different hypnotic techniques for pain relief in each session on a twice-daily basis can be especially useful.

Self-hypnosis

The ultimate aim of hypnotic techniques is for patients to be able to use them either during periods of self-hypnosis or as a particular cue (conditioned response) for pain relief, such as putting a hand on the abdomen and feeling warmth. Patients are trained in self-hypnosis and asked to practice hypnotic skills and techniques for pain relief on their own or with the aid of an audiotape. With persistent practice, they gradually find it is possible to achieve reduction of pain more easily and automatically.

Hypnotherapy and chronic abdominal pain

Hypnotherapy has proved unequivocally successful in improving the symptoms and quality of life in IBS patients, including abdominal pain, and the beneficial effects are long lasting (Houghton et al 1996). Just how and why pain relief is achieved is uncertain. In IBS, it could be due to changes in colonic motility or rectal sensitivity (Prior et al 1990, Whorwell et al 1992), perhaps depending on how the pain is initiated in the first place. Pain is a subjective experience and therefore it is likely that relief of pain from any source occurs mainly at a central level. Hypnotic analgesia of experimental pain is accompanied by increased cerebral blood flow in the frontal cortex, at least in high hypnotizables, suggesting that it may be a function of cognitive processing (Crawford et al 1993).

Although the authenticity of hypnotic phenomena, including pain relief, has been taken for granted by those working in the field, the overall efficacy of clinical hypnosis, particularly in the treatment of pain, has not been firmly established in terms of well-controlled research. The clinical literature remains largely anecdotal and particular interventions are not always described (Chaves 1993). In addition, experience has shown that the traditional hypnotic techniques for relief of chronic pain are not always successful or perhaps only in the short term. In recent years, however, hypnosis has come to be considered by some to be effective only when placed in the cognitive-behavioral framework (Golden et al 1987, Chaves 1993). The patient's pain phenomenology in terms of beliefs, cognitions and coping strategies must be taken into account. These can be modified as necessary and developed into therapeutically relevant suggestions which can then be delivered during the hypnotic state to facilitate their full incorporation into the patient's cognitive structure (Kirsch 1993).

Hypnotherapy can have several advantages over the conventional psychodynamic and cognitive-behavioral approaches already mentioned. Firstly, it allows psychological techniques to be introduced to a chronic pain patient from a physical standpoint, since most patients attribute a somatic basis to their complaint (Van Dulmen et al 1994). Patients with chronic abdominal pain or IBS have often gone through the mill of investigations, perhaps surgery, medication, even conventional psychotherapy or psychiatric referral. By this time, especially when no pathological cause has been identified, the patient has often been told 'It's all in the mind'. Emphasis can be placed on hypnosis as a way for the patient to learn to control the pain, with examples of its use for pain relief during surgery and childbirth. It is quite useful to use the concept of 'mind over matter' to explain the capacity to modify physiological mechanisms not normally under conscious control. The possibility of psychological issues can be raised gradually as necessary, while respecting the patient's own belief system. This is easier to do once the patient's trust has been gained. It is the authors' conviction that to attempt to tackle psychological issues before the patient is ready to do so carries the risk of losing the patient's confidence and cooperation. In keeping with this, Pilowsky and colleagues, using dynamic psychotherapy for chronic pain, reported that most patients found the idea of a 'talking' treatment for chronic pain difficult to accept. Poor outcome correlated with a preoccupation with physical symptoms, somatic illness and disease conviction. Indeed, it has been observed that when pain is psychogenic or part of a somatization disorder, the patient adamantly denies the possibility of a psychological cause (Pilowsky & Barrow 1992).

Not only can hypnotherapy encompass other psychological approaches, which allows an eclectic approach appropriate for the individual, but it has also been found to make these more effective (Eisen 1993, Kirsch 1994). Several factors are probably involved which account for this, including the belief of many patients that hypnosis can work, so that expectation of efficacy, reinforced by the confident demeanor of the therapist, allows greater improvement. However, it is also essential that any myths and misconceptions about hypnosis are dispelled, to eliminate any apprehensions as well as unrealistic, and therefore potentially unobtainable, expectations patients may have (Kirsch 1994). It has been argued that pain relief during hypnosis is just a placebo effect. Whilst this may partly be the case for low hypnotizables, high hypnotizables are able to achieve far greater levels of pain reduction than can be accounted for by placebo effect alone. Furthermore, the placebo effect itself is a very complex phenomenon accounting for up to 50% of the benefit of all painkillers including aspirin, codeine and morphine. Thus, it should be harnessed where possible and it is important to realize that the efficacy of any treatment can be influenced by factors such as the way the clinician or therapist conveys enthusiasm and expectation of success to the patient (Evans 1987, Kirsch 1994).

Hypnosis is viewed by some from the cognitive-behavioral perspective (Kirsch 1993) and indeed many of the techniques used, such as relaxation, imagery and distraction techniques, are common to both. However, therapy which carries the label of 'hypnosis' provides a very special context for behaviors which neither patient nor therapist would display in another context. For instance, the expectation of trance induction allows patients to be quietly comfortable and inwardly reflective and thus more able to recognize and consider issues that they otherwise would be unwilling or unable to do. Furthermore, the therapist is able to use different voice tones, emphasize different words and deliver suggestions in a repetitive way, which would sound entirely inappropriate or abnormal in any other setting. Repetition of restructured cognitions is important for these to become assimilated within the patient's cognitive repertoire (Kirsch 1993). Cognitive-behavioral interventions, such as cognitive restructuring, modifying beliefs and coping strategies, can be incorporated into the hypnotic session in various ways, for example, in the form of repetitive posthypnotic suggestions or imaginal rehearsal to try out different strategies and behaviors, as well as becoming future orientated to a successful outcome. Typically, part of the hypnotherapeutic style is to incorporate 'ego-strengthening' suggestions which increase the patient's overall confidence, sense of well-being and ability to cope, all of which are necessary in the chronic pain patient.

Limitations and possible barriers to successful outcome of psychological treatments

Certain factors need to be borne in mind which may prevent improvement when using any psychologically based treatment. Some of these have been discussed already and others will be considered here.

The first involves patient selection. Psychological interventions are not passive treatments but require the patient's active participation, both during therapy sessions and to carry out homework tasks such as achieving set goals and activities and practicing pain relief techniques. These types of treatment are not for patients who are in search of a 'quick fix' or who expect that others should make them better. However, as long as such issues are recognized, it is often possible to work to improve a patient's sense of self-efficacy and responsibility for improvement.

The presence of secondary gain, which stems from any benefits the patient has or may stand to gain from being ill, will get in the way of recovery. This includes reinforcers of pain behavior described earlier, such as love and attention from others or being able to avoid unpleasant or difficult situations. Financial benefits such as disability allowances or from impending ligitation procedures are also very important factors. These may act at a subconscious level so that the patient may not be aware that the continuation of the illness is serving some purpose and needs careful handling. In addition, because of the chronicity of the condition, some patients find it difficult to give up their pain, almost as though they have become so used to it and built their life around it that 'loss' of pain leaves a void. It is therefore important for the patient (and those around them) to learn new ways of functioning. Exploring the possibility of secondary gain may not be easy and even when patients are conscious of this, they may not willingly divulge it.

Finally, the meaning the patient attaches to the pain is important. Some are very concerned and can be entrenched in the belief that the clinicians have missed something, despite often repeated investigations. This is another reason why patients can be unwilling, usually subconsciously, to let go of the pain, since it represents the only signal to them and others that something could be wrong. This can dictate which strategies to use with this type of patient and one would probably not attempt techniques directly aimed at pain relief.

Evaluation and assessment of the patient

An initial interview with the patient before embarking on any psychological approach serves several purposes. These include eliciting information about the patient's condition and patient education, in terms of giving the patient a physiological model for the symptoms and how the particular psychological interventions are expected to help. This is also the time to establish rapport with the patient. Patients who feel comfortable in the therapist's presence are more likely to reveal and examine sensitive issues and are also more able to cooperate and be influenced during therapy. As much information as possible should be gathered about the patient's symptom(s), in terms of history, characteristics, any antecedents, the effect on lifestyle and relationships. In addition, the patient's patterns of response, beliefs and cognitions should be explored, as well as any potential benefits and secondary gain issues. Identifying a positive goal and motivation for getting well is also important as these orientate the patient to the future and new possibilities for change. Evans (1987), for example, has posed four questions to elicit the possible presence of depression, secondary gain and motivation. These are:

1. What difference would it make to your life if your pain suddenly disappeared?
2. Do you want to get better? (An unequivocal 'yes' is unlikely if depression and secondary gain are present.)
3. Would you be satisfied if your pain could be reduced to half its present intensity?
4. Will you work *with* me to get better?

CONCLUSION

The conventional approaches to pain control described herein should always be tried initially but often fail because of the complexities associated with pain perception and suffering. Thus, psychological interventions are becoming increasingly used, most commonly employing a cognitive-behavioral approach. However, if the expertise is available then hypnosis can have a powerful potentiating effect on these techniques. It is likely that

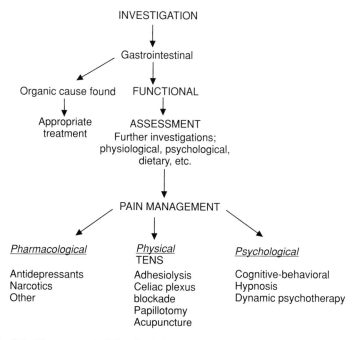

Fig. 6.1 Management of chronic abdominal pain.

the successful outcome of any particular intervention depends on the individual, their needs and preferences. Psychological approaches are not for everyone as some individuals need to view their treatment in much more 'physical' terms. For patients with chronic abdominal pain, a 'quick fix' is an unrealistic expectation but a surprising amount of progress can be made using a multimodal approach (Fig. 6.1) delivered in a sympathetic and understanding fashion.

REFERENCES

Alexander-Williams J 1987 Do adhesions cause pain? British Medical Journal 294: 659–660

Alun Jones V, Shorthouse M, McLaughlan P, Workman E, Hunter JO 1982 Food intolerance: a major factor in the pathogenesis of irritable bowel syndrome. Lancet ii: 1115–1117

Carasso RL, Arnon G, Yehuda S, Mostofsky DI 1988 Hypnotic techniques for the management of pain. Journal of the Royal Society of Health 5: 176–179

Chaves JF 1993 Hypnosis in pain management. In: Rhue JW, Lynn SJ, Kirsch I (eds) Handbook of clinical hypnosis. American Psychological Association, Washington, DC, pp 511–532

Choudhry U, Ruffolo T, Jamidar P, Hawes R, Lehman G 1993 Sphincter of Oddi dysfunction in patients with an intact gallbladder: therapeutic response to endoscopic sphincterotomy. Gastrointestinal Endoscopy 39: 492–495

Corney RH, Stanton R, Newell R, Clare A, Fairclough P 1991 Behavioural psychotherapy in the treatment of irritable bowel syndrome. Journal of Psychosomatic Research 35: 461–469

Crasilneck HB 1995 The use of the Crasilneck Bombardment Technique in problems of intractable organic pain. American Journal of Clinical Hypnosis 35: 255–266

Crawford HJ, Gur RC, Skolnick B, Gur RE, Benson BM 1993 Effects of hypnosis on regional blood flow during ischaemic pain with and without suggested hypnotic analgesia. International Journal of Psychophysiology 15: 181–195

Dolce JJ 1987 Self-efficacy and disability beliefs in behavioral treatment of pain. Behavioural Research and Therapy 25: 289–299

Drossman, DA, Leserman J, Nachman G et al 1990 Sexual and physical abuse in women with functional or organic gastrointestinal disorders. Annals of Internal Medicine 113: 828–833

Eccleston C 1995 Chronic pain and distraction: an experimental investigation into the role of sustained and shifting attention in the processing of chronic persistent pain. Behavioral Research and Therapy 33: 391–405

Eisen MR 1993 Psychoanalytic and psychodynamic models of hypnoanalysis. In: Rhue JW, Lynn SJ, Kirsch I (eds) Handbook of Clinical Hypnosis. American Psychological Association, Washington, DC, pp 123–149

Evans FJ 1987 Hypnosis and chronic pain management. In: Burrows GD, Elton D, Stanley G (eds) Handbook of chronic pain management. Elsevier Science, Amsterdam, pp 285–299

Fernandez E 1986 A classification system of cognitive coping strategies for pain. Pain 26: 141–151

Fugere F, Lewis G 1993 Coeliac plexus block for chronic pain syndromes. Canadian Journal of Anaesthesia 40: 954–963

Golden WL, Dowd ET, Friedberg F 1987 Hypnotherapy: a modern approach. Pergamon Press, New York

Greene B, Blanchard EB 1994 Cognitive therapy for irritable bowel syndrome. Journal of Consulting and Clinical Psychology 62: 576–582

Guthrie EA, Creed FH, Dawson D, Tomenson B 1991 A controlled trial of psychological treatment for the irritable bowel syndrome. Gastroenterology 100: 450–452

Hastings RH, McKay WR 1991 Treatment of benign chronic abdominal pain with neurolytic coeliac plexus block. Anaesthesiology 75: 156–158

Houghton LA, Heyman DJ, 1996 Symptomatology, quality of life and economic features of irritable bowel syndrome – the effect of hypnotherapy. Alimentary Pharmacology and Therapeutics 10: 91–95

Ikard RW 1992 There is no current indication for laparoscopic adhesiolysis to treat abdominal pain. Southern Medical Journal 85: 939–940

Jacob MC, Kerns RD, Rosenberg R, Haythornthwaite J 1993 Chronic pain: intrusion and accommodation. Behavioral Research and Therapy 31: 519–527

Jenkins PLG 1991 Psychogenic abdominal pain. General Hospital Psychiatry 13: 27–30

Keefe FJ, Dunsmore J, Burnett R 1992 Behavioral and cognitive-behavioral approaches to chronic pain: recent advances and future directions. Journal of Consulting and Clinical Psychology 60: 528–536

Kirsch I 1993 Cognitive-behavioural hypnotherapy. In: Rhue JW, Lynn SJ, Kirsch I (eds) Handbook of Clinical Hypnosis. American Psychological Association, Washington, DC, pp 151–171

Kirsch I 1994 Clinical hypnosis as a nondeceptive placebo: empirically derived techniques. American Journal of Clinical Hypnosis 37: 95–106

Lakoff R 1983 Interpretive psychotherapy with chronic pain patients. Canadian Journal of Psychiatry 28: 650–653

Main CJ, Spanswick CC 1991 Pain: psychological and psychiatric factors. British Medical Bulletin 47: 732–742

Malone MD, Strube MJ 1988 Meta-analysis of non-medical treatments for chronic pain. Pain 34: 231–244

Mathias JR, Clench MH, Reeves-Darby VG et al 1994 Effect of leuprolide acetate in patients with moderate to severe functional bowel disease. Double blind, placebo controlled study. Digestive Diseases and Sciences 39: 1155–1162

McMeeken JH, Stillman BC 1987 Transcutaneous nerve stimulation. In: Burrows GD, Elton D, Stanley G (eds) Handbook of chronic pain management. Elsevier Science, Amsterdam, pp 259–270

Pace F, Coremans G, Dapoigny M et al 1991 Therapy of irritable bowel syndrome – an overview. Digestion 56: 433–442

Pilowsky I, Barrow G 1990 A controlled study of psychotherapy and amitriptyline used individually and in combination in the treatment of chronic intractable, 'psychogenic' pain. Pain 40: 3–19

Pilowsky I, Barrow G 1992 Predictors of outcome in the treatment of chronic 'psychogenic' pain with amitriptyline and brief psychotherapy. Clinical Journal of Pain 8: 358–362

Pither CE, Nicholas MK 1991 Psychological approaches in chronic pain management. British Medical Bulletin 47: 743–761

Prior A, Colgan SM, Whorwell PJ 1990 Changes in rectal hypersensitivity following hypnotherapy for irritable bowel syndrome. Gut 31: 896–898

Schwarz SP, Taylor AE, Scharff L, Blanchard EB 1990 Behaviorally treated irritable bowel syndrome patients: a four-year follow-up. Behavioral Research and Therapy 28: 331–335

Sylvester K, Kendall GPN, Lennard-Jones JE 1986 Treatment of functional abdominal pain by transcutaneous electrical nerve stimulation. British Medical Journal 293: 481–482

Toomey TC, Mann JD, Abashian S, Thompson-Pope S 1991 Relationship between perceived self-control of pain, pain description and functioning. Pain 45: 129–133

Turner JA, Clancy S 1986 Strategies for coping with chronic low back pain: relationships to pain and disability. Pain 24: 355–364

Van Dulmen AM, Fennis JFM, Mokkink HGA, van der Velden HGM,

Bleijenberg G 1994 Doctors' perception of patients' cognitions and complaints in irritable bowel syndrome at an outpatient clinic. Journal of Psychosomatic Research 38: 581–590

Vlaeyen JWS, Haazen IWCJ, Schuerman JA, Kole-Snijders AMJ, van Eek H 1995 Behavioural rehabilitation of chronic low back pain: comparison of an operant treatment, an operant-cognitive treatment and an operant-respondent treatment. British Journal of Clinical Psychology 34: 95–118

Wain HJ 1992 Pain as a biopsychosocial entity and its significance for treatment with hypnosis. Psychiatric Medicine 10: 101–117

Walker EA, Katon WJ, Hansom J et al 1992 Medical and psychiatric symptoms in women with childhood sexual abuse. Psychosomatic Medicine 54: 658–664

Weisenberg M 1987 Psychological intervention for the control of pain. Behavioral Research and Therapy 25: 301–312

Whitehead WE, Cromwell MD, Robinson JC, Heller BR, Schuster MM 1992 Effects of stressful life events on bowel symptoms: subjects with irritable bowel syndrome compared with subjects without bowel dysfunction. Gut 33: 825–830

Whorwell PJ, Houghton LA, Taylor EE, Maxton DG 1992 Physiological effects of emotion: assessment via hypnosis. Lancet 340: 69–72

Yapko M 1989 Trancework: an introduction to the practice of clinical hypnosis, 2nd edn. Brunner/Mazel, New York

Hypersensitivity and food intolerance

RB Scott

INTRODUCTION

The potential for adverse reactions to occur after the ingestion of specific foods has been recognized for centuries, but until recently much of the evidence supporting a connection between the ingestion of specific foods and unpleasant symptoms was based only on anecdotal experience. During the last decade, significant progress has been made in our understanding of adverse reactions to food and food additives as a result of advances in the basic and clinical sciences (Anderson 1994). From a scientific perspective, the most important enabling advance was a general acceptance of those criteria which had to be met in order that clinical trials could safely and effectively advance the diagnosis and therapy of human allergic disorders (Van Metre 1983). Foremost amongst subsequent clinical achievements was recognition of the importance of the double-blind, placebo-controlled food challenge (DBPCFC) in the investigation of adverse reactions (Bock et al 1988).

The purpose of this chapter is to briefly review the pathophysiology of hypersensitivity and food intolerance, highlight recent advances in our understanding of how hypersensitivity reactions alter gastrointestinal motility and contribute to the development of clinical symptoms and lastly, outline a clinical approach to the management of patients who present to the gastroenterologist with an adverse reaction to food. A number of recent reviews (Crowe & Perdue 1992, Burks & Sampson 1993, Bock & Sampson 1994) as well as a comprehensive reference textbook (Metcalfe et al 1991) are available and address these issues in more detail.

TERMINOLOGY

The term 'adverse reaction to food' is used to describe any abnormal response or symptom exhibited by an individual after the

Table 7.1 Differential diagnosis of adverse reactions to food

Food hypersensitivity (allergy)
Food intolerance
  Gastrointestinal disorders (vomiting and/or diarrhea)
    Structural abnormalities
      Hiatal hernia
      Pyloric stenosis
      Hirschsprung's disease
      Tracheoesophageal fistula
    Enzyme deficiencies (primary versus secondary)
      Disaccharidase deficiency (lactase, sucrase-isomaltase,
        glucose-galactose)
      Galactosemia
      Phenylketonuria
    Malignancy
    Other
      Pancreatic insufficiency (cystic fibrosis, Schwachman–Diamond
        syndrome)
      Gall bladder disease
      Peptic ulcer disease
  Contaminants and additives
    Flavorings and preservatives
      Sodium metabisulfite
      Nitrites/nitrates
      Monosodium glutamate
    Dyes
      Tartrazine, ?other azo dyes
    Toxins
      Bacterial (*Clostridium botulinum,Staphylococcus aureus*)
      Fungal (aflatoxin, trichothecenes, ergot)
      Seafood associated
        Scombroid poisoning (tuna, mackerel)
        Ciguatera poisoning (grouper, snapper, barracuda)
        Saxitoxin (shellfish)
      Infectious organisms
        Bacteria (*Salmonella, Shigella, Escherichia coli, Yersinia,*
          Campylobacter)
        Parasites (*Giardia, Trichinella*)
        Virus (hepatitis, rotavirus, enterovirus)
      Mold antigens (?)
      Accidental contaminants
        Heavy metals (mercury, copper)
        Pesticides
        Antibiotics (penicillin)
  Pharmacologic agents
    Caffeine (coffee, soft drinks)
    Histamine (fish, sauerkraut)
    Serotonin (banana, tomato)
    Glycosidal alkaloid solanine (potatoes)
    Alcohol
    Theobromine (chocolate, tea)
    Tryptamine (tomato, plum)
    Phenylethylamine (chocolate)
Psychologically based food intolerance reactions

Adapted from Burks & Sampson 1993

ingestion of a food that is otherwise tolerated by the majority of the community regardless of age, sex, health or disease status (Ferguson 1992). Adverse reactions to ingested food are relatively common and cause a wide variety of symptoms, syndromes or diseases, which may be described in very general terms as 'sensitivities' or 'intolerances'. However, these labels convey no information about the mechanism behind the reaction, which might be immunologic, the physiologic consequence of an underlying gastrointestinal disorder or due to metabolic, toxic, pharmacologic or psychologic factors (Burks & Sampson 1993; Table 7.1).

To enhance communication and promote scientific clarity, it is currently recommended (Ferguson 1992) that the term 'food allergy' or 'food hypersensitivity' be reserved for those forms of intolerance in which there is both a reproducible adverse reaction to specific foods and evidence of an underlying immunologic mechanism. 'Food intolerance' or 'food sensitivity' should be used to refer to any reproducible, adverse reaction to a specific food or food ingredient which is not immune mediated or psychologically based. Psychologically based food reactions (food aversions) are those in which the subject avoids food for psychologic reasons (psychologic avoidance) or experiences an unpleasant bodily reaction caused by emotions associated with the food, rather than the food itself, and which do not occur when the food is given in an unrecognizable form (psychologic intolerance).

PREVALENCE OF FOOD ALLERGY

Objective measurements of the prevalence of food hypersensitivity (allergy) are infrequent. Because of a failure to discriminate between food intolerance and food allergy, there is a public perception that the prevalence of food allergy is very high. Population surveys cited in recent reviews (Sampson & Metcalfe 1992, Burks & Sampson 1993) report that 15% of the population, or at least one family member in one of every three American households, believe themselves to be allergic to some food ingredient. In contrast, while parents reported one in four children as having experienced an adverse reaction to food, only 8% overall had symptoms confirmed by subsequent blinded oral food challenge. Thus, when adverse reactions to food are objectively evaluated, the 'prevalence' of true food allergy is much lower than that of all adverse reactions to food.

PATHOPHYSIOLOGY OF FOOD HYPERSENSITIVITY

Gastrointestinal antigen exposure

The main function of the gastrointestinal tract is to process ingested food so that it can be absorbed and used for energy and tissue growth. In performing this function, the intestine is routinely exposed to an enormous array of macromolecules derived from ingested food, resident bacterial flora and invasive microorganisms. Antigens are those substances capable of inducing an immune response when introduced into the tissues of an animal. Ingested food is the single largest source of antigen exposure to the human immune system. Of the enormous quantity and variety of ingested macromolecules, some exert no pathologic effect while others have the potential to act adversely (either within the gut lumen or by crossing the mucosal barrier) as toxins, biologically active peptides or antigens.

The uptake and transport of macromolecules from the intestine and the possible role of this process in disease has recently been reviewed (Sanderson & Walker 1993). Normally, the gastrointestinal tract uses both non-immunologic and immunologic measures to prevent intact foreign antigens from crossing the intestinal mucosal barrier and entering the tissues or circulation (Table 7.2). Despite the presence of this multifactorial mucosal barrier, minute amounts of intact food antigens are absorbed and transported throughout the body.

Table 7.2 Components of the mucosal barrier to intestinal pathogens, toxins and antigens

---
Non-immunologic mechanisms
Intraluminal
   Gastric acid
   Proteolytic activity of digestive enzymes
   Motility
Mucosal surface
   Mucin
   Microvillus membrane

Immunologic mechanisms
Gut-associated lymphoid tissue (GALT)
Secretory IgA
Cell-mediated immunity

Physiologic macromolecular uptake

Physiological uptake of luminal macromolecules (Sanderson & Walker 1993) is particularly important during infancy when intestinal growth and maturation are incomplete and specific mechanisms have evolved to facilitate the transepithelial uptake of important growth factors and immunoglobulin (receptor-mediated transport). However, luminal macromolecules also have the potential to act as antigens and cells specialized for their uptake (membranous or microfold epithelial 'M' cells that overlay lymphoid molecules) incorporate macromolecules into membrane-bound compartments for transport across the cell and presentation to lymphoid cells. Fortunately, the presentation of immunologically intact protein to the enteric immune system does not normally cause adverse reactions because most individuals develop tolerance to ingested food antigens.

Gut-associated lymphoid tissue – immune responsiveness and tolerance

The immunologic surveillance of antigens within the lumen of the gastrointestinal tract by gut-associated lymphoid tissue (GALT) is crucial to the development of both appropriate immune responsiveness and tolerance (Shanahan 1994). GALT is collectively the largest lymphoid organ in the body. Anatomically it consists of organized (comprising aggregated lymphoid follicles or Peyers's patches, isolated follicles and mesenteric lymph nodes) and diffuse lymphoid tissue (comprising intraepithelial lymphocytes or IELs, lamina propria mononuclear cells including lamina propria lymphocytes or LPLs). In contrast to the organized GALT which contains mainly precursor B and T lymphocytes, the diffuse GALT distributed throughout the lamina propria and epithelium consists of an infiltrate of effector cells that contains mature effector T lymphocytes (IELs and LPLs) and immunoglobulin-producing plasma cells (LPLs) and creates in the intestinal mucosa a unique state of 'controlled inflammation'. The lymphoid populations of IELs and LPLs are in close proximity to other components of the mucosal microenvironment, which includes enterocytes, neurons, smooth muscle and fibroblasts. Strong evidence is emerging in support of bidirectional communication amongst immunologic and non-immunologic tissues within the mucosa. While the precise mechanism by which tolerance develops to ingested food proteins is not well understood, it appears that antigen exposure at the intestinal mucosal surface normally results in induction of IgA-B cell precursors with simultaneous suppression of IgM, IgG and IgE-B cell subtypes, as well as cell-mediated immune responses. This reciprocal arrangement permits a protective mucosal IgA response to antigen challenge in the absence of a systemic response – a condition of systemic tolerance to ingested antigenic food proteins.

Non-specific, potentially pathophysiologic macromolecular uptake

Potentially pathologic macromolecular uptake may occur by at least two pathways (Sanderson & Walker 1993). Molecules which have adhered (in the absence of specific receptors) to the apical surface membrane of epithelial cells may be incorporated into intracellular vesicles, escape intracellular enzymatic digestion and be transported to the basolateral membrane. Secondly, paracellular transport may occur if there is disruption at the tight junctions between enterocytes. A variety of pathologic insults are known to increase the permeability of the paracellular pathway sufficiently to allow for macromolecular uptake: intestinal disorders (food allergy, celiac disease, acute gastroenteritis, chronic infectious enteritis, inflammatory bowel disease and surgery), systemic insults (radiation, burns, septic or hypovolemic shock and malnutrition) and drugs (non-steroidal antiinflammatory agents). The increased non-specific permeability of the mucosal barrier during development or in response to injury increases the potential for immune-mediated gastrointestinal disorders like food allergy, autoimmune enteropathy and perhaps inflammatory bowel disease (Crowe & Perdue 1992, Sanderson & Walker 1993, Shanahan 1994). In susceptible individuals, pathologic exposure to macromolecules or breakdown of the oral tolerance mechanism may result in allergic reactions to ingested food proteins. The classic Gell & Coombs classification provides a useful framework for their characterization.

Gell & Coombs classification of immunologic injury

There are four types of immune-mediated tissue damage and each has the potential to mediate food allergy (Burks & Sampson 1993). Types I–III are antibody mediated and are distinguished by the type of antigen recognized and the different classes of antibody involved. Type I responses are mediated by IgE, which induces mast cell activation, while types II and III are mediated by IgG which can activate either (a) complement-mediated tissue injury directed against cell-surface or matrix-associated antigen (type II) or (b) phagocytosis of antigen–antibody complexes (type III). Type IV is T cell-mediated and tissue damage may be caused by activation of inflammatory pathways by T_H1 cells or the direct effects of cytotoxic T cells.

The majority of food allergic disorders in which the immunopathophysiologic mechanisms have been clearly

Table 7.3 Disorders for which type III (antigen–antibody) or IV (cell-mediated) immune mechanisms are postulated to be involved (Burks & Sampson 1993)

Food-induced enterocolitis (protein intolerance) in infants
Food-induced colitis in infants
Celiac disease
Allergic eosinophilic gastroenteritis
Food-induced pulmonary hemosiderosis (Heiner's syndrome)
Dermatitis herpetiformis
Others (<u>some</u> cases of arthritis, epilepsy, migraine)

documented are of the type I IgE-mediated immediate hypersensitivity type, although the overall immune response may progress to involve more than one immunologic mechanism (Burks & Sampson 1993). Type II antibody-dependent thrombocytopenia has been reported in response to the ingestion of milk (Burks & Sampson 1993). Although there are a variety of disorders which are thought to be the result of antigen–antibody (type III) and cell-mediated (type IV) mechanisms, documentation of the immunopathophysiologic mechanism is incomplete (Burks & Sampson 1993; Table 7.3). The remainder of this section will focus on the pathophysiology of the most frequent and best documented form of food allergy – IgE-mediated food hypersensitivity.

TYPE I IgE-MEDIATED HYPERSENSITIVITY

Type I IgE-mediated hypersensitivity (anaphylaxis) to ingested food proteins is a specific example of immunologic intestinal injury in the absence of systemic tolerance (Sampson & Metcalfe 1992, Burks & Sampson 1993, Bock & Sampson 1994). Intestinal anaphylaxis occurs in those sensitized individuals who have preferentially synthesized reaginic antibodies (usually IgE but also IgG IV in humans) in response to an initial antigen exposure. The mechanism of its development is not entirely clear; however, it is more frequently seen in the immature and injured gut where the mucosal barrier is relatively impaired and is also greatest in the young as a result of their relatively diminished suppressor T cell activity. Atopy is the genetic predisposition to selective synthesis of IgE antibody on exposure to environmental antigens. In atopic patients, extremely small doses of antigen prime or sensitize the individual and sustain IgE antibody responses. IgE antibodies circulating in the serum or synthesized from local plasma cells become anchored to Fc receptors on the surface of tissue mast cells and basophils which are distributed throughout the body, including along the gastrointestinal tract. Mast cells to which IgE has been bound are said to be sensitized. A hypersensitivity

Table 7.4   Mast cell mediators

Preformed: intragranular
Amines
  Histamine
  Serotonin[a]
Chemotactic factors
Lysosomal enzymes
  Exoglycosidases
  Kininogenase
  Chymotrypsin/trypsin
  Peroxidase
  Superoxide dismutase
  Arylsulfatase, A and B
Superoxide anions
Proteoglycans
  Heparin
  Chondroitin sulfate

Membrane derived (newly generated)
Leukotrienes (LTB$_4$, LTC$_4$, LTD$_4$ and LTE$_4$)
Prostaglandins (PGD$_2$)
Monohydroeicosatetraenoic acids
Hydroperoxyeicosatetraenoic acids
Thromboxanes
Platelet-activating factor (PAF)

Cytokines[b]
Interleukins 1–6
Interferon γ (IFN-γ)
Tumor necrosis factor α (TNF-α)
Transforming growth factor β (TGF-β)
Macrophage inflammatory protein 1 (MIP-1) family
Granulocyte-macrophage colony-stimulating factor (GM-CSF)

[a] Found in some rodent species, but not present in human mast cells
[b] Present in various mast cell populations
Adapted from Crowe & Perdue 1992

reaction requires reexposure to antigen. When the allergen to which the individual has been previously sensitized crosslinks cell-bound IgE molecules, a series of membrane and intracellular events result in mast cell degranulation and the release of a wide variety of preformed and newly synthesized pharmacologic mediators (Crowe & Perdue 1992; Table 7.4).

The mast cell, leukocyte, cytokine cascade and the late-phase reaction

Mast cells are a heterogeneous population of cells, best studied in the rat, where intestinal mucosal mast cells have been shown to possess different properties (morphology, staining characteristics, mediator content, response to secretagogues or 'stabilizers') from connective tissue mast cells (Crowe & Perdue 1992). The preformed amines (e.g. histamines) and membrane-derived mediators (e.g. prostaglandins and leukotrienes) released from activated mast cells cause the vasodilation, smooth muscle contraction and mucus secretion that result in the clinical symptoms which characterize immediate hypersensitivity reactions (e.g. allergic rhinitis and asthma). However, activated mast cells also release chemotactic factors and cytokines (especially TNF-α) which recruit leukocytes that may themselves contribute to the amplification of the immediate anaphylactic reaction and progression of a late-phase reaction through the release of additional mediators. The late-phase response may result in inflammation and symptomatology much greater than that directly related to the initial antigen challenge. Not only is the immediate anaphylactic response augmented, but both immune complex and delayed-hypersensitivity reactions may be initiated (Galli 1993).

Clinical manifestations of food-induced IgE-mediated hypersensitivity

The clinical presentation of IgE-mediated allergic reactions to food is directly related to the site and extent of antigen–IgE-mediated mast cell degranulation (Sampson & Metcalfe 1992, Burks & Sampson 1993, Bock & Sampson 1994; Table 7.5). As the development of clinical symptoms depends upon the activation of a cascade of events resulting in the release of inflammatory mediators, a multiplicity of factors can modify the response to an individual exposure to antigen (e.g. amount of antigen, acute versus repeated or chronic exposure, concurrent pharmacotherapy with antihistamines or 'mast cell stabilizers', etc.).

The signs and symptoms of an anaphylactic reaction to food may be limited to the gastrointestinal tract with localized pruritus

Table 7.5 Clinical manifestations of IgE-mediated, food-induced hypersensitivity

Gastrointestinal	Extraintestinal	Systemic anaphylaxis

Pruritus and angioedema of the lips, tongue, palate and pharynx
Nausea
Vomiting
Bloating
Abdominal pain or cramping
Diarrhea
	Dermatologic
	  Pruritus
	  Erythema
	  Urticaria
	  Angioedema
	  Eczema
	
	Ocular
	  Conjunctivitis
	
	Respiratory
	  Rhinitis
	  Asthma
		Oropharyngeal pruritus and angioedema
		Urticaria, angioedema
		Dyspnea, wheezing and cyanosis
		Abdominal pain
		Vomiting and diarrhea
		Chest pain
		Hypotension/shock
		Death

and swelling of the oropharynx, nausea, vomiting, bloating, abdominal pain and/or diarrhea. More extensive spread of antigen through the blood stream can lead to activation of mast cells in the skin causing pruritus, erythema, urticaria, angioedema and eczema; in the respiratory tree causing rhinitis and asthma; or in the eyes resulting in conjunctivitis. When significant systemic mast cell degranulation takes place the massive release of mediators provokes the acute and potentially fatal reaction of systemic anaphylaxis. These patients may experience the dermatologic, gastrointestinal and respiratory symptoms mentioned above as well as the cardiovascular complaints of chest pain, hypotension and shock. Laryngeal edema, severe reversible obstructive airway disease or shock may be fatal. Unfortunately, there is nothing characteristic of the initial symptoms of patients experiencing exclusively oral or gastrointestinal anaphylaxis that can predict whether or not there will be progression to systemic anaphylaxis.

Food hypersensitivity alters gastrointestinal function

Because of inaccessibility of the target organ, a lack of objective tests and ethical issues, most human studies of gastrointestinal food-induced hypersensitivity (anaphylaxis) have been descriptive in nature (Crowe & Perdue 1992), suggesting that enteric mucosal inflammation or altered motility could occur in response to challenge of sensitized individuals, confirming the potential for enteric mucosal anaphylaxis in passive transfer experiments, implicating mast cell degranulation and histamine release, suggesting altered mucosal permeability and demonstrating increased levels of IgE in the lumen or feces of allergic individuals. Most of the research on pathophysiologic mechanisms and the effects of anaphylaxis on intestinal function has been performed in animal models.

Several recent comprehensive reviews detail what is known regarding the effects and mediation of anaphylaxis-induced alterations of intestinal electrolyte transport, nutrient absorption, smooth muscle contractility or motility in the stomach, jejunum, ileum or colon of rat, mouse, guinea pig, piglet and canine animal models (Crowe & Perdue 1992, Castro & Powell 1994). In these studies, animals were sensitized by oral feeding (β-lactoglobulin), parenteral injection (ovalbumin) or infection with an enteric nematode (*T. spiralis* or *N. brasiliensis*). Despite diversity in the methods of sensitization, the antigenic stimuli evoking the responses, the region of gut or species of mammal studied and the mediators implicated in functional transduction of the immune response, investigators made a number of common observations.

1. In vitro and acute in vivo studies implicated a type I hypersensitivity (anaphylactic) response as the mechanism behind the immune-mediated inflammatory response observed after antigenic challenge of the gastrointestinal tract or tissues from sensitized animals.

2. When gastrointestinal water and electrolyte transport, smooth muscle contractility or motility were assessed, antigen-induced anaphylaxis was associated with chloride secretion, smooth muscle contraction and alterations in the pattern of motor activity and transit respectively.

3. The enteric nervous system was often implicated in the anaphylaxis-induced alterations in gastrointestinal function.

The current consensus of opinion is that the functional effects of gastrointestinal anaphylaxis observed in these models reflect an integrated response of the intestinal mucosal immune system, the enteric nervous system (ENS) with input from the autonomic and central nervous system (CNS) and intestinal effector tissues controlling circulation, secretion, absorption and motor activity (Crowe & Perdue 1992, Castro & Powell 1994; Fig. 7.1). It is speculated that the clinical signs and symptoms reported by individuals who have experienced food protein-induced intestinal anaphylaxis (abdominal cramping, emesis and diarrhea) may reflect secretion of water and electrolytes, intense local contraction of intestinal smooth muscle and/or alterations in the normal pattern of intestinal motility. Considerable data in support of this hypothesis have been accumulated in the Hooded–Lister rat model of IgE-mediated food hypersensitivity (anaphylaxis).

The Hooded–Lister rat model of food protein-induced gastrointestinal anaphylaxis

The Hooded–Lister rat preferentially produces specific IgE antibodies in response to sensitization with foreign protein (Jarrett & Stewart 1974). Once sensitized with ovalbumin, animals can subsequently be challenged with the allergen and their response studied as a model of the changes in mucosal structure (Perdue et al 1984a,b; Patrick et al 1988), water and electrolyte transport (Perdue et al 1984a, Forbes et al 1988, Catto-Smith et al 1989b) and motility (Scott et al 1988, Diamant et al 1989, Maric et al 1989, Catto-Smith et al 1989a, Fargeas et al 1992, 1993 Scott &

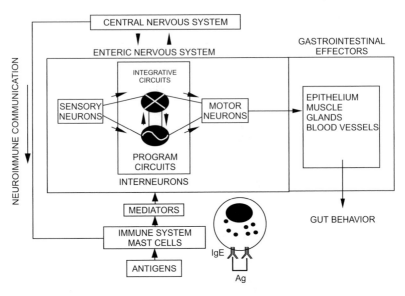

Fig. 7.1 Model of enteric neuroimmune communication. The enteric nervous system (ENS) is a 'minibrain' in close proximity to the gastrointestinal effectors it controls. Mast cells of the enteric immune system are anatomically positioned to both detect foreign antigens and signal their presence to the ENS or to be activated by neural signals. A variety of mediators have been implicated in this bidirectional transmission of information. The ENS is also in two-way communication with the central nervous system. The nervous system responds to immune signals by initiating coordinated motor output to the various gastrointestinal effectors responsible for gut behavior. In the case of food hypersensitivity, gastrointestinal secretory and motility responses are coordinated to destroy and expel the offending antigenic stimulus. (Modified from Castro & Powell 1994.)

Maric 1993, Catto-Smith et al 1994, Scott & Tan 1996, Oliver et al 1995a,b, Oliver et al 1996) that occur in food protein-induced hypersensitivity reactions. The alterations in gastrointestinal function observed in this model are present only after antigen (Ag) challenge of animals specifically sensitized to egg albumin, as evidenced by specific IgE antiegg albumin antibody titers of $\geq$ 1:64. Following Ag exposure, these animals exhibit a systemic elevation of rat mast cell protease II and significantly fewer granulated mast cells are present in the mucosa of sensitized compared to control animals, suggesting that mast cell degranulation has occurred. Furthermore, pharmacologic treatment with agents that cause mast cell degranulation mimic the anaphylaxis-induced functional response, while agents that prevent mast cell degranulation or antagonists of specific mast cell mediators inhibit the functional response.

Morphologic Injury

In sensitized animals, intraluminal exposure to specific Ag results in morphologic injury characterized by mucosal edema, enterocyte shedding and diffuse ultrastructural disruption of the basement membrane and the underlying collagenous matrix of the lamina propria (Perdue et al 1984a,b, Patrick et al 1988). It is postulated that this physical disruption of the mucosal barrier, together with the vasoactive effects of released mast cell mediators (e.g. histamine), may account for the increased permeability of the mucosa and increased absorption of Ag during hypersensitivity reactions.

Secretion

Ovalbumin challenge of the stomach of the sensitized rat provokes mucosal mast cell degranulation with a rise in intraluminal histamine concentration and a sharp increase in gastric acid output (Catto-Smith et al 1989a). Specific Ag challenge of the jejunum (Perdue et al 1984a) and colon (Forbes et al 1988) of sensitized animals is associated with active mucosal chloride secretion mediated by activated mucosal mast cells that release 5-hydroxytryptamine and synthesize prostaglandins (Catto-Smith et al 1989b).

Motility

From a motility point of view, and quite apart from similar capabilities it subserves in the regulation of the circulation, secretion and absorption, the ENS is capable of independent and coordinated reflex activity (e.g. the peristaltic reflex) or complex patterned motor activity such as the fasting migrating myoelectric complex (MMC) and the fed pattern.

In the Hooded–Lister rat, just as in humans, small intestinal motility is characterized by migrating myoelectric (or motor) complexes (MMCs) during fasting and a continuous irregular pattern of myoelectric spike and associated contractile activity (the fed pattern) postprandially (Diamant & Scott 1987).

Antigen challenge of the stomach of sensitized animals and the resultant mucosal mast cell activation leads not only to histamine release and increased gastric acid output, but to a significant delay in emptying (Catto-Smith et al 1989a, 1994). The combination of increased acid output and delayed emptying acts as a protective mechanism promoting denaturation of the offending antigen.

In the <u>small intestine</u>, in vitro studies show that Ag challenge of sensitized jejunal segments provokes an IgE-mediated mucosal and connective tissue mast cell degranulation, 5-hydroxytryptamine release, prostaglandin synthesis and a direct contractile effect of these agents on circular and longitudinal smooth muscle (Scott et al 1990, Scott & Maric 1993). This would be expected to lead to reductions in luminal diameter, gut length and luminal volume, all factors which might favor an increased rate of transit. Exposure of sensitized jejunum to egg albumin in vivo alters both fasting (Scott et al 1988) and postprandial (Diamant et al 1989) small intestinal myoelectric and motor activity and is associated with an increased rate of aboral transit and diarrhea (Maric et al 1989) – a response which would tend to rid the organ of the offending allergen. In fasting rats, the MMC is temporarily abolished by Ag challenge of sensitized animals and replaced by a continuous, irregular myoelectric and motor activity (Fig. 7.2), which comprises a succession of aborally migrating clusters of action potentials and their motor correlate, migrating clusters of contractions (MCCs). MCCs are a normal feature of phase II of the MMC and of the postprandial period (Fig. 7.3). However, after Ag challenge of a sensitized animal, in either the interdigestive or postprandial period, MCCs are more frequent and of different character (Fig. 7.4). The phasic activity persists, but is superimposed on a high-amplitude prolonged tonic elevation in pressure, the whole complex resembling the giant migrating contraction

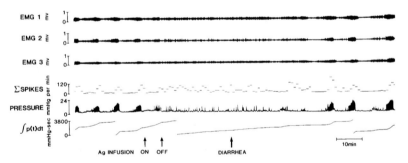

Fig. 7.2 Fasting jejunal myoelectric and motor activity associated with antigen (Ag) challenge of a sensitized rat. Phase III of 4 MMCs appear in the most proximal electromyogram (EMG) and propagate aborally through EMG 2 and 3. The fourth trace records the sum of myoelectric spike activity in EMG 2 for the previous minute. Jejunal motility recorded from a manometry catheter adjacent to EMG 2 is shown in the fifth trace and the cumulative area under the jejunal pressure recording [integral $p(t)dt$] is shown in the sixth trace. The motility index resets to 0 each time area under the curve reaches 3800 mmHg X s. Within minutes of Ag challenge, MMCs were abolished and replaced by a continuous pattern of irregular myoelectric spike and associated contractile activity that lasted 63 min before MMCs were again identified.

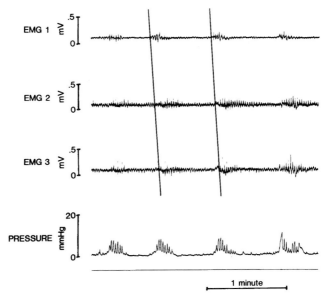

Fig. 7.3 An expanded segment of postprandial myoelectric and motor activity recorded from a rat. Four aborally migrating clustered spike bursts and their motor correlate, four groups of aborally migrating clusters of contractions (MCCs) occurring at the slow wave frequency, are shown in detail. MCCs are defined as discrete groups of 3–15 contractions that occur at the slow wave frequency and their myoelectric correlate is a discrete group of 3–15 slow waves with spike bursts superimposed on each depolarization. The slope of the solid lines superimposed on clustered spike bursts, as they appear in successively more distal electromyogram (EMG) leads, represents a propagation velocity of 1 cm/s. MCCs are a normal feature of phase II activity of the fasting MMC and of postprandial motility in the rat. (Reproduced with permission from Diamant & Scott 1987.)

(GMC) (Scott & Tan 1996). GMCs are large-amplitude and long-duration propulsive contractions that usually propagate uninterruptedly from the point of their origin in the small intestine to the terminal ileum at a velocity of ~ 1 cm/s (Quigley et al 1984, Sarna 1987). These alterations in motility are dependent upon mast cell degranulation and the activation of neuronal circuitry (Fargeas et al 1992, 1993, Scott & Tan 1996). 5-HT$_{2,3}$ antagonists partially inhibit and indomethacin most effectively blocks the response, suggesting that activated mast cells release prostaglandins and perhaps 5-HT which stimulate the neuronal pathway controlling the motor response (Fargeas et al 1992, Scott & Tan 1996).

It is probably the increased number of GMCs (not the disruption or the presence of MCCs) that is responsible for the diarrhea in this model. Diarrhea is not associated with the normal appearance of MCCs during phase II of the MMC, nor with the

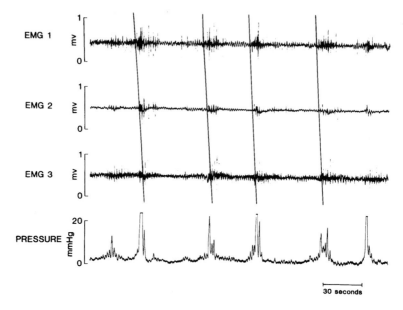

Fig. 7.4 An expanded segment of fasting myoelectric and motor activity recorded from a sensitized animal after antigen (Ag) challenge. Four aborally migrating clustered spike bursts and their motor correlate, four groups of aborally migrating clusters of contractions (MCCs) occurring at the slow wave frequency, are shown in detail. The slope of the solid lines superimposed on clustered spike bursts, as they appear in successively more distal electromyogram (EMG) leads, represents a propagation velocity of 1 cm/s. While MCCs are a normal feature of phase II activity of the MMC or of postprandial motility in the rat (Diamant & Scott 1987; Fig. 7.3), those observed after Ag challenge of a sensitized animal are more frequent and of different character. The phasic contractile activity persists but is superimposed upon a high-amplitude prolonged tonic elevation in pressure (the contractions which exceed 20 mmHg and 'topout' in this figure), the whole complex resembling the giant migrating contraction (GMC). (Reproduced with permission from Scott et al 1988.)

postprandial disruption of the MMC by continuous MCC activity (Diamant & Scott 1987). GMCs normally occur in the terminal ileum once or twice daily during fasting and are not associated with diarrhea (Quigley et al 1984). However, during trichinosis, after irradiation or after pharmacological stimulation there is a significant increase in the frequency of small intestinal GMCs; they originate from more proximal locations and are associated with diarrhea (Otterson & Sarna 1994). Their high lumen-occluding amplitude and rapid, uninterrupted propagation make them highly propulsive (Kruis et al 1985, Sarna 1987). The abdominal discomfort reported in association with GMCs (Kellow & Phillips 1987, Sarna 1987) may be due to the amplitude of the contraction itself or the movement of intestinal secretions and undigested food into the colon, thereby causing both distension and osmotic overload (Otterson & Sarna 1994).

In the sensitized rat colon, the Ag-induced release of mast cell-derived leukotrienes and platelet-activating factor exerts a direct contractile effect on colonic longitudinal (Oliver et al 1995a) and circular (Oliver et al 1996) muscle and, through the activation of neural pathways, is associated with increased colonic myoelectric spike activity, an increased rate of aboral colonic transit and diarrhea (Oliver et al 1995b).

Neuroimmune regulation of anaphylaxis-induced alterations in gastrointestinal secretion

Neural involvement in intestinal anaphylaxis is supported by an extensive literature on anaphylaxis-induced alterations of mucosal ion transport. Not only is there a close anatomical relationship between mast cells and peptidergic nerves in the intestinal mucosa (Stead et al 1987), but there is evidence of a bidirectional functional relationship. In food protein-sensitized rat models (Crowe et al 1990, Catto-Smith et al 1994), the antigen-induced secretory response is significantly inhibited by tetrodotoxin and the muscarinic receptor antagonist atropine has no effect, whereas in the parasite-sensitized rat or the parasite or food protein-sensitized guinea pig, cholinergic nerves have been shown to be involved in the secretory response (Castro et al 1987, Wang et al 1991, Jared et al 1992). In addition, neural output (Pavlovian conditioning of sensitized rats to psychologic cues (MacQueen et al 1989)) can degranulate mast cells and, in an egg albumin-sensitized rat model of intestinal anaphylaxis, induce mucosal chloride secretion that can be inhibited by diphenhydramine and ketanserin (Perdue et al 1991). The converse has also been demonstrated – mast cell mediators appear to modulate neural activity controlling intestinal ion transport (Perdue et al 1991, Frieling et al 1994). Thus, intestinal mast cells can be activated by nerve stimulation and mast cell stimulation of intestinal nerves is an intrinsic part of the effector response. As the mucosa is in the closest proximity to luminal Ag exposure, contains the greatest concentration of mast cells and in sensitized animals reacts to Ag challenge with Cl⁻ secretion that is at least partially neurally mediated (Castro et al 1987, Crowe et al 1990, Wang et al 1991, Jared et al 1992, Catto-Smith et al 1994), it is very possible that it is the submucosal ganglia that both regulate secretory activity of the epithelium and recruit neuronal circuit within the myenteric plexus to control contractile activity in the muscular layers.

Neuroimmune regulation of anaphylaxis-induced alterations in motility

Mast cell-mediated neuromodulation has been characterized in several different animal models of hypersensitivity; however, there are fewer electrophysiologic data supporting the potential for antigen-induced, IgE and mast cell-mediated activation of myenteric neurons involved in the control of intestinal motor activity (Palmer 1991).

In the Hooded–Lister rat model, in vivo, atropine and hexamethonium block the antigen-induced disruption of MMCs, the increase in MCCs and GMCs and diarrhea in sensitized rats, suggesting that these alterations are dependent upon the mast cell-mediated activation of neuronal circuitry (Fargeas et al 1993, Scott & Tan 1996). This is consistent with a report that the duration of the antigen-induced alterations in motility was shortened by systemic capsaicin pretreatment and substance P antagonists, suggesting that substance P and capsaicin-sensitive afferent nerves also play a role in the anaphylaxis-induced disturbances of intestinal motility (Fargeas et al 1992). Recently, Castex et al (1995) reported that pretreatment with the selective 5- HT_3 antagonist ondansetron, or perivagal capsaicin treatment, blocked both brainstem Fos expression (in the nucleus tractus solitarii, lateral parabrachial nucleus and paraventricular nucleus) and MMC disruption in sensitized animals challenged with antigen. This suggests that vagal afferents at least monitor the intestinal response to food protein-induced intestinal anaphylaxis or might be the afferent limb of a centrally programmed intestinal motor response.

IRRITABLE BOWEL SYNDROME AND FOOD ALLERGY

Irritable bowel syndrome (IBS) is a chronic intestinal disorder of unknown origin characterized by recurring symptoms of abdominal pain and altered bowel habit (constipation and/or diarrhea). As the symptoms of IBS are often manifest after meals, there has been speculation that it might represent the response of the gastrointestinal tract to food allergy.

In 1982, Jones et al approached 25 consecutive patients with IBS to participate in an investigation of the potential role of food intolerance in their symptomatology. Fourteen of 21 patients who consented to participate noted resolution of their symptomatology on a 1-week exclusion diet and identified one or more foods (wheat (nine patients), corn (five patients), dairy products (four patients), coffee (four patients), tea (three patients) and citrus fruits (two patients)) which reproducibly provoked symptoms. All patients intolerant of wheat had a histologically normal jejunal biopsy and showed no increase in breath hydrogen production after ingestion of test meals. Six patients who had reproducible food intolerance in the open challenge were then involved in a double-blind, placebo-controlled, randomized challenge (two exposures to placebo and two to the test food) and successfully identified 10 of the 12 test days and 11 of the 12 controls days (p<0.01). Five additional patients underwent a single-blind, placebo-controlled, non-randomized challenge (two days of exposure to the placebo followed by two days of exposure to the test food) and all patients correctly identified the test period. While the single or double-blind challenges data support a diagnosis of food intolerance, the authors present no immunologic evidence for food allergy.

Bentley et al (1983) evaluated 27 patients with IBS. Open exclusion and reintroduction dietary testing lead to no change in symptoms in seven patients, no consistent exacerbation with reintroduction in four and consistent exacerbation in 10. Six patients did not complete the dietary trial. Of the 10 patients who reported consistent exacerbation, two refused double-blind testing and in only three of the remaining eight patients did double-blind challenge confirm the presence of a food intolerance (one yeast-sensitive patient with a positive skin test and two milk-sensitive patients, neither of whom was lactose intolerant or had a positive skin test to milk). Thus, objective evidence for food intolerance as a cause of abdominal symptoms was obtained in only 3/21 patients, but only one of whom had a positive skin test supportive of an IgE-mediated hypersensitivity reaction.

Initial open exclusion and reintroduction dietary testing was used by Petitpierre et al (1985) to screen 24 IBS patients (18 recruited from an outpatient allergy clinic) for potential food intolerance. Patients reporting exacerbation with open reintroduction underwent a blind provocative test. Seven patients experienced no change in their symptomatology during the initial exclusion and reintroduction phase. Of 17 patients reporting consistent exacerbation of symptoms after exposure to one or more foods, the response was reproduced in 14 after a blind challenge. Of these 14 patients, only seven indicated that specific foods or additives induced typical symptoms of IBS. While skin-prick tests and RAST were performed, the data are not presented in a way that permits correlation of those patients who experienced an exacerbation of IBS symptoms on double-blind food challenge with positive skin-prick tests or RAST results. Thus, even in this highly selected population of atopic patients, in only seven of 24 individuals were foods shown to induce typical symptoms of IBS, presumably because of hypersensitivity.

Zwetchkenbaum & Burakoff (1988) studied 10 patients with IBS, of whom six had positive skin scratch results and 10 had RAST IgG antibodies to a variety of foods. Despite this potential for immune responsiveness, six patients showed no significant change in symptoms during open exclusion and rechallenge, three reported improvement during the open elimination diet but had no exacerbation of symptoms with rechallenge and one patient dropped out of the study.

The largest study evaluating the proportion of IBS patients who respond to an exclusion diet is that of Nanda et al (1989). Of 189 patients who completed 3 weeks of a very restricted open exclusion diet, 91 (48.1%) claimed symptomatic improvement and the majority reported long-term improvement with persistent exclusion, but no objective confirmation of intolerance (double-blind challenge) or evidence of an allergic mechanism was provided. The remaining 98 patients (51.9%) showed no improvement. A history of atopy was present in 22.8% of the whole group and there were no differences in demography or symptoms between the responders and non-responders. Interestingly, after the 3-week period of strict dietary exclusion the mean weight loss of those patients with symptomatic improvement was 3.5 kg compared to 2.1 kg in the non-responders (p<0.0001), suggesting that psychologic variables, dietary compliance and factors such as reduced carbohydrate load may have contributed to the symptomatic improvement of the responding patients.

Thus, the studies which have been performed to evaluate the role of food hypersensitivity in IBS patients are few in number, generally involve small numbers of patients and have had major methodologic problems including a bias towards selection of atopic patients, failure to confirm food intolerance by double-blind, placebo-controlled food challenges or failure to perform or appropriately report data that would support an immune response as the mechanism responsible for the patient's symptomatology. The limited available data in the literature suggest that in only a small minority of often atopic individuals will double-blind, placebo-controlled food challenges and immunologic testing support an allergy to specific foods as the cause of the symptoms of IBS patients.

DIAGNOSTIC CRITERIA AND THE APPROACH TO INVESTIGATION

Clinical assessment

As with any medical condition, the initial step in the evaluation of an adverse reaction to food is a full medical history, physical examination and relevant general investigations to identify:

- underlying disorders with symptoms that cannot be attributed to the ingestion of specific foods;
- non-immunologically based food intolerances due to the ingestion of food additives, toxins or pharmacologic agents within specific foods;
- psychologic reactions to foods;
- information supportive of a potential immunologically based reaction to specific foods (Burks & Sampson 1992, 1993; Table 7.6).

Obviously, diet, lifestyle and activities, other medical conditions and drug therapy, as well as personal and family features of atopy, allergy and immune status are particularly important. Burks & Sampson (1992, 1993) suggest that to assist in establishing that a food reaction has occurred, the history should clearly identify the following:

1. the food suspected to have provoked the challenge;
2. the quantity of the food ingested;
3. the length of time between the ingestion and development of symptoms;
4. a description of the symptoms provoked;
5. whether similar symptoms developed on other occasions when the food was eaten;

Table 7.6 Methods used in the evaluation of adverse reactions to foods

Medical history, physical examination, relevant general investigations – diet, lifestyle (activities), medical conditions and pharmacotherapy with attention to personal and family history of atopy, allergy, immune status
Dietary diary
Elimination diet until well
Skin-prick test
Radioallergosorbent tests (RAST)
Basophil histamine release assay
Intestinal mast cell histamine release
Intragastric provocation under endoscopy
Double-blind, placebo-controlled food challenge (DBPCFC)
Intestinal biopsy after allergen exclusion and challenge

Adapted from Burks & Sampson 1993

6. whether other factors (e.g. exercise) are necessary;

7. the length of time since the last reaction.

When an adverse reaction is suspected but the patient's or parents' recall of the dietary history is unclear, a diet diary may prospectively establish an association between a food and the patient's symptoms.

Elimination diets and common food allergens

When certain foods are suspected of provoking a reaction, they should be eliminated from the diet to permit resolution of symptoms. Resolution is supportive but not diagnostic of a cause and effect association. In an effort to obtain a clear response, undiminished by recent challenge, avoidance of suspected food allergens is recommended prior to a blinded food challenge.

Most true food allergies occur in children, primarily infants, and 93% of the acute hypersensitivity reactions occur to only eight foods (Bock et al 1988; Table 7.7). In infants, reactions that occur to milk, egg, soy and wheat have a relatively short natural history and patients will often develop clinical tolerance over a period of months, generally before the age of 3 years. The process which underlies the development of this tolerance is not known as patients frequently persist in having in vivo (skin) and in vitro (radioallergosorbent test) reactions to these foods. In contrast, patients who have survived life-threatening reactions to peanuts, fish, crustacean shellfish and tree nuts usually exhibit prolonged clinical sensitivity and must be considered to have a lifelong natural history (Burks & Sampson 1993).

Skin testing

Skin testing with food extracts, done by the prick or puncture method, is a highly reproducible method of screening patients

Table 7.7 Foods responsible for the majority of IgE-mediated hypersensitivity reactions (listed in order of frequency)

Egg†
Peanut*
Milk†
Soy†
Tree nuts* (e.g. pecans)
Crustacean type of shellfish* (e.g. crab)
Fish*
Wheat†

*Lifelong natural history of sensitivity
†Tendency to a shorter natural history of sensitivity

with suspected IgE-mediated food allergy (Burks & Sampson 1992, 1993, Sampson & Metcalfe 1992). Briefly, glycerinated food extracts (1:10 or 1:20), an appropriate positive control substance (histamine) and an appropriate negative control substance (saline) are applied by the prick or puncture technique and any allergen eliciting a wheal of at least 3 mm greater than that elicited by the negative control substance is considered to be an allergen; anything less is considered negative. A positive skin test result indicates that the patient is sensitized to the allergen and that there is a potential for symptomatic reactivity to that specific food (the positive predictive accuracy is $> 50\%$). A negative skin test result confirms the absence of an IgE-mediated hypersensitivity reaction (overall negative predictive accuracy $< 95\%$). Thus, the skin-prick test can be considered an excellent means of excluding IgE-mediated food allergies but is only 'suggestive' of the presence of clinical food allergies. Burks & Sampson (1992, 1993) note that there are several exceptions to this general statement.

1. IgE-mediated sensitivity to several fruits and vegetables (apples, oranges, bananas, pears, melons, potatoes, carrots, celery, etc.) can frequently not be detected with commercial reagents apparently as a result of the lability of responsible allergen in the food.

2. Children less than 1 year old may have IgE-mediated allergy without a positive skin test and children less than 2 years old may have small wheals, perhaps because of a lack of skin reactivity.

3. A positive skin test to a food ingested in isolation that has provoked a serious systemic anaphylactic reaction may be taken as diagnostic.

In vitro tests of sensitization

In patients with extensive skin disease, dermatographism or in whom exposure to minute quantities of a specific food has resulted in a life-threatening reaction, in vitro diagnostic tests are preferred to in vivo skin testing (Burks & Sampson 1992, 1993). Radioallergosorbent tests and the enzyme link immunosorbent assay provide in vitro measurements of food-specific IgE and are only slightly less sensitive than the skin-prick test. The assays of basophil histamine release in small amounts of whole blood or of intestinal mast cell histamine release from dispersed intestinal mast cells obtained from intestinal biopsy specimens are additional in vitro methods of screening for IgE-mediated food sensitivity, but are generally only available in research settings.

Endoscopic gastric mucosal food challenge

Small quantities of food extract applied to the gastric mucosa under endoscopy appear to be a highly sensitive indicator of patient sensitization; however, the specificity of this text for predicting responses in patients with positive skin tests and nonreactivity has never been evaluated and the method may be no safer than oral challenge itself (Burks & Sampson 1992, 1993).

Double-blind, placebo-controlled food challenge

The double-blind, placebo-controlled food challenge (DBPCFC) has become accepted as the 'gold standard' for the diagnosis of food allergies in patients of all ages (Bock et al 1988, Burks & Sampson 1992, 1993, Anderson 1994). Considerations for performing a standardized DBPCFC are summarized in Table 7.8 and have been expanded upon elsewhere (Burks & Sampson 1992, 1993). The DBPCFC is the best means of controlling for the variability of chronic disorders (e.g. atopic dermatitis), potential temporal effects and acute exacerbations as a result of reducing or discontinuing medications and of eliminating psychogenic factors or observer bias. The choice of foods to be tested in the oral challenge is based on the history and/or skin-prick test or RAST results. While foods which are unlikely to provoke a food allergic reaction may be screened by open or single-blind challenges, it is important, except in very young infants, to then confirm a positive reaction by DBPCFC. In the case of suspect foods in which

Table 7.8 Considerations for performing a standardized double-blind, placebo-controlled food challenge

Eliminate suspected foods for 7–14 days before challenge
Discontinue antihistamines; minimize other medications
Administer challenge to patient on an empty stomach
Administer equal number of food and placebo challenges; randomize by non-interested party (dietitian)
Give lyophilized food in liquid or capsules (blind procedure)
Administer 10 g for 1 h; first dose <500 mg
Use standardized scoring system
Duration of observation period depends on type of reaction being studied
Have appropriate equipment available to treat systemic anaphylaxis

All negative challenge results must be confirmed by an open feeding under observation
Adapted from Burks & Sampson 1992

sensitization has been demonstrated, negative DBPCFC results should also be confirmed under observed open feeding conditions to exclude the rare possibility of false-negative results. DBPCFC should generally be conducted in a clinic or hospital setting, especially if an IgE-mediated reaction is suspected. Trained personnel and appropriate equipment for managing systemic anaphylaxis should be present (Patel et al 1994). Patients with a positive skin test and a clear history of severe anaphylaxis following the isolated ingestion of specific foods should not be challenged (Burks & Sampson 1992, 1993).

TREATMENT OF FOOD HYPERSENSITIVITY

Burks & Sampson (1992, 1993) have suggested an algorithm for the clinical evaluation of patients with adverse food reactions (Fig. 7.5). When the clinical history, skin-prick test or RAST results and the response to appropriate exclusion diets and DBPCFC confirm an IgE-mediated food hypersensitivity, <u>strict elimination of the offending allergen is the only therapy of proven value</u>. When prescribing an elimination diet the physician should ensure that the patient and/or parents receive sufficient instruction that they can read food labels appropriately and avoid hidden food allergen and also that the diet does not result in

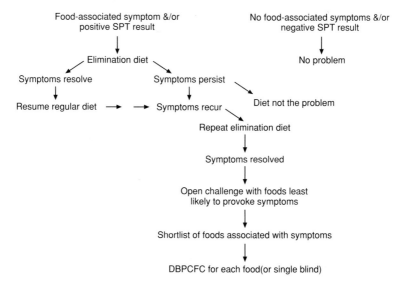

Fig. 7.5 Algorithm for the evaluation of an adverse reaction to food. SPT, skin-prick test; DBPCFC, double-blind, placebo-controlled food challenge. (Modified from Burks & Sampson 1992.)

unwanted side-effects (malnutrition, eating disorders) due to the inappropriate or excessive exclusion of multiple foods for extended periods of time. Symptomatic reactivity to food allergens is typically quite specific and patients rarely react to more than one member of a botanical family or animal species. Lastly, studies in both children and adults indicate that symptomatic reactivity to some food allergens is lost over time and cautious reintroduction may be appropriate in the future.

A variety of drugs have been employed in attempts to prevent or reduce the clinical symptomatology of patients with food hypersensitivity (e.g. H_1 and H_2 antihistamines, ketotifen, cromolyn sodium, corticosteroids and prostaglandin synthase inhibitors). While these drugs have the potential to modify symptoms and some studies support a therapeutic role, other studies have reported minimal efficacy and unacceptable side-effects (Burks & Sampson 1993). Many of the clinical studies suffer from methodologic deficiencies (Burks & Sampson 1993). Lastly, a growing basic science literature in this field shows that a multiplicity of mast cell mediators are involved and that there is a heterogeneity of mast cell types and the potential for progression and involvement of more than one immunologic mechanism (Crowe & Perdue 1992). These are all factors which make it less likely that single pharmacologic agents will be efficacious in therapy. In contrast, initial reports suggest that there may be some prophylactic effect of exclusive breastfeeding and delaying the introduction of multiple foods early in life, particularly in the atopic infant at increased risk of developing food hypersensitivity (Burks & Sampson 1993, Bock & Sampson 1994).

SUMMARY

As physicians, we very commonly encounter patients who believe that they have food allergy and relate histories of often non-specific symptoms in response to the single or repeated adverse reaction to the exposure to one or more foods. Fortunately, recent advances in the basic and clinical sciences have lead to a greater awareness of the numerous potential mechanisms by which patients might experience adverse reactions to food (Table 7.1), increased our understanding of the pathophysiology of the much less frequent allergic responses to food (particularly IgE-mediated hypersensitivity) and validated investigative approaches and clinical tools (e.g. the double-blind, placebo-controlled food challenge and skin-prick testing) to begin objectively evaluating our patients. The current foundation of basic scientific knowledge of allergic disease and the availability of objective methods which legitimize clinical evaluation make it likely that we will see an ever-increasing amount of research and even greater advances in the coming decade.

Given our current understanding of the field, food hypersensitivity is a relatively infrequent disorder with a spectrum of symptoms ranging from mild local oropharyngeal through significant gastrointestinal and/or extraintestinal to potentially fatal systemic anaphylaxis. Food hypersensitivity is not an etiologic explanation for more than a small fraction of the very large numbers of patients with irritable bowel syndrome. Strict elimination of the offending allergen remains the only effective preventive therapy for gastrointestinal or systemic symptoms due to food hypersensitivity.

REFERENCES

Anderson JA 1994 Establishing double-blind, placebo-controlled food challenge (DBPCFC) as the 'gold standard' for defining specific patient populations to be used in scientific studies. Annals of Allergy 72: 143–154

Bentley SJ, Pearson DJ, Rix KJB 1983 Food hypersensitivity in irritable bowel syndrome. Lancet ii: 295–297

Bock SA, Sampson HA 1994 Food allergy in infancy. Pediatric Clinics of North America 41(5): 1047–1067

Bock SA, Sampson HA, Atkins FM et al 1988 Double-blind, placebo-controlled food challenge (DBPCFC) as an office procedure: a manual. Journal of Allergy and Clinical Immunology 82: 986–987

Burks AW, Sampson HA 1992 Diagnostic approaches to the patient with suspected food allergies. Journal of Pediatrics 121: S64–S71

Burks AW, Sampson HA 1993 Food allergies in children. Current Problems in Pediatrics 23: 230–252

Castex N, Fioramonti J, Fargeas MJ, Bueno L 1995 c-fos expression in specific rat brain nuclei after intestinal anaphylaxis; involvement of 5-HT$_3$ receptor and vagal afferent fibres. Brain Research 688: 149–160

Castro GA, Powell DW 1994 The physiology of the mucosal immune system and immune-mediated responses in the gastrointestinal tract. In: Johnson LR (ed.) Physiology of the gastrointestinal tract. Raven Press, New York, pp. 709–750

Castro GA, Harari Y, Russell D 1987 Mediators of anaphylaxis-induced ion transport changes in small intestine. American Journal of Physiology 253: G540–G548

Catto-Smith AG, Patrick MK, Scott RB, Davison JS, Gall DG 1989a Gastric response to mucosal IgE mediated reactions. American Journal of Physiology 257: G704–G708

Catto-Smith AG, Patrick MK, Hardin JA, Gall DG 1989b Intestinal anaphylaxis in the rat: mediators responsible for the ion transport abnormalities. Agents and Actions 28: 185–191

Catto-Smith AG, Tan DTM, Gall DG, Scott RB 1994 Rat gastric motor response to food protein-induced anaphylaxis. Gastroenterology 106: 1505–1513

Crowe SE, Perdue MH 1992 Gastrointestinal food hypersensitivity: basic mechanisms of pathophysiology. Gastroenterology 103: 1075–1095

Crowe SE, Sestini P, Perdue MH 1990 Allergic reactions of rat jejunal mucosa. Ion transport responses to luminal antigen and inflammatory mediators. Gastroenterology 99: 74–82

Diamant SC, Scott RB 1987 MAPCs, a feature of normal jejunal myoelectric activity in the rat. Canadian Journal of Physiology and Pharmacology 65: 2269–2273

Diamant SC, Gall DG, Scott RB 1989 The effect of intestinal anaphylaxis on postprandial motility in the rat. Canadian Journal of Physiology and Pharmacology 67: 1326–1330

Fargeas MJ, Theodourou V, Fioramonti J, Bueno L 1992 Relationship between mast cell degranulation and jejunal myoelectric alterations in intestinal anaphylaxis in rats. Gastroenterology 102: 157–162

Fargeas MJ, Fioramonti J, Bueno L 1993 Involvement of capsaicin-sensitive afferent nerves in the intestinal motor alterations induced by intestinal anaphylaxis in rats. International Archives of Allergy and Immunology 101: 190–195

Ferguson A 1992 Definitions and diagnosis of food intolerance and food allergy: consensus and controversy. Journal of Pediatrics 121: S7–S11

Forbes D, Patrick M, Perdue M, Buret A, Gall DG 1988 Intestinal anaphylaxis: in vivo and in vitro studies of the rat proximal colon. American Journal of Physiology 255: G201–G205

Frieling T, Cooke HJ, Wood JD 1994 Neuroimmune communication in the submucous plexus of guinea pig colon after sensitization to milk antigen. American Journal of Physiology 267: G1087–1093

Galli SJ 1993 New concepts about the mast cell. New England Journal of Medicine 328: 257–265

Jared NH, Wang YZ, Cooke HJ 1992 Neuroimmune reactions: role for cholinergic neurons in intestinal anaphylaxis. American Journal of Physiology 263: G847–G852

Jarrett EEE, Stewart DC 1974 Rat IgE production. I. Effect of dose of antigen on primary and secondary reaginic antibody response. Immunology 27: 365–381

Jones VA, Shorthouse M, McLaughlan P, Workman E, Hunter JO 1982 Food intolerance: a major factor in the pathogenesis of irritable bowel syndrome. Lancet ii: 1115–1117

Kellow JE, Phillips SF 1987 Altered small bowel motility in irritable bowel syndrome is correlated with symptoms. Gastroenterology 92: 1885–1893

Kruis W, Azpiroz F, Phillips SF 1985 Contractile patterns and transit of fluid in canine terminal ileum. American Journal of Physiology 249: G264–G270

MacQueen G, Marshall JS, Siegal S, Perdue MH, Bienenstock J 1989 Conditioned secretion of rat mast cell protease II release by mucosal mast cells. Science 243: 83–85

Maric MD, Gall DG, Scott RB 1989 The effect of IgE-mediated intestinal anaphylaxis on intestinal transit. Canadian Journal of Physiology and Pharmacology 67: 1437–1441

Metcalfe DD, Sampson HA, Simon RA 1991 Food allergy – adverse reactions to food and food additives. Blackwell Scientific, Cambridge, MA.

Nanda R, James R, Smith H, Dudley CRK, Jewell DP 1989 Food intolerance and the irritable bowel syndrome. Gut 30: 1099–1104

Oliver MR, Tan DTM, Scott RB 1995a Intestinal anaphylaxis: mediation of the response of colonic longitudinal muscle in rat. American Journal of Physiology 268: G764–G771

Oliver MR, Tan DTM, Kirk DR, Rioux KP, Scott RB 1995b Colonic antigen challenge results in both local and jejunal motor alterations: the role of a mast cell–neural interaction. Gastroenterology 108: A661

Oliver MR, Tan DTM, Scott RB 1996 Colonic motor response to IgE-mediated mast cell degranulation in the Hooded—Lister rat. Neurogastroenterology and Motility (in press)

Otterson MF, Sarna SK 1994 Neural control of small intestinal giant migrating contractions. American Journal of Physiology 266: G576–G584

Palmer JM 1991 Immunomodulation of electrical and synaptic behaviour of myenteric neurons of guinea pig small intestine during infection with

Trichinella spiralis. In: Snape W, Collins S, (eds) Effects of immune cells and inflammation on smooth muscle and enteric nerves. CRC, Boca Raton, FL, pp. 181–195

Patel L, Radivan FS, David TJ 1994 Management of anaphylactic reactions to food. Archives of Disease in Childhood 71: 370–375

Patrick MK, Dunn IJ, Buret A et al 1988 Mast cell protease release and mucosal ultrastructure during intestinal anaphylaxis in the rat. Gastroenterology 94: 1–9

Perdue MH, Chung M, Gall DG 1984a Effect of intestinal anaphylaxis on gut function in the rat. Gastroenterology 86: 391–397

Perdue MH, Forstner JF, Roomi NW, Gall DG 1984b Epithelial response to intestinal anaphylaxis in rats: goblet cell secretion and enterocyte damage. American Journal of Physiology 247: G632–G637

Perdue MH, Masson S, Wershil BK, Galli SJ 1991 Role of mast cells in ion transport abnormalities associated with intestinal anaphylaxis. Correction of the diminished secretory response in genetically mast cell-deficient W/Wv mice by bone marrow transplantation. Journal of Clinical Investigation 87: 687–693

Petitpierre M, Gumowski P, Girard J-P 1985 Irritable bowel syndrome and hypersensitivity to food. Annals of Allergy 54: 538–540

Quigley EM, Phillips SF, Dent J 1984 Distinctive patterns of interdigestive motility at the canine ileocolonic junction. Gastroenterology 87: 836–844

Sampson HA, Metcalfe DA 1992 Food allergies. Journal of the American Medical Association 268(20): 2840–2844

Sanderson IR, Walker WA 1993 Uptake and transport of macromolecules by the intestine: possible role in clinical disorders (an update). Gastroenterology 104: 622–639

Sarna SK 1987 Giant migrating contractions and their myoelectric correlates in the small intestine. American Journal of Physiology 253: G697–G705

Scott RB, Maric M 1993 Mediation of anaphylaxis induced jejunal circular smooth muscle contraction in rats. Digestive Diseases and Sciences 38 (suppl. 3): 396–402

Scott RB, Tan DTM 1996 Enteric neural mediation of altered motility in intestinal anaphylaxis in the rat. Canadian Journal of Physiology and Pharmacology

Scott RB, Diamant SC, Gall DG 1988 The motility effects of IgE-mediated intestinal anaphylaxis in the rat. American Journal of Physiology 255: G505–G511

Scott RB, Gall DG, Maric M 1990 Mediation of food protein-induced jejunal smooth muscle contraction in sensitized rats. American Journal of Physiology 259: G6-G14

Shanahan F 1994 The intestinal immune system. In: Johnson LR (ed.), Physiology of the gastrointestinal tract. Raven Press, New York, pp 643–670

Stead RH, Tomioka M, Qunonez G, Simon GT, Felten SY, Bienenstock J 1987 Intestinal mucosal mast cells in normal and nematode infected rat intestines are in intimate contact with peptidergic nerves. Proceedings of the National Academy of Sciences USA 84: 2975–2979

Van Metre T 1983 Critique of controversial and unproven procedures for diagnosis and therapy of allergic disorders. Pediatric Clinics of North America 30: 807–813

Wang Y, Palmer JM, Cooke HJ 1991 Neuroimmune regulation of colonic secretion in guinea pigs. American Journal of Physiology 260: G307–G314

Zwetchkenbaum J, Burakoff R 1988 The irritable bowel syndrome and food hypersensitivity. Annals of Allergy 61: 47–49

Regional syndromes: clinical physiology and clinical management

The esophagus: clinical physiology

DF Evans

INTRODUCTION

The primary function of the esophagus is to transport ingested nutrient from the mouth to the stomach. Its physiology is simple in some respects but complex in others. Its pathology relates to abnormalities of organic and non-organic (functional) diseases which result in impairment of its primary function (i.e. transport). This includes the most comon motility disorder in gastroenterology, reflux of gastric content back into the esophagus caused by failure of the antireflux mechanism (ARM). It was Franz Ingelfinger who coined the phrase, 'The sphincter is a sphinx' and likened the lower esophageal sphincter to the Egyptian sphinx (Ingelfinger 1971) in hiding its mysteries.

This chapter will describe the normal function of the esophagus in terms of anatomy and the physiology of nutrient transport.

STRUCTURE

The esophagus is a muscular tube approximately 25 cm in length connecting the pharynx and the stomach and lies in loose connective tissue in the posterior mediastinum. The distal 3–5 cm is normally intraabdominal, having passed through the diaphragmatic hiatus in the left hemidiaphragm formed by the crura, just anterior to the aorta and posterior to the left lobe of the liver. The esophagus terminates at the gastroesophageal junction (GEJ) or cardia. Internally, the squamous epithelium also terminates close to the GEJ where it joins the columnar-lined epithelium of the stomach (Z line) (Fig. 8.1).

The blood supply to the esophagus in the neck is principally from the inferior thyroid arteries and in the throat from branches directly from the aorta and bronchial arteries. Venous drainage is via the azygos vein. The lymphatic drainage is to paraesophageal

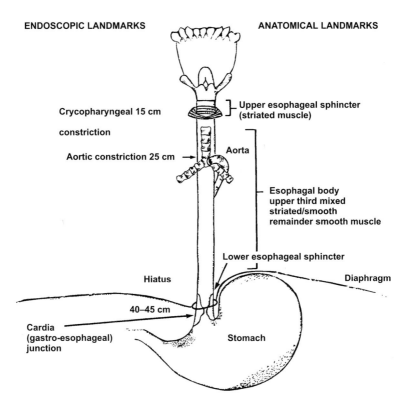

ENDOSCOPIC LANDMARKS

ANATOMICAL LANDMARKS

Crycopharyngeal 15 cm

constriction

Upper esophageal sphincter
(striated muscle)

Aortic constriction 25 cm

Aorta

Esophagal body
upper third mixed
striated/smooth
remainder smooth muscle

Lower esophageal sphincter

Hiatus

Diaphragm

40–45 cm

Cardia
(gastro-esophageal)
junction

Stomach

Fig. 8.1 Normal structure of the esophagus – endoscopic and anatomical landmarks.

nodes and then into the thoracic duct which lies to the left of the esophagus and vertebral column.

Histologically, the esophagus can be separated into the following regions.

1. *The innermost layer.* Here, the mucosa consists of non-keratinized stratified epithelium, lamina propria and muscularis mucosae. Mucus-secreting glands are also present close to the GEJ. There are no other secreted substances within the esophageal mucosa as its entire function relates to maintaining a state of emptiness.
2. *The submucosa,* which contains connective tissue, blood vessels and mucus glands.
3. *The muscularis layer,* which contains two layers of muscle – an inner circular layer and an outer longitudinal layer. This is similar to the remainder of the GI tract.

The most proximal 5% of the esophageal body, distal to the upper sphincter, is composed entirely of striated muscle fibers. The next 35–40% is mixed striated and smooth muscle with an increasing proportion of smooth to striated muscle moving distally. The most distal 35–40% is composed entirely of smooth muscle fibers (Arey & Tremaine 1933, Meyer et al 1986). The outer adventitial layer is composed of connective tissue which merges with adjacent structures within the thorax.

Extrinsic innervation is via the vagus nerve (Cannon 1907, Roman & Gonella 1987) which forms a plexus of mixed sympathetic and parasympathetic nerve fibers on the outer surface of the esophagus which coalesce in the distal third to form the anterior and posterior vagal trunks. Intrinsic innervation is controlled by the two ganglionated neural plexi (Mukhopadyhyay & Weisbrodt 1975, Christensen 1978). The submucosal or Meissner's plexus lies between the submucosal and circular muscle layer and the myenteric or Auerbach's plexus lies between the circular and longitudinal muscle layers. The function of the submucosal plexus is mainly control of secretion and blood flow in the epithelium and submucosa. The myenteric plexus controls motor function, including sphincter activity during deglutition. Extrinsic neural modulation is also via these nerve plexi and this is important in the regulation of deglutitive reflex activity (Diamant & Sharkawy 1977, Furness & Costa 1987).

The esophageal sphincters

The esophagus contains two sphincters.

The upper esophageal sphincter (UES) is situated at the junction of the pharynx and esophageal body and lies behind the hyoid bone. It is a slit-like structure, having a high pressure (50–100 mmHg) manometrically, predominantly in the anterior and posterior orientation with lower pressures laterally. Functionally, the UES protects the esophagus from the oral cavity and prevents aerophagia and esophagopharyngeal reflux.

The lower esophageal sphincter (LES) is found at the GEJ and within the hiatus. Anatomically and histologically, no major distinction is evident at the LES and the remainder of the muscle layers, although there is slight thickening of the wall at this region. Functionally, a high pressure zone exists in the most distal 2–5 cm of the circular smooth muscle. The LES exhibits both radial and axial asymmetry from extrinsic and intrinsic influences and also shows diurnal, postural and prandial variations in

Table 8.1 Factors affecting the function of the LES and esophageal body

	Decrease LES activity	Increase LES activity
Hormones & peptides	Glucagon Secretin Cholecystokinin VIP GIP Progesterone Estrogens Serotonin Histamines Enkephalins	Gastrin Motilin Bombesin Histamine (H_1 receptors) Serotonin (M receptors)
Prostaglandins	E1, E2, A2	F2
Drugs	Atropine Ca^{2+} inhibitors Ganglion inhibitors Tricyclic antidepressants	Metoclopramide Domperidone Cisapride Cholinergic drugs Anticholinesterases
Foods	Caffeine Fats Chocolate Alcohol	Protein meal
Other	Smoking	

pressure. Many external factors have been shown to affect the overall pressure in the LES and esophageal body motility and these are illustrated in Table 8.1.

The LES acts as a non-return valve and is a weak sphincter with an intrinsic pressure of only 10–25 mmHg. The LES is a major component of the antireflux mechanism (ARM) and is under both neural and hormonal control. The intrinsic basal tone has to resist reflux of gastric contents under the challenge of a wide range of intrathoracic (down to –60 mmHg) and intraabdominal pressures (up to 100 mmHg). Not surprisingly, LES dysfunction is very common.

NORMAL SWALLOWING

Swallowing can be initiated voluntarily or as part of a reflex following stimulation of the mouth and pharynx. However, once initiated, the act of swallowing become an involuntary act. The sensory nerves for this reflux are the glossopharyngeal and superior laryngeal branches of the vagus. Stimuli reach the swallowing center in the medulla and pons where swallowing is coordinated. Efferent impulses travel via the fifth, seventh, 10th, 11th and 12th cranial nerves as well as the motor neurons from C1–C3. There are three phases to normal swallowing.

Oral phase

Food is broken up and lubricated with saliva by mastication. The bolus is moved into the posterior oropharynx by the tongue and forced into the hypopharynx.

Pharyngeal phase

Simultaneously with the posterior movement of the tongue, the soft palate is raised to close the nasopharynx and prevent nasal regurgitation. The hyoid is pulled upwards, elevating the larynx to bring the epiglottis under the tongue. This backward tilt of the epiglottis covers the opening of the larynx and, with adduction of the vocal cords and the inhibition of respiration, prevents the passage of food into the airway. The pressure in the hypopharynx rises abruptly during swallowing to reach at least 60 mmHg. A pressure differential develops between the pharynx and the subatmospheric pressure of the intrathoracic esophagus which results in movement of the bolus into the esophagus when the crycopharyngeus relaxes. Once the bolus enters the esophagus proper, the crycopharyngeus closes with an immediate closing pressure of double the resting pressure (100 mmHg). The peristaltic wave initiated in the proximal esophageal body is initiated at the time of the highest crycopharyngeal pressure to prevent reflux into the pharynx. Once the peristaltic wave progresses distally, the UES returns to its resting pressure.

Esophageal phase

The pharyngeal activity in swallowing initiates the esophageal phase. The transmission of the food bolus from the distal esophagus into the stomach is accomplished over a pressure gradient of 5–50 mmHg below atmospheric pressure in the thorax to 5–30 mmHg above atmospheric pressure in the abdomen. A primary peristaltic wave is initiated by a pharyngeal swallow and consists of an occlusive pressure rise varying from 30 to 160 mmHg. The peak wave of contraction moves down the esophagus at a velocity ranging from 2 to 5 cm/s and reaches the distal esophagus between 4 and 10 s after the initial pharyngeal stimulus. Once the bolus reaches the lower esophagus, a further peristaltic wave may be initiated by a reflex secondary to lower esophageal distension and this is termed secondary peristalsis. At the time the bolus is approaching the stomach and after the initial pharyngeal stimulus, the LES relaxes completely to the level of the gastric baseline pressure to allow the passage of luminal content. The relaxation phase exists for up to 4 s. The LES undergoes an aftercontraction with a pressure rise of up to 50–100 mmHg in some cases before returning to its basal tone of 15–20 mmHg. The function of the aftercontraction is suggested to be a clearing contraction to ensure that any remaining content is moved into the stomach. Table 8.2 lists the normal physiological pressure values derived from manometry for the normal swallowing sequence.

Table 8.2 Normal pressure parameters developed in the esophagus during swallowing

	Range
Lower esophageal sphincter	
Position	38–48 cm
Length	2–4 cm
Intraabdominal length	> 1 cm
Resting pressure	6–25 mmHg
Relaxation on swallowing	< 5 mmHg above gastric baseline
Esophageal body motility	
Peristalsis	80–100%
Wave type	Monophasic
Simultaneous contractions	< 20%
Peak contractile amplitudes	30–160 mmHg
Duration of contractions	2–6 s
Peristaltic velocity	1.8–5 cm/s
Upper esophageal sphincter	
Position	15–20 cm
Pressure	30–150 mmHg
Relaxation	< 5 mmHg of thoracic baseline

A third type of contraction can sometimes be present in the esophageal body. These tertiary contractions may be seen as isolated contractions at any site in the esophageal body that are not preceded by a voluntary swallow or secondary peristalsis. The function of tertiary contractions is unknown but may be related to localized stimulation of stretch or chemoreceptors in the wall. Figure 8.2 illustrates the different patterns of esophageal body motility detectable by manometry.

THE NORMAL ANTIREFLUX MECHANISM (ARM)

Infrequent, short-lived periods of gastroesophageal reflux (GER) of gastric juice are common and are regarded as physiological.

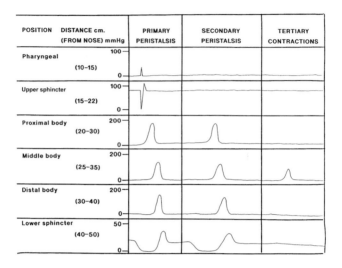

POSITION	DISTANCE cm. (FROM NOSE) mmHg	PRIMARY PERISTALSIS	SECONDARY PERISTALSIS	TERTIARY CONTRACTIONS
Pharyngeal	(10–15)			
Upper sphincter	(15–22)			
Proximal body	(20–30)			
Middle body	(25–35)			
Distal body	(30–40)			
Lower sphincter	(40–50)			

Fig. 8.2   Normal esophageal motility profiles during swallowing.

Physiological GER is often associated with eating and is most commonly experienced in the prandial period, sometimes in conjunction with eructation (belching). Physiological GER is rarely experienced during sleep unless a meal has been taken shortly before retiring or there has been some dietary abuse (large volume intake, high fat content, alcohol excess, hot spices, etc.). Pathological GER is associated with symptoms and is usually caused by more frequent reflux episodes, including some at night. This type of GER can give rise to esophageal damage (esophagitis) by gastric juice.

The majority of episodes of GER occur during transient periods of LES relaxation. Transient relaxations of the LES (TLESRs) were first described by Dent (Dent et al 1988) and are termed 'inappropriate' as they are not preceded by a corresponding primary peristaltic wave in the esophageal body initiated by a voluntary swallow. TLESRs have been shown to account for a significant proportion of GER.

Although the LES in itself is an important barrier to GER, it is one of only a number of other factors that are likely to be important in the overall ARM. Failure of one or more of these factors may result in reflux which, when also giving rise to symptoms, precipitates the disease entity of gastroesophageal reflux disease (GERD). The following factors have been proposed as being important in maintaining an effective reflux barrier. Although some have been unequivocally proven as being important in reflux control others, although based on sound phyiological principles, have not been sufficiently well defined or the order of importance classified.

Esophageal factors

LES Length

An important physical factor relating to valve function is the length of the valve closure. The resistance to opening pressure is related to the total length of the valve where the opening pressure exerts a dividing force, as in the shortening of the neck of a balloon on expansion.

Intraabdominal length

In addition to total length, the intraabdominal part of the LES may be important. For example, in the case of a hiatus hernia the LES is entirely in the thorax so no intraabdominal segment exists. A hiatus hernia is said to exist if part of the proximal stomach lies in the chest. This is caused by an anatomical defect in the hiatus, allowing either temporary or permanent displacement of the LES into the thorax. Any augmentation of LOSP by the abdominal pressure is therefore lost.

Anatomical factors

In addition to sphincter tone and length, other mechanical factors present at the gastroesophageal junction will influence overall LES competence.

Angle of His

The 'flap valve' mechanism caused by the acute angle of the esophagus and cardia (angle of His) has been shown to be an effective barrier to reflux (Atkinson & Summerling 1954). In hiatus hernia, this angle is absent and Steiner (1977) found that, compared to adults, the cardioesophageal angle in infants with hiatus hernia was virtually absent and the esophagus and stomach formed a straight tube, a possible explanation for GER in the newborn.

Diaphragmatic crus

The 'pinchcock' action of the right crus of the diaphragm is also a contributory factor in the overall valvelike action of the LES.

Indeed, the radial asymmetry of the LES may be a direct result of the pinchcock action of the crus (Kaye & Showalter 1971). Anatomically, other extraluminal factors associated with the ARM may be contributions from the oblique gastric sling fibers and the phrenoesophageal ligament.

Mucosal rosette

The convoluted folds of the esophageal mucosa, held in apposition by the surface tension of mucosal secretions, form a mucosal 'rosette' or 'choke', which acts as a reflux barrier (Petterson 1980). In esophagitis, where the integrity of the distal esophageal mucosa is compromised, it is likely that this factor will be absent, thus enhancing the reflux problem.

LES vagal reflex

The esophagus is extrinsically innervated by the vagus nerve although the majority of neural activity is controlled by the intramural myenteric plexus. Even so, a vagovagal reflux has been described (Ogilvie & Atkinson 1984) which may play an important role in reflux prevention. A reflex rise in LES pressure has been shown to exist in response to an increase in intraabdominal pressure. This is thought to be a physiological mechanism to protect the esophageal mucosa from acid when gastric pressure exceeds LES pressure. This reflex can be abolished by atropine and vagotomy and has shown to be impaired in chronic reflux patients with esophagitis (Ogilvie et al 1985). This is an important finding and may help to explain why some patients with apparently good LES tone and esophageal body peristalsis have severe reflux.

Esophageal motility

Esophageal passage of swallowed food is normally effected by coordinated contraction of the esophageal smooth muscle to project the food bolus distally. This peristalsis is essential in quadrupeds, where the stomach is often higher than the mouth (the giraffe, for example), and desirable in bipeds, even though gravity helps the passage of the bolus into the stomach. Where peristalsis is absent or impaired (as in diseases like scleroderma or achalasia), esophageal clearance is affected and dysphagia and regurgitation are common symptoms. Therefore, any dysfunction of normal esophageal motility may give rise to or worsen GER.

Many studies have shown that GER is possible when esophageal motility is impaired and acid clearance is delayed under these conditions (Karihlas et al 1988). Other important motility factors in the efficiency of esophageal contractility are amplitude, propagation velocity and coordination of the passage of the peristaltic wave and LES opening and closure.

Saliva

In man, saliva is produced by the salivary glands in the mouth to lubricate food and contains a number of substances including bicarbonate, mucus and salivary enzymes which initiate the first stages of digestion. Salivary output varies widely from a minimal basal state to a maximum secretion when stimulated by mastication. Swallowed saliva is thought to be important in GERD as the volume and composition of saliva plays an important role in the neutralization of GER of refluxed acid. Many papers have been produced which show the importance of saliva in GERD (Helm et al 1984, 1987).

Gastric factors

Motility and transit

Esophageal symptoms may be a result of gastric dysfunction if its consequences relate to 'backing up' of gastric content into the esophagus.

Food entering the stomach undergoes partial and mechanical breakdown prior to its further digestion in the small intestine. The stomach, like the esophagus, relies to some degree on coordinated contraction of its smooth muscle walls to propel chyme into the small intestine although liquids can be passively emptied by a pressure gradient across the pylorus. Unlike the esophagus, gastric motility is composed of two major types – mixing and peristaltic waves. In order to facilitate mechanical and chemical breakdown of ingested food, the stomach has the ability to mix its contents with secretions produced by the gastric wall, including acid and pepsin which initiate the process of digestion. When the mixture has attained the appropriate consistency for passage into the duodenum, a series of antral peristaltic waves propel small quantities of chyme across the pylorus, which opens reflexly to accommodate the passage. Any impairment of contractility or coordination may lead to gastric stasis. As volume and pressure rise in the stomach (caused by secretion and chemical breakdown) GER may be a consequence and esophageal symptoms may be produced. Gastric function therefore also has to be taken into account when assessing esophageal physiology.

Gastric acid secretion

The logical importance of acid secretion in the pathophysiology of esophageal physiology is also important for the reasons outlined above. The evidence for acid being a contributory factor in esophageal dysfunction is, on the surface, strong. Esophageal acidification may give rise to a variety of symptoms: heartburn and pain from mucosal irritation and sometimes also dysphagia as a secondary symptom. Regurgitation, caused by GER, and chest pain from esophageal spasm may also be symptoms associated with esophageal acidification. The most efficacious medical treatment for GERD is powerful acid suppression and even the 'softer', i.e. non-systemic, GER therapies incorporate some form of acid suppression in the form of neutralization with alkaline substances. Whether the esophageal symptoms are related to hypersecretion of gastric acid is in some doubt.

A large number of studies have been performed to examine acid secretor status in GERD and although some have shown significant differences in basal and peak acid outputs in symptomatic patients, the majority of studies show little difference in overall acid secretory levels against controls (Cadiot et al 1994). Other secretions in the stomach include pepsin, the proteolytic enzyme and, in a few patients, duodenogastric refluxate, including bile acids. Again, overall, there is no clearcut evidence that pepsinergic activity is implicated in the pathogenesis of GERD but bile acids in substantial quantities have certainly been found in some patients with complicated GERD, for example Barrett's esophagus (Gillen et al 1988, Gotley et al 1991, Iftikhar et al 1993). Figure 8.3 summarizes the factors which contribute to the ARM.

DISRUPTION OF NORMAL PHYSIOLOGY

Given that the role of the esophagus is simply that of transport, it is difficult to understand why esophageal disorders account for such a high proportion of gastroenterological consultations. The disorders can be divided into organic and functional and affecting the upper and lower sphincters and the esophageal body. Detailed discussion of such disorders is covered in the next section but the pathophysiology is outlined below.

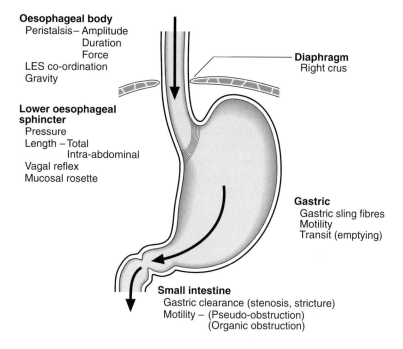

Oesophageal body
   Peristalsis– Amplitude
              Duration
              Force
   LES co-ordination
   Gravity

Diaphragm
   Right crus

Lower oesophageal sphincter
   Pressure
   Length – Total
              Intra-abdominal
   Vagal reflex
   Mucosal rosette

Gastric
   Gastric sling fibres
   Motility
   Transit (emptying)

Small intestine
   Gastric clearance (stenosis, stricture)
   Motility – (Pseudo-obstruction)
                (Organic obstruction)

Fig. 8.3   Putative esophagus antireflux mechanisms.

Sphincters

Disorders of the sphincters can be broadly divided into those where pressure is either too high or too low or where the coordination required to facilitate the normal passage of luminal content is impaired or compromised.

Upper sphincter

The upper sphincter is controlled by the cranial nerves and comprises striated muscle fibers and as such is spared whenever dysfunction of the smooth muscle part of the esophagus is involved (body and LES). Disorders of the upper sphincter are either caused by obstruction due to ingrowth of benign or malignant lesions (e.g. thyroid goiter, pharyngeal cancers, etc.) or by neurological impairment affecting the nervous system (e.g. cerebrovascular accident, cord lesions, multiple sclerosis, motor neuron disease). Disorders of the UES are therefore rare. If the UES is impaired, resolution of the problem is significantly more difficult to treat than when other parts of the esophagus are affected.

Lower sphincter

Disorders of the LES are, as for the UES, related to pressures which are either too high or too low. This can be caused by functional changes (achalasia, GERD) or organic problems (obstruction of the cardia from tumor growth of the GI tract or thoracic tumors invading extrinsically). Functional disorders that affect pressure are usually limited to diseases which result in degeneration of the myenteric plexus and therefore also affect the esophageal body (e.g. achalasia). Neurodegenerative disorders cannot be 'cured' but the symptoms can be treated. Disorders which reduce LES tone result in GERD which is generally treated with acid suppression in spite of being a disease of motility.

Esophageal body

Disorders of the esophageal body can be divided into those that affect muscle function and those that compromise neurological control. Disorders of muscle function include those that either reduce, increase or abolish contractile activity. Disorders that affect the myenteric plexus are those that impair peristalsis, affect sphincter coordination or destroy the normal propagation phenomena required for active luminal transport.

As symptoms are such a poor marker of specific esophageal disease, detailed objective investigation is required to obtain an accurate diagnosis.

INVESTIGATIONS

In order to examine the function of the esophagus and to investigate possible pathology, a number of new investigations have been developed over the years. These have been devised to examine structure and function and when used appropriately, help the clinician to obtain a clearer picture with regard to the causes of symptoms.

Radiology

Radiology continues to be of major importance in the investigation of the esophagus. Barium-based studies yield vital information regarding structure and function although in recent years other methods such as manometry and pH have replaced some radiological techniques.

Barium swallow

Examination of the esophagus with the lumen outlined with barium-based contrast media allows identification of normal structure. The mucosa can be identified and the esophageal lumen examined for any abnormalities. Irregularities of the mucosal surface seen in esophagitis are sometimes reported and major mucosal changes can be identified. Esophageal body luminal changes such as diverticula, rings and webs can be identified. Luminal obstruction, benign strictures, carcinoma and LES abnormalities (tight, lax) can also be identified. Motility abnormalities are more usually assessed using dynamic techniques.

Video fluoroscopy

Video fluoroscopy is used to assess dynamic function. Barium-based liquids or coated solids are swallowed whilst the radiologist follows the passage of the medium along the esophageal length. This type of radiology remains the best means of examination of the upper sphincter and is also useful in detection of motility abnormalities of the esophageal body and lower sphincter.

Marshmallow or bread swallows

In order to examine the response of the esophagus in as near a physiological way as possible, it is desirable to 'stress' the normal function with a normal load. In view of this, a barium-soaked marshmallow or bread bolus has been used to demonstrate pathology where a normal liquid barium bolus has failed.

Endoscopy and biopsy

The introduction of flexible endoscopes in the 1950s and 1960s revolutionized the investigation of the GI tract and was the single most important development that lead to the recognition of gastroenterology as a medical specialty in its own right. Flexible fiberoptic endoscopes are long tubes containing two glass fiber bundles, one with coherent fibers for viewing and a second non-coherent bundle for illumination by an external light source. The tip of the endoscope is controllable via external control wheels and air and water channels with valves are used to enhance the view during use. A magnifying eyepiece gives the operator direct magnified vision of the tip of the endoscope. In recent years, new developments in optics and television have seen the introduction of videoscopes which give full color, high-fidelity images, transmitted directly to a television monitor. Therapeutic advances have also been made with the use of lasers and other advanced cautery devices for tissue ablation and hemostasis.

Examination of the esophagus

Direct visual examination is performed under sedation or with topical lignocaine. The patient is positioned in the left or right lateral position with a mouthguard in place to protect the endoscope. The endoscope is passed into the pharynx and visual examination of the oropharynx, esophageal mucosa, sphincters and gastroesophageal junction is undertaken. Measurements of LES position and the Z line are documented. The presence of esophageal pathology including diverticula, webs, rings, hiatus hernia and any obvious obstructive pathology can be identified. Occasionally, the presence of a motility abnormality may be detected, either by the existence of hyperperistalsis or absence or irregularity of esophageal contractions.

Mucosal abnormalities, including esophagitis, proximal columnar epithelial migration (Barrett's esophagus), the presence of peptic strictures and mucosal infection or other damage, may be identified. Esophagitis is graded according to severity of mucosal damage and there have been numerous grading criteria published in recent years. The basis of grading is subjective but can be standardized by adherence to published guidelines describing the extent and severity of acid damage to the distal esophagus.

Tissue samples of the mucosa or deeper layers can be obtained to support visual or macroscopic findings and to examine other pathology. Tissue samples can be fixed, sectioned and histologically prepared using various techniques and graded by the pathologist with respect to cellular and morphological abnormalities. Tissue samples are obtained using special tools introduced through the biopsy channel of the endoscope. They include needle aspiration, punch or biopsy forceps and brush cytology. Vital stains are occasionally used in diagnostic endoscopy to aid recognition of mucosal abnormalities. For example, methylene blue or Indian ink can be sprayed on to the esophageal mucosa to identify areas of tissue damage or necrosis. Intravital stains such as methylene blue, Lugol's iodine and Congo red have also been used to demonstrate preferential uptake by diseased tissue.

Manometry

Esophageal manometry was first developed in its present form in the 1950s. The major role for esophageal manometry in clinical use is the investigation of dysphagia and chest pain and other symptoms undiagnosed by radiology, endoscopy or pH monitoring. The development of ambulatory manometry is also proving useful in patients with intermittent or infrequent symptoms suggestive of esophageal spasm.

Static perfused tube

The main technique for measurement of esophageal motility is the water-perfused tube. A soft, plastic, multilumen tube with side holes placed along its length is positioned at the desired site by nasal or oral intubation. Each port is perfused with water by a pneumohydraulic pump at a flow rate determined by the desired frequency response of the system. Occlusion of the side hole in any pressure channel by contraction of the esophageal wall causes a rise in pressure in that channel. The pressure rise is detected by an inline pressure transducer connected to a recording device (analog pen recorder or computer-driven system supported by an analog-to-digital conversion unit).

Strain gauge microtransducers

Miniature strain gauges mounted on small, flexible catheters are becoming increasingly popular in the measurement of esophageal motility. Although expensive (£500–1000 per sensor), they obviate the need for water perfusion and can be used more easily in ambulatory measurements.

Sleeve sensors

The tendency for the position of the LES to alter in relation to a fixed point makes accurate siting of a pressure sensor in the LES difficult, especially for prolonged measurements. To overcome this problem, Dent devised a thin, 6 cm, open-ended, silastic sleeve which surrounded the most distal perfused port of a multiumen catheter, specifically to facilitate LES measurements (Dent et al 1988). The function of the sleeve was to straddle the high pressure zone of the LES and record the average circumferential and axial pressure caused by all forces acting on the sleeve.

For prolonged ambulatory studies of LES pressure, a device called a sphinctometer has been developed (Barham et al 1992) and subsequently commercially manufactured (Gaeltec Ltd, Isle of Skye, Scotland). This device is sited at the most distal port of a multichannel microtransducer catheter and consists of a side-mounted strain gauge surrounded by a silicone oil-filled Silastic tube 6 cm in length and the same diameter as the catheter.

Measurement techniques

Static sensor Transducers are sited in the relevant part of the esophagus and tethered from without. Recordings of function are made for the required period on suitable recording devices, while ambulatory.

Pull-Through These techniques are most useful for sphincter measurements. This is achieved with either radially mounted sensors at the same level (minimum three (120°), maximum eight (45°)) or staggered along the length of the catheter where the radial LES measurement is achieved during station pull-through. These catheters are essential to accurately map LES pressure as it is well known that the LES is radially asymmetric.

Station Pull-Through The recording ports are passed beyond the LES and withdrawn in small increments (usually 0.5–1 cm),

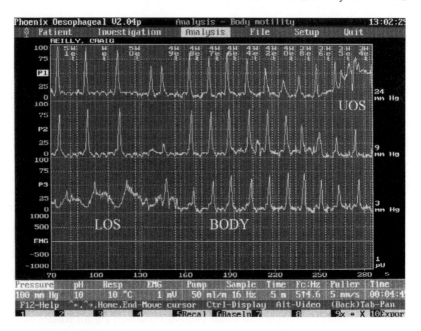

Fig. 8.4 Station pull-through manometry – normal.

recordings being made at each station for a sufficient period to give a stable reading. Figure 8.4 illustrates a typical station pull-through manometry in a normal subject. LES and UES function are measured as part of the procedure and peristalis in the esophageal body is demonstrated by multiple wet swallows with water.

Rapid Pull-Through This technique, using similar equipment to that above, requires a steady, continuous withdrawal of the recording ports through the sphincter. This is best achieved by a mechanical puller. The technique is to pull the catheter through the LES at a continuous steady rate (0.5–1 cm/s) whilst the patient holds their breath. This allows LES pressures to be measured without the interference of respiration.

Sphincter measurements – LES

LES pressure measurements are used to document pressure, length and relaxation and as such give the majority of information required to characterize the sphincter functionally. The recording of radial pressures from many ports at the same level has facilitated the production of three-dimensional images of LES morphology in addition to the other data and is called 'vector volume'. The technique, first developed in the anorectum, can be used to produce three-dimensional visual images of LES pressure profiles which may be useful where sphincter defects are to be corrected, for example, where reconstruction of the LES is planned for hiatus hernia repair and fundoplication.

Sphincter measurement – UES

Manometric assessment of the UES comprises measurements of position and intrinsic tone with due attention paid to radial asymmetry, relaxation and the relationship of relaxation to pharyngeal and esophageal contractions. The perfused tube catheter does not have a frequency response fast enough to follow UES dynamics so micro strain gauge transducers are recommended for the accurate assessment of this sphincter. Static and station pull-through protocols are the most widely used methods to examine the function of the UES and detailed information regarding the equipment and methodology is available (Wilson & Heading 1993).

Prolonged ambulatory recordings

In recent years, gastroenterologists have recognized that the symptoms of disordered GI function are often intermittent and that representative measurements may be better obtained by prolonged recordings. Furthermore, circadian changes in gut biorhythms require that measurements span a normal daily cycle, i.e. in most cases for a minimum of 24 h. This requirement, together with rapid development in computer technology, has seen the introduction of digital recording systems. Equipment is battery powered, lightweight and portable and allows for almost total ambulation during measurement. Patients can therefore undergo studies in their homes and workplaces. Event markers also allow for correlation between symptoms and measured abnormalities.

Such technology has also added the ability to analyze recordings with sophisticated computer software programs. Further benefits are both time saving and the rapid acquisition of accurate, repeatable, unbiased information derived from large quantities of data.

Esophageal pH measurements

Intraesophageal pH measurement is used to investigate GER which gives rise to esophageal symptoms. Table 8.3 outlines such symptoms and it can be seen that there is a great deal of overlap between the typical symptoms and those which might mimic other diseases. An accurate diagnosis of GERD can be complicated by the absence of visible esophagitis in up to 40% of patients (Richter & Castell 1982) and in some cases, a poor correlation with symptoms. Many investigations have been developed to aid diagnosis, including manometry and endoscopy but neither of these detects the presence of gastric juice in the esophagus. Intraesophageal pH was first described in the late 1960s, refined by Demeester and colleagues (DeMeester et al 1976) and subsequently developed as an ambulatory technique (Evans 1987). Ambulatory pH measurement is now held to be the best discriminator

Table 8.3 Common symptoms of GER

	Adult	Pediatric
Typical	Heartburn Regurgitation Epigastric pain Retrosternal pain	Vomiting Hematemesis Pain??
Atypical	Angina-like chest pain Dysphagia Nocturnal wheeze/asthma Laryngeal symptoms Rumination Toothwear halitosis	Chronic wheeze Chest infection Bronchodysplasia Pneumonia Stridor Failure to thrive Near sudden infant death

between physiological and pathological reflux and is regarded as the gold standard in the diagnosis of reflux disease.

Methodology

Sensors   Miniature ($<$ 2 mm) glass or antimony electrodes are available with either combined or external reference electrodes. Electrodes may be disposable or reusable depending on the manufacturing process and their sterilizability. Some electrodes are semidisposable and are inexpensive but reusable glass electrodes with a combined reference are probably more accurate, especially in a highly acidic environment such as the stomach and the esophagus.

Recorders   Recorders are digital, portable and solid state. Ambulatory outpatient recordings are desirable in order to express acid states physiologically. Most recorders incorporate event markers to document symptoms, meals and upright and supine periods.

Procedure

The pH sensor is introduced transnasally or orally and the distal esophageal sensor (or tip sensor if more than one sensor is used) is positioned 5 cm proximal to the lower esophageal sphincter, this being determined ideally by manometry.

pH measurements should ideally be performed for 24 h but shorter periods are permitted. It is essential to include at least two meals and the night period. This is to ensure that postprandial and nocturnal GER is assessed. Studies should be performed under near physiological conditions and patients should be encouraged to perform normal daily activities where possible. During diagnostic tests, free access to normal meals is encouraged, and patients are asked to document relevant events (activity, sleep, etc). Symptom markers are also included to correlate reflux symptoms with pH changes. Antireflux medication is usually withdrawn for up to 5 days prior to study (5 days proton pump inhibitors, 2 days H_2 receptor antagonists and prokinetics, 24 h antacids and alginates), but in some circumstances may be continued, in which case the investigation may be useful in assessing the efficacy of treatment. Dual esophageal and gastric pH recordings are useful to detect failure of acid inhibitors and to document alkaline reflux, although the latter is rare.

Figure 8.5 is a 24 h recording taken from patients with symptoms of GER. The trace illustrates the degree of GER that can be found in patients with severe GERD. GER is seen during both day

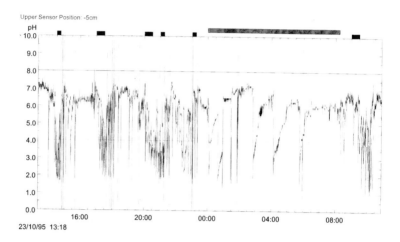

Fig. 8.5 24-h pH trace showing severe GER.

and night and acid clearance is also poor. Symptom correlation is also very high as indicated by the symptom marker and coincident GER. This patient is a possible candidate for surgery.

pH measurement with pressure

The last few years have seen the introduction of data loggers with high-capacity solid-state memory and multichannel recording facilities. This type of equipment is useful in investigations of unexplained, non-cardiac chest pain (NCCP). The objective of such recordings is the simultaneous monitoring of esophageal motility, LES function and pH. This enables a comparison of abnormalities of motility and GER and any correlation with symptoms.

Technically, the recordings can be achieved easily, using solid-state multichannel microtransducers, either combined with one or two pH channels or, as is more common, separate from the pH electrode. The investigation is more demanding for the patient due to the presence of a larger catheter and for the investigator because of the more complex analysis and interpretation of the recording. Figure 8.6 is an example of one such recording and illustrates GER and pressure abnormalities which are related to symptoms.

Provocation tests

Provocation tests have been devised to simulate symptoms in a controlled setting. Acid-related symptoms may be provoked with

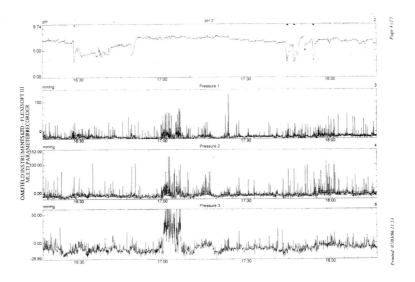

Fig. 8.6   Combined manometry with ambulatory pH.

instillation of hydrochloric acid into the esophagus to mimic the pain induced by acid reflux (Bernstein & Baker 1958) or by inducing reflux by structured activities such as raising intraabdominal pressure or inversion of the patient (standard acid reflux test (SART), acid reflux provocation test (ARPT). However, these test have mostly been abandoned since the introduction of 24-h pH monitoring.

Provocation of pain by spasm

Atypical chest pain of non-cardiac origin thought to be caused by esophageal spasm may be provoked by various means in an attempt to effect a diagnosis, especially where symptoms are intermittent.

Balloon distension   This test involves inflating a latex balloon in the esophageal body to elicit pain. The volume which initiates pain has been shown to be significantly lower in patients with various motility disorders than in controls (Richter et al 1986).

Pharmacological provocation   There are a number of pharmacological methods that have been developed in an attempt to elicit esophageal pain. Parasympathomimetic substances including ergometrine and bethanechol were initially advocated, being injected intravenously (randomized with saline to avoid false positives) and recording any symptoms produced. The side-effects of cholinomimetics (bradycardia and hypotension) led to alternatives being sought. Edrophonium (Tensilon), an anti-cholinesterase (DeCaestecker et al 1986), was advocated as a safer stimulant with fewer side-effects and the 'Tensilon test' was coined to describe almost any pharmacological provocation test.

Pharmacological provocation is not widely used today and has largely been superseded by balloon distension and prolonged pH and manometry recording. It remains useful in the investigation of the difficult patient.

Esophageal scintigraphy

Esophageal scintigraphy has been adapted to investigate the esophagus as an alternative to radiological investigation. Although scintigraphy lacks the fidelity of radiology as an imaging technique, it has the advantage of yielding dynamic data with objective measurements of esophageal transit. Two techniques have been developed.

The basic technique involves labeling a liquid or solid meal with a short half-life γ isotope, the most commonly used isotope being Technetium-99m. A γ camera with a large diameter head is required so that the whole of the esophagus can be imaged simultaneously. Aqueous liquids (water, orange juice) or solids (egg) are mixed with a standard dose of isotope and swallowed by the patient during rapid acquisition of images (200–500 ms over the first 2 min, longer after this if stasis or GER is being investigated). Data are stored in a computer and replayed in sequence to measure the transit characteristics of the swallow. Condensed images can be simultaneously displayed and graphs generated to examine the bolus transit of the test meal and identify areas of hold-up or reflux (Blackwell et al 1983, Kjelan et al 1984). γ scintigraphy is useful in the examination of achalasia and other disorders of esophageal motility and GERD, especially where complications may be suspected (Barrett's or stricture).

Prolonged, ambulatory scintigraphy has been described (Washington et al 1993) which utilizes a portable selenium detector strapped to the chest over the epigastrium connected to a portable recorder. The technique is currently mainly a research tool but can examine the differential reflux of food against acid by simultaneous isotope detection and pH monitoring.

SUMMARY

The physiology of the esophagus presents as a series of neurological and myogenic events resulting in the transport of ingesta
from the mouth to the stomach on demand. In itself, the malfunction of the mechanisms controlling these events does not
pose a life-threatening problem but in time, the starvation ensu-
ing from the inability to deliver nutrient to the body would eventually lead to death. Esophageal function is therefore regarded as
a primary function to support life. Disorders of the esophagus are
therefore important and notwithstanding the alterations to quality of life, the diseases which affect esophageal function are actively investigated and treated accordingly by gastroenterologists
and physicians alike.

REFERENCES

Arey LB, Tremaine MJ 1933 The muscle content of the lower oesophagus of man. Anatomical Record 56: 315–320

Atkinson M, Summerling MD 1954, The competence of the cardia after cardiomyotomy. Gastroenterology 92: 23–134

Barham CP, Gotley DC, Miller R, Mills A, Alderson D 1992 Ambulatory measurement of oesophageal function: clinical use of a new pH and motility recording system. British Journal of Surgery 79: 1056

Bernstein LM, Baker LA 1958 A clinical test for the oesophagitis. Gastroenterology 34: 760–781

Blackwell JN, Hannan WJ, Adam RD, Heading RC 1983 Radionuclide transit studies in the detection of oesophageal dysmotility. Gut 24: 421–426

Cadiot G, Sekera E, Mignon M 1994 Gastric secretion in GORD. In: Scarpignato C, Galmiche JP (eds) Functional evaluation in esophageal disease. Frontiers. Gastrointestinal Research; 22: 209–222

Cannon WB 1907 Oesophageal peristalsis after bilateral vagotomy. American Journal of Physiology 19: 436–444

Christensen J 1978 The innervation and motility of the esophagus. Frontiers of Gastrointestinal Research 3: 18–32

DeCaestecker JS, Pryde A, Heading RC 1986 Comparison of intravenous edrophonium and oesophageal acid perfusion during esophageal manometry in patients with non-cardiac chest pain. Gut 29: 1029–1034

DeMeester TR, Johnson LR, Joseph GJ, Toscano MS, Hall AW, Skinner DB 1976 Patterns of gastroesophageal reflux in health and disease. Annals of Surgery 184: 459–469

Dent J, Hollaway RH, Toouli J, Dodds WJ 1988 Mechanism of lower oesophageal sphincter incompetence in patients with symptomatic gastro-oesophageal reflux. Gut 29: 1020–1028

Diamant NE, Sharkawy TY 1977 Neural control of oesophageal peristalsis. A conceptual analysis. Gastroenterology 72: 546–556

Evans DF 1987 Twenty-four hour ambulatory oesophageal pH monitoring: an update. British Journal of Surgery 74: 157–161

Furness JB, Costa M 1987 Arrangement of the enteric plexuses. In: Furness JB, Costa M (eds) The enteric nervous system. Churchill Livingstone, London.

Gillen P, Keeling P, Byrne PJ, Hennessy TPJ 1988 Implications of duodenogastric reflux in the pathogenesis of Barrett's oesophagus. British Journal of Surgery 75: 540–543

Gotley DC, Morgan AP, Ball D, Owen RW, Cooper MJ 1991 Composition of gastro-oesophageal reflux. Gut 32: 1093–1099

Helm JF, Dodds WJ, Pele L, Palmer DW, Hogan WJ, Teeter BC 1984 Effect of esophageal emptying and saliva on acid clearance. New England Journal of Medicine 310: 284–288

Helm JF, Dodds WJ, Hogan WJ 1987 Salivary response to esophageal acid in normal subjects and patients with reflux esophagitis. Gastroenterology 93; 1393–1397

Iftikhar YF, Ledingham SJ, Evans DF et al 1993 Bile reflux in columnar lined Barrett's oesophagus. Annals of the Royal College of Surgeons of England 75: 411–416

Kaye MD, Showalter JP 1971 Manometric configuration of the lower oesophageal sphincter in normal human subjects. Gastroenterology 61: 213–223

Kjelan G, Svedberg JB, Tibbling L 1984 Solid bolus transit by esophageal transit scintigraphy in patients with dysphagia and normal manometry and radiography. Digestive Diseases and Sciences 29: 1–5

Meyer GW, Austin RM, Brady CE, Castell DO 1986 Muscle anatomy of the human oesophagus. Journal of Clinical Gastroenterology 8: 13

Mukhopadyhyay AK, Weisbrodt NW 1975 Neural organisation of esophageal peristalsis: role of the vagus nerve. Gastroenterology 68: 444–447

Ogilvie A, Atkinson M 1984 Influence of the vagus nerve on reflux control of the lower oesophageal sphincter. Gut 25: 253–258

Ogilvie A, James PD, Atkinson M 1985 Impairment of vagal function in reflex oesophagitis. Quarterly Journal of Medicine 54: 61–74

Petterson GB, Bombech CT, Nyhus LM 1980 The lower oesophageal sphincter mechanism of opening and closure. Surgery 88: 307–314

Richter JE, Castell DO 1982 Gastroesophageal reflux. Pathogenesis, diagnosis and therapy. Annals of Internal Medicine 97: 93–103

Richter JE, Barish CF, Castell DO 1986 Abnormal sensory perception in patients with esophageal chest pain. Gastroenterology 91: 845–852

Roman C, Gonella J 1987 Extrinsic control of digestive tract motility. In: Johnson LR (ed.) Physiology of the gastrointestinal tract, 2nd edn. Raven Press, New York, pp 507–553

Steiner GM 1977 Gastro-oesophageal reflux. Hiatus hernia and the radiologist with special reference to children. British Journal of Radiology 50: 164–174

Washington N, Moss HA, Washington C, Greaves JL, Steele RJC, Wilson GG 1993 Non-invasive detection of GOR using an ambulatory system. Gut 34: 1482–1486

Wilson J, Heading R 1993 The upper oesophageal sphincter. In: Kumar D, Wingate DL (eds) Illustrated guide to gastrointestinal motility. Churchill Livingstone, London

The esophagus: disorders of swallowing and chest pain. Clinical management

RW Tobin, CE Pope II

Disturbances in function of the esophagus can present with either characteristic (dysphagia) or non-specific (chest pain) symptoms. This chapter will confine itself to such manifestations and not discuss symptoms due to structural abnormalities of the esophagus such as odynophagia of mucosal origin or pain due to carcinoma. Occasionally the detection of the cause for functional esophageal symptoms can be relatively easy; more often, the search for a cause of symptoms and their alleviation will be a much more difficult task.

DYSPHAGIA

Introduction

Dysphagia is a symptom which always points to dysfunction of the oropharynx or esophagus. It is never a manifestation of hysteria or psychic stress, although such stress can often exacerbate an underlying motor problem of the esophagus. There are three basic categories of dysphagia: oropharyngeal dysphagia, dysphagia secondary to structural abnormalities of the esophagus and dysphagia produced by malfunction of the muscular body and sphincters of the esophagus. This chapter will focus primarily on the latter; the other two categories can usually be distinguished from motor disorders by careful history, taking or simple investigations.

Oropharyngeal dysphagia

Oropharyngeal dysphagia occurs either when the patient cannot initiate a swallow or when the bolus travels to an alternative destination such as the nasopharynx or the trachea. Patients often describe an inability to begin the act of swallowing or to transfer a bolus to the back of the mouth. Symptoms can include a feeling of food sticking in the throat, a cough on swallowing liquids or nasal regurgitation of a liquid bolus. Oropharyngeal dysphagia can be accompanied by dysarthria, increased snoring or nasal speech. Although a mechanical obstruction must be excluded, oropharyngeal dysphagia is usually due to a lesion proximal to the body of the esophagus and often involves an abnormality in the neuromuscular control of the mouth, tongue, pharynx, hypopharynx or upper esophageal sphincter. Most commonly, these neuromuscular abnormalities are only part of a more global disease process and dysphagia is only one of the manifestations of this process. Evaluation of oropharyngeal dysphagia is best done by video fluoroscopy to which manometry can be added in some research centers. A speech pathologist can also be helpful in the evaluation of such patients. Treatment consists of improving the underlying condition (if possible), changing the food consistency to maximize swallowing ability and instructing the patient in modifying the technique of swallowing.

Structural abnormalities of the esophagus

Patients with a structural lesion of the esophagus producing dysphagia, such as a stricture or obstructing cancer, usually have certain clinical characteristics which help in identifying the dysphagia as structural in origin. Patients with structural abnormalities note dysphagia for solids and usually not for liquids. If liquid dysphagia is present, careful questioning will reveal that a solid bolus has usually preceded the liquid; it is unusual to begin a meal with a liquid and experience dysphagia if an organic narrowing is present. Dysphagia is usually relieved by bringing up the offending bolus – attempts to wash it down with fluid often end with regurgitation of the fluid by an obstructed esophagus. Structural dysphagia tends to be constant rather than varying from week to week whereas a cancer tends to be relentlessly progressive. History alone is a fairly good determinant when trying to decide between structural and dysmotility causes. A discriminant analysis was able to differentiate between them with a sensitivity of 77% and a specificity of 80% (Kim et al 1993).

A structural esophageal abnormality will usually be identified by a carefully performed barium esophagram, perhaps supplemented by a barium-soaked solid bolus of bread or marshmallow. Endoscopy will also be useful in visualizing and possibly treating an obstructing lesion. It is always important to rule out an obstructing lesion before moving on to a consideration of a possible motility problem, as the prognosis and therapy of structural lesions are very different from those of dysmotility.

Motor dysfunction of the esophagus

With some notable exceptions to be discussed, the symptoms of functional disorders of the esophagus tend to be less marked than those of structural problems. The dysphagia of functional disease is caused by both solids and liquids and is often dependent on the temperature of the ingested material, cold being the worst offender. The patient may complain only of a transient arrest which is easily solved by reswallowing or, in the case of an arrested solid bolus, by taking fluid. Compared to structural dysphagia, there is much more variation in both the frequency and intensity of dysphagia over time, the patient having good weeks and bad weeks. Pressing chest pain may accompany swallowing or may occur at other times of the day or night. Rare manifestations of dysmotility include regurgitation of fluid back up into the nasopharynx after it has been swallowed into the esophagus and audible gurgling after ingestion of fluid. Prolonged retention of food and fluid in the esophageal body is unusual except in the case of patients with achalasia. Ropy mucus can also be regurgitated by some patients with motor disorders.

There are three main diagnostic categories into which patients with motor dysfunction fall. First is achalasia, a syndrome whose pathophysiology, clinical manifestations, diagnosis and therapeutic options are fairly well understood. Another category is a group of illnesses in which the main problem is esophageal muscle weakness. The third and largest group, and the one which is least understood, is the non-specific esophageal motor disorders or NEMD. Some authors try to subdivide NEMD with such terms as 'diffuse esophageal spasm', 'hypertensive lower esophageal sphincter', 'nutcracker esophagus' and 'hypercontracting lower esophageal sphincter'. Since many of these distinctions are blurred and definitive pathophysiological information, diagnostic criteria and therapeutic options remain unknown, we would prefer to consider all these as variants under the title of NEMD with qualifying phrases such as high-amplitude, long-duration waves when applicable. Each of the main three categories (achalasia, primary muscle disease and NEMD) will be considered separately.

Achalasia

Unlike the other entities to be discussed, the pathophysiology, diagnostic tests and therapy of achalasia have been fairly well established. It is a disorder manifesting two disturbances in function: inability of the lower esophageal sphincter to relax in response to a swallow and failure of a peristaltic wave to traverse the smooth muscle of the esophagus after deglutition. Myenteric nerve bodies in the lower esophageal sphincter muscle zone, which presumably release inhibitory neurotransmitters such as nitrous oxide and vasoinhibitory peptide, are absent or markedly reduced. This causes the tone of the LES to be increased and food and fluid are retained in the esophagus, leading not only to dysphagia but also to aspiration.

Diagnosis is usually made by a barium esophagram showing a dilated esophagus and a 'bird beak' appearance of the gastro-esophageal junction. In a study in which manometry was used as the gold standard, X-ray was only 41% sensitive in establishing the diagnosis (Stacher et al 1994). If the X-ray appearance is inconclusive, the manometric finding of a lower esophageal sphincter that does not completely relax upon swallowing combined with simultaneous low-amplitude pressure waves recorded from the esophageal body will confirm the diagnosis of achalasia.

Therapy is aimed at weakening the tonically contracted lower esophageal sphincter by local injection of botulinum toxin (Pasricha et al 1995), balloon dilation (Parkman et al 1993), esophagomyotomy by open surgery, laparoscopy (Ancona et al 1995) or thoracoscopy (Pellegrini et al 1993). The only randomized series of dilation versus surgery suggested that surgery is more effective than balloon dilation in both the short and long term (Csendes et al 1989).

Primary muscle disease

Patients with scleroderma or other collagen-vascular diseases may occasionally suffer with dysphagia. This dysphagia may be intensified by reflux damage, as these patients will also suffer from sphincter insufficiency as well as loss of muscle strength in the body of the esophagus. The clinical situation usually makes diagnosis very easy and intraluminal manometry offers a quick explanation for the symptom of dysphagia. Either total aperistalsis or very reduced peristaltic amplitudes are encountered on manometry. In control subjects, amplitudes of 30 mmHg or less are associated with inadequate bolus transport (Kahrilas et al 1988). The dysphagia is usually mild and not the major problem for the patient.

Treatment of the primary muscle diseases is not effective with the present state of knowledge. Attempts to increase the amplitude of peristaltic waves pharmacologically have not been successful. Treatment of associated reflux damage should be undertaken as it may improve swallowing function. This can be done with the proton pump inhibitors; antireflux surgery is not often employed because of the fear of postoperative dysphagia.

Non-specific esophageal motor disorders (NEMD)

This category contains an extremely heterogeneous group of disorders. Most of them have been defined by their manometric patterns (Table 9.1), but their pathophysiology, anatomic correlates, constancy and interconvertability remain unknown. Dysphagia is for both liquids and solids and rarely leads to profound weight loss. Patients with NEMD may also complain of chest pain which clinically resembles the pain of coronary artery disease (see below).

Manometry is currently employed to detect and define motor abnormalities of the esophagus. If scintigraphy or radiology is used, another group of patients will be identified. Approximately 50% of a group of patients with severe reflux disease will have dysphagia (Russell et al 1982, Triadafilopoulos 1989). Many of these will have normal manometric patterns; a subset will also show abnormalities in the transport of a radioisotope. Other patients will complain of dysphagia, yet all our current technologies will not be able to explain this symptom. In a referral practice at the Mayo Clinic, current technology could not explain the dysphagia in nearly 40% of patients without structural lesions (Kim et al 1993).

Therapy for these miscellaneous but very common disorders is empirical. There is scant evidence that any pharmacologic therapy is useful in this group of disorders. If reflux is associated with the dysphagia, then a vigorous trial of proton pump inhibitors seems to be in order. If manometry reveals high-amplitude, long-duration waves, then a trial of diltiazem 90 mg q.i.d. would be worth a try. Low-amplitude waves do not seem to have a pharmacologic treatment. Often the best treatment seems to be an explanation to the patient, stressing that the dysphagia will

Table 9.1 Classification of non-specific esophageal motor disorders

Diffuse spasm	Multiple simultaneous contractions interposed with peristaltic contractions
Low-amplitude waves	Peristaltic waves less than 30 mmHg in amplitude
Failed peristalsis	Peristalsis not transmitted entire length of esophagus
Multiple peaks	Three or more peaks in one wave form
Hypertensive LES	LES pressure > 40 mmHg with relaxation on swallowing
Aperistalsis	No contraction in response to a wet swallow

probably not progress and will not usually lead to marked weight loss. Long myotomy would not seem to be indicated for dysphagia due to NEMD.

Figure 9.1 summarizes the diagnostic and therapeutic considerations in the management of dysphagia. Oropharyngeal dysphagia can usually be suspected clinically and evaluated cinefluorographically. Evaluation of eosphageal dysphagia can begin with a barium esophagram, although many experts prefer to go directly to endoscopy. If a structural abnormality is detected by either X-ray or endoscopy, appropriate therapy can be directed to the cause of obstruction. If the endoscopy is not revealing, then manometry can be obtained, although some clinicians might choose a diagnostic trial of proton pump inhibitors, hoping to treat reflux-induced dysphagia. Manometry will show either achalasia, NEMD, evidence for primary muscle disorders, be within normal limits. In the latter case, it may be desirable to obtain a scintigram to document the presence of a transport

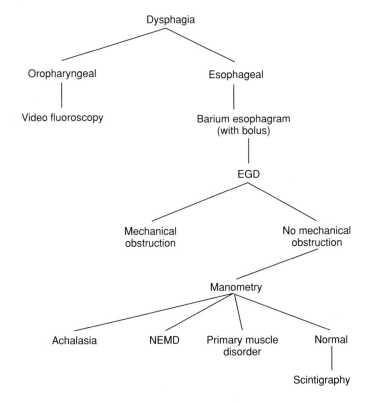

Fig. 9.1 Diagnostic and therapeutic considerations in the management of dysphagia.

abnormality, even though the therapeutic approaches for this at the present time are limited.

Globus sensation

Another functional symptom, globus sensation, can sometimes be confused with dysphagia. It is usually described by the patient as a lump or a pressing sensation deep in the base of the neck. Unlike dysphagia, which is always temporally associated with the act of swallowing, globus is present constantly and may be accompanied by a need to clear the throat repeatedly. This symptom can occur in the setting of gastroesophageal reflux disease with acid laryngitis. This relationship can be confirmed by treating the reflux by pharmacological or surgical methods. Other workers are less impressed with the relationship between reflux and globus sensation and have detected an increased amplitude of pharyngeal contraction pressures in patients with globus (Wilson et al 1989).

CHEST PAIN

Chest pain from abnormal motor activity of the esophagus has been postulated for over 100 years. Osler's textbook of medicine published at the beginning of the century talked of 'oesophagismus' or spasm of the gullet. The idea of spasm became more firmly rooted in the 1950s when barium studies showed abnormal contractions in patients with chest pain whose electrocardiograms were normal (Evans 1952). The concept that acid irritation of the esophagus could produce not only heartburn but crushing chest pain is a much later concept of the 1970s and 1980s. If left to their own devices, most patients will not choose the term 'pain' to describe the sensation caused by acid stimulation of the esophagus; they prefer the term 'burning'. Yet acid-induced chest pain indistinguishable from the pain of coronary artery disease is a real entity which does not have to be accompanied by the more mundane symptom of heartburn.

In the 1990s, the possibility that chest pain from the esophagus might be caused by abnormalities of the esophageal afferent enteric nervous system was raised after it was shown that some subjects with chest pain were abnormally sensitive to balloon stimulation of the esophagus (Barish et al 1986, Cannon & Benjamin 1993, Paterson et al 1995). This situation seems analogous to the lowered threshold to balloon stimulation demonstrated in patients with irritable bowel syndrome.

It is still unclear how often each of these three mechanisms (contraction abnormalities, acid sensitivity or disturbances in the perception of afferent impulses) is present in an individual patient with chest pain of unknown origin. Some of the reasons leading to this uncertainty will be discussed under the headings of the diagnosis and therapy of chest pain secondary to functional disease of the esophagus.

Clinical features

Before discussing the clinical features of chest pain of esophageal origin, it is worthwhile to differentiate the symptom of heartburn from that of chest pain. Heartburn, the most common clinical manifestation of gastroesophageal reflux, is usually described as a burning sensation, located substernally and radiating up into the neck. 'Burning', 'hot', 'on fire' are common descriptors. The other essential component of heartburn is relief by antacids (even transiently). Heartburn is usually triggered in susceptible individuals by large meals containing fat, alcoholic beverages, chocolate and/or onions. It may be accompanied by regurgitation of sour or bitter fluid into the mouth. Chest pain of esophageal origin and heartburn can be found in the same patient who is usually quite capable of telling one sensation from the other. Heartburn does not usually intensify to become chest pain; the two sensations may come and go independently.

Heartburn tends to respond to simple measures (Table 9.2) whereas chest pain of esophageal origin rarely does. Sometimes in patients in whom heartburn and chest pain coexist, the lifestyle changes of Table 9.2 or addition of standard doses of H_2 blockers will cause the heartburn to disappear while the chest pain continues unabated.

Chest pain of esophageal origin is most often confused with cardiac pain. This is, of course, the most important distinction to draw since the prognosis and treatment options of the two conditions are entirely different. Pain from the chest wall or abdominal wall can be difficult to distinguish from chest pain of esophageal

Table 9.2 Simple measures to treat heartburn

1. Elevate the head of the bed from four to six inches with blocks.
2. Avoid food and drink before retiring.
3. Avoid fat, chocolate, alcohol, citrus fruits and onions.
4. Eat small meals.
5. Take antacids as necessary.
6. Lose weight.

origin. The thoracic outlet syndrome or gall bladder disease may have pain referred to the chest.

Differentiation between cardiac and esophageal pain can be extremely difficult. The most reliable differentiator is the radiation directly through to the back found in pain of esophageal origin. In an informal poll of local cardiologists, most agreed that although both cardiac and esophageal pain can radiate to the neck, jaw and left arm, radiation to the back is distinctly uncommon in cardiac pain. This is also the opinion of other cardiologists (Hanshaw 1992).

Many patients shown to have an esophageal origin of their chest pain will state that exercise will tend to bring on their chest pain (which usually increases the confusion as to whether chest pain is of cardiac or esophageal origin). Closer questioning will often reveal that there is a variable relationship between the amount of exercise and the onset of chest pain. Patients with chest pain of esophageal origin will note wide variability in the amount of exercise which is followed by chest pain, whereas patients with coronary artery disease will feel chest pain after the same amount of exercise on different occasions.

In patients who present with chest pain, the presence of dysphagia suggests an esophageal origin of the pain. Chest pain and dysphagia do not often occur simultaneously; patients experiencing chest pain do not usually feel like eating or drinking at that moment. More commonly, the patient with chest pain of esophageal origin will notice very mild dysphagia at times totally unrelated to episodes of chest pain. The dysphagia will be of a motor type, i.e. usually for solids and relieved by reswallowing or washing down the bolus with liquids. The dysphagia is not intense enough to cause the patient to seek medical attention for this symptom and is rarely pronounced enough to cause weight loss. Its presence can be sought by asking whether bread or meat ever 'hangs up', 'hesitates' or 'sticks on the way down'. Merely asking the patient whether they have trouble with swallowing will not produce a positive answer very often.

Nevertheless, clinical distinction between chest pain of cardiac and esophageal origin can be extremely difficult, especially when the pain is of central location not radiating to the back or accompanied by dysphagia. Without these clues, differentiation between pain of cardiac and esophageal origin should be approached by evaluating risk factors for coronary artery disease such as hypertension or lipid disorders. If there is a high probability of coronary artery disease, then a cardiac diagnostic testing sequence ranging from treadmill tests to coronary arteriography should be undertaken. The degree of invasiveness will depend on the clinical probability of coronary artery disease in the individual patient under investigation. If the clinical probability of coronary artery disease is very low because of the patient's lack of risk factors, then testing for pain of esophageal origin can begin.

Diagnostic testing in esophageal pain

Before launching into a discussion of the sensitivity and specificity of various diagnostic tests, it is well to pause and examine some of the methodological pitfalls lurking for those studying the relationship between a test of esophageal function and chest pain.

The first problem is that most test procedures do not have an absolute answer in terms of 'yes' or 'no'. A prime example is 24-h pH testing in which all 'normal' control subjects have a certain number of reflux episodes, usually in the postprandial period. This problem has been addressed by the construction of receptor-operator curves (ROC) which allow a clinical evaluation of the importance of a test result to determine whether a test is 'normal' or 'abnormal'. If it is important that a positive test result identifies every individual with the condition under evaluation, then a larger number of false-positive tests can be tolerated in order to make certain of including all patients with the condition. If it is very expensive to evaluate false positives and the condition is not life threatening, then a different point on the ROC curve can be selected which will pick up most of the patients with the condition and avoid the extra effort necessary to evaluate a large number of false positives.

Another problem specific to the evaluation of chest pain of unknown origin is that a new test or diagnostic fact is evaluated using a group suspected of suffering from an esophageal origin of pain. These patients are usually chosen because they have a 'negative' cardiac evaluation. The extent of cardiac evaluation varies; most series do not uniformly use coronary artery angiography. Clinical evaluation of the presence of coronary artery disease is notoriously unreliable. Therefore, the 'chest pain of esophageal origin' group against which the sensitivity and specificity of a given test are being evaluated includes an unknown number of patients who actually have unrecognized cardiac disease.

This problem can be approached by refining the group with chest pain to include only patients whose treatment of the putative esophageal cause has led to complete symptom relief. This approach is especially valuable for chest pain due to mucosal acid sensitivity as acid can temporarily be ablated with proton pump inhibitors. However, it is occasionally necessary to use very high doses of the proton pump inhibitors to attain a therapeutic result (Schindlbeck et al 1995). Since there are no consistently effective methods of treating motor disorders or afferent sensation disorders responsible for pain, this approach can only be partially successful.

Yet a third problem exists when it is necessary to determine if an event (episode of reflux or an abnormal esophageal contraction) is related to an episode of chest pain. If every episode of reflux is followed shortly by esophageal distress or, conversely, if an episode of chest pain occurs when the pH meter shows no acid to be present, then it is easy to determine whether a causal relationship exists. More commonly, chest pain will follow some but not all episodes of a reflux of acid or an abnormal contraction. How close does this relationship between an event (acid reflux) and a symptom (chest pain) need to be in order to assign a causal relationship? This question has been approached by calculating several types of indices. A symptom index divides the number of reflux-related symptom episodes by the total number of symptom episodes (a measure of specificity). Alternatively, the number of reflux episodes associated with symptoms divided by the total number of reflux episodes, the symptom sensitivity index, is a measure of sensitivity. Another approach is to divide the monitoring period into short segments and then construct a 2 x 2 table showing the relationship between event and symptom. From this, Fisher's Exact Test can be applied to provide a statistical probability that the two are related (Weusten et al 1994). However, there is no clinical agreement as to what value of what index must be reached to assign a patient to a 'test positive' or 'test negative' status.

With these caveats in mind, it is instructive to examine the results of testing esophageal function in patients with chest pain of uncertain origin. Such studies can be divided into three types: short-term testing, 24-h ambulatory testing and provocative testing.

The results of short-term testing suggest that a manometric abnormality can be demonstrated in approximately 30% of patients. This, of course, does not prove causation. Such studies most frequently identify high-amplitude, long-duration waves (nutcracker esophagus) as being the most common manometric finding. Doubt has been expressed as to whether such high-amplitude waves have any clinical importance as they are often present in periods in which no symptoms are reported. Non-specific motor disorders are the next most common diagnostic abnormality, while diffuse spasm is quite uncommon in most series. In a study of patients with chest pain and NEMD on manometry, there was not a close correlation between improvement in symptoms and change in manometric patterns over time (Achem et al 1992).

The advent of 24-h pH recording allowed a more physiologic appraisal of the relationship between acid reflux and symptoms than did short-term pH monitoring with its requisite loading of the stomach with acid. Several studies have shown that abnormal pH scores were recorded from approximately half of the patients with chest pain of unknown origin. One of these studies also pointed out that in some patients with a normal total exposure time to acid, a high correlation existed between episodes of reflux and episodes of pain (Hewson et al 1991).

Advances in technology now allow prolonged monitoring of both pH and motor activity of the esophagus. It was originally hoped that being able to study patients for a prolonged period in their usual environment would lead to a higher diagnostic yield than that obtained from laboratory-based studies. Even though combined studies have been done in patients complaining of daily chest pain, the diagnostic yield has not been as high as expected. If patients with very intermittent pain are studied with ambulatory equipment, the yield is even lower. In a group of patients with chest pain not felt to be cardiac in origin, 24-h monitoring showed reflux-associated pain in 5%, motility-associated pain in 5%, both causes in 9% and no association with either acid or motility in 81% (Breumelhof et al 1990). However, the same laboratory reported a much higher yield when patients were studied soon after a cardiac cause for pain was ruled out (Lam et al 1992). In this instance, reflux-associated pain was demonstrated in 32%, pain with motor abnormalities in 24% while 44% of patients had neither. A group of cardiologists, using similar techniques in a group of patients with normal coronary angiograms, found essentially no relationship between either acid reflux or motor abnormalities and their patients' pain episodes (Hick et al 1992). Even ST changes observed during cardiac monitoring during the same study did not correlate well with chest pain.

Efforts to provoke chest pain using various stimuli have met with limited success. Chest pain due to acid sensitivity of the esophagus has been sought with an intraesophageal acid drip (Bernstein test). In one series, 16 of 71 patients developed chest pain after a 10-min infusion of acid, producing a positive predictive value of only 38% (Hewson et al 1991). Attempts to correlate a positive acid infusion test with a positive 24-h pH test or with a positive symptom index were not very successful. In another series 16 of 60 patients thought to have an esophageal origin of chest pain had a positive Bernstein test (Janssen et al 1986). Approximately half of these patients with a positive acid infusion test had a positive 24-h pH monitor result. The same authors reported a positive acid perfusion test in 14 of 50 chest pain patients (Ghillebert et al 1990). As in the prior series, these acid infusion-positive patients did not often have a positive 24-h pH monitor test.

Cholinergic stimuli have been used in an attempt to provoke abnormal motor activity. Bethanechol and edrophonium are the two drugs used most often, with edrophonium being the favored agent because of a shorter duration of action. Edrophonium causes an increase in peristaltic amplitude in both control subjects and patients with non-cardiac chest pain; only the latter group develops chest pain to accompany the increased amplitude. In a study in which acid infusion and edrophonium were compared, acid was more effective in inducing chest pain (35% yield) than was edrophonium (20% yield) (DeCaestecker et al 1988). Eleven of the 12 patients responding to edrophonium also had a positive response when exposed to acid. In patients who respond to multiple provocative agents, it is difficult to assign a particular etiology for their chest pain. An even bigger problem is when the results of provocation are compared to test results obtained during 24-h monitoring. In DeCaestecker's study mentioned above, only seven of 18 patients with a positive acid infusion test had chest pain during spontaneous acid reflux during 24-h monitoring.

Balloon stimulation of the esophagus is another provocative test that may offer some insight into the mechanism(s) of chest pain. In a group of 50 patients suspected of an esophageal source of pain, gradually increasing balloon inflation produced pain identical to that felt spontaneously in 28; only 12 of these patients responded to either acid or edrophonium infusion (Barish et al 1986). The balloon volume necessary to produce discomfort was much smaller in the patient group than in the control subjects. This result has led the authors to suggest that the patients with balloon-stimulated chest pain have an altered sensory threshold and may therefore perceive stimuli which control subjects do not sense. A possible objection to balloon stimulation is that distension is not a usual condition when chest pain occurs – patients are rarely eating during chest pain attacks. An intriguing paper showed that patients with chest pain and a positive balloon response do not belch easily when air is infused into their esophagus (Gignoux 1995). Perhaps air refluxed from the stomach and not cleared by a belch might stretch the esophagus and stimulate pain. Another group of investigators working with balloon stimulation found a yield of 26 positive results in 62 patients; only nine of these patients responded to either acid drip or edrophonium (Deschner et al 1990). Yet in another group of patients with chest pain, balloon stimulation reproduced pain in only one of 20 patients tested (Ghillebert et al 1990). Perhaps use of a balloon whose actual dimensions can be measured with impedance changes will refine this technique (Orvar et al 1993).

In summary, abnormalities in muscular function and acid reflux can be demonstrated in many patients with chest pain of presumed esophageal origin, but it is difficult to assign a causal role in many of these patients. Some patients tend to respond with the same kind of pain to both acid reflux and to abnormal esophageal contractions. There is not a constant relationship between stimulus and response; acid will cause pain at one time in the record but not at another. Provocation with cholinergic compounds or with an acid infusion can reproduce the symptoms of chest pain; however, the results of a positive provocation test and events detected during spontaneous pain often do not agree. Very few of the papers on the diagnostic accuracy of testing for causes of chest pain provide data on the results when the putative cause is treated. Balloon stimulation appears to be a promising method of esophageal testing, suggesting that the afferent pathway in the esophageal–brain system needs to be examined more closely. At the present time, there is no diagnostic test or combination of tests which can unequivocally demonstrate that the esophagus is the source of the chest pain.

With this somewhat gloomy assessment in mind, is there any place for esophageal testing in the evaluation of chest pain of uncertain etiology? A possible scheme is presented in Figure 9.2. In this sequence, cardiac disease is excluded and the intensity and invasiveness of the evaluation are driven by the level of positive risk factors for coronary artery disease. Ultrasound follows to rule out gall stone disease. Depending on availability, either an acid suppression test with 40 mg of omeprazole or a 24-h pH probe test can be applied. The latter will pick up both individuals with increased acid exposure and another group whose exposure times are normal but who react with chest pain with each burst of reflux.

If the pH probe result is normal, then a standard manometry test might be considered. This will have a very low yield of

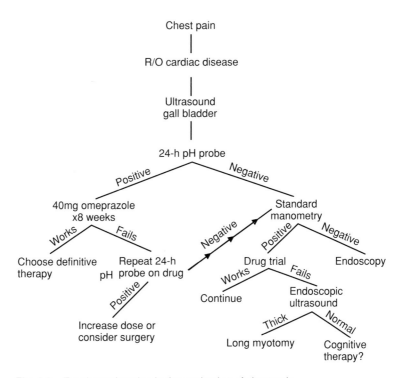

Fig. 9.2   Esophageal testing in the evaluation of chest pain.

definitive results, as the patient must have an attack of chest pain during the manometric procedure in order to establish a causal relationship. In an early series, this only occurred 14% of the time (Brand 1978). If high-amplitude, long-duration waves are found on the stationary manometry, a drug trial might be worth while. If the manometric exam is negative, an endoscopy could be done to make certain that erosive esophagitis or a peptic ulcer has not been overlooked. This will also tend to be a low-yield procedure. Further therapy and diagnostic evaluation will be deferred until after a discussion of the therapeutic options.

Therapy

The type of therapy offered will depend on the presumed pathophysiology of the chest pain. The three major hypotheses – acid-induced, motor-induced or altered afferent information processing – will lead to different modalities of therapy. With the advent of the proton pump inhibitors such as omeprazole or lansoprazole, effective control of acid secretion is possible. Omeprazole 40 mg per day is a good starting dose, although some individuals might require a higher dose for symptomatic relief. In a recent trial of patients with ordinary reflux, some required 60–80 mg of omeprazole for control of symptoms (Schindlbeck et al 1995). The risk of such a trial is minimal, although it is moderately expensive. If a positive outcome is obtained, then a decision is taken on whether permanent pharmacotherapy or an antireflux operation will be undertaken, using the usual considerations.

The therapy of motor disorders of the esophagus producing chest pain is more problematic. Table 9.3 lists some agents which have been recommended. Most of them have no placebo-controlled studies to support the recommendation. One trial suggests that diltiazem 90 mg q.i.d. is effective in patients with high-amplitude, long-duration contractions (Cattau et al 1991). It also seems possible that some patients who have been given nitroglycerine or calcium channel-blocking drugs for presumed coronary artery disease have had a good result because their unrecognized esophageal motor disorder has inadvertently been treated.

Drugs which might modulate afferent sensitivity have not been thoroughly tested for this indication. In a controlled trial of trazodone, patients with chest pain felt better even though the drug did not reduce the frequency of chest pain (Clouse et al 1987). Imipramine in low dose was also effective in a trial of therapy for patients with non-coronary chest pain, many of whom had motor abnormalities of the esophagus (Cannon et al 1994). Although patients with chest pain of unknown origin have a high degree of psychological abnormality when tested (Clouse 1991), there have been few attempts to treat chest pain with psychological techniques. One interesting study from Oxford reports good short-term results with cognitive therapy in a trial which was placebo controlled (Klimes et al 1990).

Long myotomy has been utilized in a very few patients, but most reported series are in single figures. It is possible that the advent of thoracoscopic laparoscopy may increase this form of treatment (Shimi et al 1992, Patti et al 1995). However, the sur-

Table 9.3 Agents recommended for chest pain of esophageal origin

Nitroglycerine
Isosorbide
Hydralazine
Diltiazem
Nifedipine
Imipramine
Trazodone

geon should be as certain as possible that the esophagus is the source of the difficulty before doing a long myotomy.

In summary, the diagnosis and treatment of chest pain of esophageal origin continues to frustrate the medical and surgical establishment. The diagnosis of acid-induced pain and its therapy are on a fairly secure footing. Pain secondary to motor abnormalities undoubtedly exists, but there is no consensus as to mechanism or treatment. Studies of increased afferent sensitivity as a cause of chest pain are in their infancy. There still remain a significant number of patients with chest pain in whom no cause can be found. It is hoped that other methods of evaluating esophageal muscle function and sensation will be developed and will explain these patients who elude a definitive diagnosis at the present time.

REFERENCES

Achem SR, Crittenden J, Kolts B, Burton L 1992 Long-term clinical and manometric follow-up of patients with nonspecific esophageal motor disorder. American Journal of Gastroenterology 87: 825–830

Ancona E, Anselmino M, Zaninotto G et al 1995 Esophageal achalasia; laparoscopic versus conventional open Heller-Dor operations. American Journal of Surgery 170: 265–270

Barish CF, Castell DO, Richter JE 1986 Graded esophageal balloon distension. Digestive Diseases and Sciences 31: 1292–1298

Brand DL, Martin D, Pope CE II 1977 Esophageal manometrics in patients with angina-like chest pain. Digestive Diseases and Sciences 22: 300–304

Breumelhof R, Nadorp JHSM, Akkermans LMA, Smout AJPM 1990 Analysis of 24-hour esophageal pressure and pH data in unselected patients with noncardiac chest pain. Gastroenterology 99: 1257–1264

Cannon RO, Benjamin SB 1993 Chest pain as a consequence of abnormal visceral nociception. Digestive Diseases and Sciences 38: 193–196

Cannon RO, Quyyumi AA, Mincemoyer R et al 1994 Imipramine in patients with chest pain despite normal coronary angiograms. New England Journal of Medicine 330: 1411–1417

Cattau EL, Castell DO, Johnson DA et al 1991 Diltiazem therapy for symptoms associated with nutcracker esophagus. American Journal of Gastroenterology 86: 272–276

Clouse RE 1991 Psychiatric disorders in patients with esophageal disease. Medical Clinics of North America 75: 1081–1096

Clouse RE, Lustman PJ, Eckert TC, Ferney DM, Griffith LS 1987 Low-dose trazodone for symptomatic patients with esophageal contraction abnormalities. Gastroenterology 92: 1027–1036

Csendes A, Braghetto I, Henriquez A, Cortes C 1989 Late results of a prospective randomized study comparing forceful dilatation and oesophagomyotomy in patients with achalasia. Gut 30: 299–304

DeCaestecker JS, Pryde A, Heading RC 1988 Comparison of intravenous edrophonium and oesophageal acid perfusion during oesophageal manometry in patients with non-cardiac chest pain. Gut 29: 1029–1034

Deschner WK, Maher KA, Cattau EL, Benjamin SB 1990 Intraesophageal balloon distension versus drug provocation in the evaluation of noncardiac chest pain. American Journal of Gastroenterology 85: 938–943

Evans W 1952 Oesophageal contraction and cardiac pain. Lancet ii: 1091–1097

Ghillebert G, Janssens J, Vantrappen G, Piessens J 1990 Ambulatory 24 hour intraoesophageal pH and pressure recordings v provocation tests in the diagnosis of chest pain of oesophageal origin. Gut 31: 738–744

Gignoux C, Bost R, Hostein J et al 1993 Role of upper esophageal reflex and belch reflex dysfunctions in noncardiac chest pain. Digestive Diseases and Sciences 38: 1909–1914

Hanshaw BT 1992 Excluding heart disease in the patient with chest pain. American Journal of Medicine 92 (suppl. 5A): 46S–51S

Hewson EG, Sinclair JW, Dalton CB, Richter JE 1991 Twenty-four-hour esophageal pH monitoring: the most useful test for evaluating noncardiac chest pain. American Journal of Medicine 90: 576–583

Hick DG, Morrison JFB, Casey JF, Al-Ashhab W, Williams GJ, Davies GA 1992 Oesophageal motility, luminal pH, and electrocardiographic-ST segment analysis during spontaneous episodes of angina like chest pain. Gut 33: 79–86

Howard PJ, Maher L, Pryde A, Cameron EWJ, Heading RC 1992 Five year prospective study of the incidence, clinical features and diagnosis of achalasia in Edinburgh. Gut 33: 1011–1015

Janssen J, Vantrappen G, Ghillebert G 1986 24-hour recording of esophageal pressure and pH in patients with noncardiac chest pain. Gastroenterology 90: 1978–1984

Kahrilas PJ, Dodds WJ, Hogan WJ 1988 Effect of peristaltic dysfunction on esophageal volume clearance. Gastroenterology 94: 73–80

Kim CH, Weaver AL, Hsu JJ, Rainwater L, Zinsmeister AR 1993 Discriminate value of esophageal symptoms: a study of the initial clinical findings in 499 patients with dysphagia of various causes. Mayo Clinic Proceedings 68: 948–954

Klimes I, Mayou RA, Pearce MJ, Coles L, Fagg JR 1990 Psychological treatment for atypical non-cardiac chest pain: a controlled observation. Psychological Medicine 20: 605–611

Lam HGT, Dekker W, Kan G, Breedijk M, Smout AJPM 1992 Acute noncardiac chest pain in a coronary care unit: evaluation by 24-hour pressure and pH recordings of the esophagus. Gastroenterology 102: 453–460

Orvar KB, Gregersen H, Christensen J 1993 Biomechanical characteristics of the human esophagus. Digestive Diseases and Sciences 38: 197–205

Parkman HP, Reynolds JC, Ouyang A, Rosato EF, Eisenberg JM, Cohen S 1993 Pneumatic dilatation or esophagomyotomy treatment for idiopathic achalasia: clinical outcomes and cost analysis. Digestive Diseases and Sciences 38: 75–85

Pasricha PJ, Ravich WJ, Hendrix TR, Sostr S, Jones B, Kallo AN 1995 Intrasphincteric botulinum toxin for the treatment of achalasia. New England Journal of Medicine 332: 774–778

Paterson WG, Wang H, Vanner SJ 1995 Increasing pain sensation to repeated esophageal balloon distension in patients with chest pain of undetermined etiology. Digestive Diseases and Sciences 40: 1325–1331

Patti MG, Pellegrini CA, Arcerito M, Tong J, Mulvihill SJ, Way LW 1995 Comparison of medical and minimally invasive surgical therapy for primary esophageal motility disorders. Archives of Surgery 130: 609–615

Pellegrini C, Wetter LA, Patti M et al 1992 Thoracoscopic esophagomyotomy: initial experience with a new approach for the treatment of achalasia. Annals of Surgery 216: 291–299

Russell COH, Pope II CE, Gannan RM, Allen FD, Velasco N, Hill LD 1982 Does surgery correct esophageal motor dysfunction in gastroesophageal reflux? Annals of Surgery 194: 290–296

Schindlbeck NE, Klauser AG, Voderholzer WA, Muller-Lissner SA 1995 Empiric therapy for gastroesophageal reflux disease. Archives of Internal Medicine 155: 1808–1812

Shimi SM, Nathanson LK, Cuschieri A 1992 Thoracoscopic long myotomy for nutcracker oesophagus: initial experience of a new surgical approach. British Journal of Surgery 79: 533–536

Stacher G, Schima W, Bergmann H 1994 Sensitivity of radionuclide bolus transport and videofluoroscopic studies compared with manometry in the detection of achalasia. American Journal of Gastroenterology 89: 1484–1488

Triadafilopoulos G 1989 Nonobstructive dysphagia in reflux esophagitis. American Journal of Gastroenterology 84: 614–618

Weusten BLAM, Roelofs JMM, Akkermans LMA, Van Berge-Henegouwen GP, Smout AJPM 1994 The symptom-association probability: an improved method for symptom analysis of 24-hour esophageal pH data. Gastroenterology 107: 1741–1745

Wilson JA, Pryde A, Piris J et al 1989 Pharyngoesophageal dysmotility in globus sensation. Archives of Otolaryngology and Head and Neck Surgery 115: 1086–1090

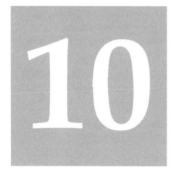

The stomach: nausea, vomiting and other food-related symptoms. Clinical physiology

AJPM Smout

SYMPTOMS ATTRIBUTED TO GASTRIC DISORDERS

A wide range

Diseases of the stomach may manifest themselves through a wide range of symptoms. Unlike the esophagus where dysphagia and retrosternal pain are relatively simple and rather specific signals of lesions or dysfunction of the organ, the stomach uses a complicated and unspecific repertoire of symptoms to express its distress. The symptoms usually thought to be referable to the stomach are listed in Table 10.1. Most of these occur postprandially, i.e. within minutes to hours after ingestion of food, but some of the gastric symptoms may also occur when the stomach is empty.

In a subset of patients with these symptoms structural abnormalities, such as peptic ulcer disease, erosive gastritis or carcinoma of the stomach, may be found but much more often no organic substrate is demonstrable. Gastric symptoms may also be caused by disorders in organs or organ systems other than the stomach.

Table 10.1 Symptoms of gastric disease or dysfunction

Nausea
Vomiting
Early satiety
Fullness
Bloating
Upper abdominal discomfort
Upper abdominal pain
Waterbrash
Belching
Heartburn
Regurgitation

196

Nausea and vomiting

Nausea and vomiting are strongly interrelated symptoms. Usually nausea precedes vomiting and the best description of nausea probably is the sensation of impending vomiting. Nausea is often accompanied by systemic symptoms such as sweating, pallor, tachycardia, paleness and excessive saliva production. Vomiting is a rather complicated act, controlled by specialized centers in the central nervous system. The powerful expulsion of gastric contents is brought about by strong contractions of the abdominal wall muscles and the diaphragm. In contrast to popular belief, the stomach is relaxed during vomiting.

Although nausea and vomiting mostly occur in association, vomiting without preceding nausea may occur, as can nausea without vomiting. Both symptoms may be meal related but may also occur when the stomach is empty.

Early satiety, fullness and bloating

The phenomenon of early satiety typically occurs postprandially. After having eaten a small amount of food (often after a few bites) the patient experiences a sensation as if a full meal were eaten. The symptom may or may not be associated with nausea and be followed by vomiting. The sense of having a full stomach for a prolonged period after eating or even before eating is often indistinguishable from early satiety.

The term 'bloating' appears to be poorly defined. Usually, upper abdominal distension is felt to be one of the components of bloating. If an abnormal amount of gas is thought to be present in the abdomen, the patient may report the symptom as gas bloating. In the latter case, belching may be present as well.

Upper abdominal discomfort and pain

Unpleasant or painful sensations in the upper abdomen, in particular when localized in the epigastric region, are almost invariably attributed (by both patient and doctor) to the stomach. The intensity of the discomfort may vary from hardly noticeable unease to excruciating pain. Pain or discomfort may be present when the stomach is empty (classically thought to be highly indicative of duodenal ulcer disease) or after a meal or may be unrelated to food.

Waterbrash

Waterbrash is the term used for a short-lived inappropriate excessive saliva secretion that may accompany upper abdominal symptoms, including those that originate in the stomach. Waterbrash often precedes nausea and vomiting, but is otherwise a rather uncommon symptom.

Belching

Belching, the passage of gaseous material from the stomach to the mouth, is a physiological phenomenon. It protects the stomach against overdistension and could thus be compared to the function of a safety valve on a high-pressure cooker. However, many diseases of the stomach lead to excessive belching. A special form of belching is the aerophagia syndrome in which the patient swallows too much air through a semivoluntary act. In aerophagia, the patient usually believes that the excessive belching is caused by a gastric disorder.

Heartburn and regurgitation

Heartburn (pyrosis) is usually described as a burning sensation in the lower part of the chest or upper abdomen. This is the key symptom of gastroesophageal reflux disease (GERD) and there is ample evidence that it is usually caused by acidification of the distal esophagus (Klauser et al 1990). It is not impossible, however, that abnormalities other than esophageal may generate heartburn; some patients report heartburn but do not have identifiable GERD. Likewise, regurgitation, the retrograde movement of small amounts of gastric contents to the oral cavity, is a symptom of GERD rather than of gastric disease. Although the symptom definitely is not generated in the stomach, it may be associated with and confounded with gastric symptoms.

THE 'DYSPEPSIA' CONCEPT

The term 'dyspepsia', originating from the Greek words for 'bad' and 'digestion', is often used to denote any combination of upper abdominal symptoms, occurring either postprandially or without relation to meals. In an attempt to define the term better, it has been recommended that dyspepsia should be used only when upper abdominal discomfort or pain is prominent among the symptoms (Colin-Jones et al 1988, Talley et al 1991). Even with this restriction, dyspepsia is an umbrella term applied to a wide range of symptoms that may either be caused by organic abnormalities or be brought about by disordered function of the upper gastrointestinal tract. When organic abnormalities are found to be absent, as appears to be the case in up to 80% of patients investigated because of dyspeptic symptoms, the term 'functional' dyspepsia or 'non-ulcer' dyspepsia is applicable. The use of these terms may be helpful not only in research but also in clinical practice. It should be realized, however, that they are merely descriptive tools and not diagnostic entities. Functional dyspepsia is not a single functional disorder; many functional abnormalities may cause a patient to present with symptoms that can be labelled as dyspeptic.

EXTRAGASTRIC CAUSES OF DYSPEPSIA

Patients and doctors too often assume that the cause of gastric symptoms should be sought in the stomach. Frequently, however, dyspeptic symptoms are not referable to a disorder of the stomach or even to the gastrointestinal tract.

Many diseases within the abdomen or outside it may lead to nausea and vomiting through stimulation of the vomiting center in the area postrema of the brain. Examples of these are the nausea and vomiting that occur in association with gall stone disease and that occurring during an attack of migraine. Numerous other disorders, in particular electrolyte imbalance and hormonal disorders, and many drugs may induce nausea and vomiting. A chemoreceptor trigger zone in the medulla oblongata senses the presence of potentially toxic substances in the blood stream. From this zone information is sent to the vomiting centers. In this chapter the extraintestinal causes of nausea and vomiting will not be discussed in detail, but awareness of these is of particular importance in the management of dyspeptic patients. Dyspeptic symptoms other than nausea and vomiting may also arise from extragastric and extraintestinal causes. Although many doctors encounter examples of this on an almost daily basis, formal studies into the relationships between dyspepsia and other illnesses have seldom been performed.

A very common but often overlooked cause of dyspeptic symptoms is constipation. Constipation may give rise to upper abdominal symptoms such as fullness, discomfort and pain, but also to nausea and vomiting, which may initially be ascribed, by both patient and doctor, to a gastric disorder. Treatment by means of laxatives cures the gastric symptoms in this condition.

ORGANIC VERSUS FUNCTIONAL CAUSES OF DYSPEPSIA

Organic lesions of the stomach may be the cause of any combination of the gastric symptoms described above. However, several studies have shown that organic abnormalities, such as peptic ulcer disease, erosive gastritis or carcinoma of the stomach, are found only in a small subgroup of patients with dyspeptic symptoms. For instance, in a Scandinavian study in patients with dyspepsia a peptic ulcer prevalence of only 10% was found (Bernersen et al 1996). Obviously, it is important to recognize an organic cause when present, but in most dyspeptic patients an overextensive search for organic abnormalities is not desirable.

FUNCTIONS OF THE STOMACH

Four functions

Classically, the stomach is considered to have two main functions, secretion and motility. In the context of functional dyspeptic symptoms, a third function, namely perception, should be added to these. Abnormalities of each of these functions may cause upper abdominal symptoms. In the context of this chapter on gastric symptoms, the prevention of gastroesophageal reflux should be included in the list of gastric functions. In the following paragraphs these four functions of the stomach will be summarized. Relatively little attention will be paid to the secretory function, since neither hypersecretion nor hyposecretion of gastric acid has been found to play an important role in the pathogenesis of dyspeptic symptoms.

Gastric secretion

The proximal part of the stomach (fundus and corpus) is an exocrine organ secreting hydrogen, chloride, sodium and potassium ions and pepsin. The vagus nerve mediates central nervous control of gastric acid secretion through the release of acetylcholine and gastrin-releasing peptide. Acid secretion is stimulated by eating, through the mechanisms described above, but in the first hour after a meal intragastric pH may be high, due to acid-buffering properties of the food.

Gastric motility and emptying

As far as its motor function is concerned, the stomach should be considered as consisting of two parts, the proximal and the distal stomach. As illustrated in Figure 10.1, the boundary between these two parts lies in the proximal corpus and thus is not identical to the boundary between the acid-secreting and non-secreting parts of the stomach.

Motility of the proximal stomach

The motility of the proximal stomach (fundus and upper third of the corpus) is characterized by slow, tonic contractions and relaxations. In this part of the stomach peristaltic contractions do not occur. Upon swallowing, the proximal stomach relaxes synchronously with the relaxation of the lower esophageal sphincter (LES). This relaxation, which lasts for about 10 s, is called 'receptive relaxation'. In this relaxation, efferent vagal fibers are involved that are neither adrenergic nor cholinergic (NANC). It is now clear that at least some of these inhibitory neurons use nitrous oxide (NO) as the transmitter.

With increasing filling of the proximal stomach a more prolonged relaxation takes place, which allows larger amounts of food to be accommodated in the stomach without a significant rise in intraluminal pressure. This phenomenon is called 'adaptive relaxation' and also involves NANC vagal efferents. The process of adaptive relaxation not only requires intact efferent innervation but also afferent information relayed from stretch or

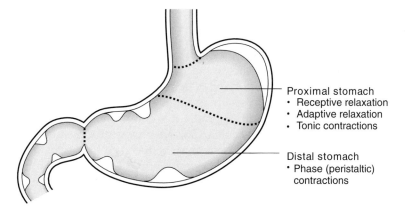

Fig. 10.1 The proximal and distal stomach have different motor functions. The proximal stomach relaxes and contracts slowly (tonically). In the distal stomach, peristaltic contractions occur.

tension receptors in the proximal stomach to the central nervous system.

Motility of the distal stomach

The motility of the distal stomach is dominated by phasic peristaltic contractions that propagate towards the pylorus. Most of the phasic contractions of the pylorus are related to those of the antrum. Others, however, appear to occur in concert with the contractions of the proximal duodenum. In humans, the peristaltic contractions of the distal stomach have a maximum frequency of three per minute. Their occurrence is controlled by two myogenic electrical phenomena, one of which is called 'slow waves' or 'electrical control activity' (ECA) and the other 'electrical response activity' (ERA). ECA is a relentless periodic activity with a frequency of three cycles per minute. ERA occurs episodically, in association with phasic contractions. ERA and contractions can only occur in the second quarter of the ECA cycle and are thus time locked to the ECA.

The most important function of the distal stomach is to grind solid food particles. This grinding action of the antral 'mill', combined with acid peptic digestion, reduces digestible solid particles to a chyme. The grinding process has to be completed before passage of the gastric contents into duodenum is allowed. In order to achieve this, the pylorus closes in concert with each antral peristaltic contraction. When the pylorus functions normally, only a few milliliters of chyme are transported to the duodenum with each antral peristaltic wave.

Gastric emptying

Components of a meal with different consistencies are selectively emptied from the stomach, with liquids being evacuated most rapidly. The emptying of liquids is believed to be a function primarily of the pressure gradient between the stomach and the duodenum and this gradient is determined largely by the tone of the proximal stomach. The emptying of digestible solids starts after the particles have been reduced to a sufficiently small size (< 1 mm). The preemptying phase (or lag phase) is thus defined as the period between meal ingestion and the appearance of food in the small intestine.

The rate of gastric emptying is adapted to the composition of the gastric chyme. In general, carbohydrates empty faster than proteins, which in turn are evacuated faster than fats. Putative receptors in the proximal small bowel, including receptors for osmolarity, fatty acids and some amino acids, continuously sense the quality of the chyme that is evacuated from the stomach. Complex and incompletely understood control mechanisms delay gastric emptying when the rate of delivery to the duodenum is too high. The regulation is such that isocaloric concentrations of fat, protein and carbohydrate are emptied from the stomach at comparable rates. The acidity of the gastric chyme also influences the rate of gastric emptying, with high acid concentrations causing a more profound inhibition of emptying than lower concentrations.

Interdigestive motility and emptying

These motor and emptying patterns persist for several hours after a normal meal but when the stomach is empty, or almost empty, a characteristic fasting motor pattern sets in. This is a cyclically recurring motor pattern which begins in the proximal stomach and lower esophageal Sphincter (LES) and migrates slowly through the small bowel. The cycle duration of this activity is approximately 90 min but there is considerable intra- and interindividual variability in cycle duration. The phenomenon, called interdigestive motor complex (IMC) or migrating motor complex (MMC), is composed of three sequential phases: phase 1 is a period of motor quiescence lasting for approximately 45 min, phase 2 is characterized by intermittent contractions resembling those seen in the digestive state and lasts for about 40 min, and phase 3 is a period of intense regular peristaltic contractions lasting for about 5 min. During phase 3 the gastric antrum contracts at its maximum frequency, three contractions per minute. During this phase indigestible solid particles are removed from the stomach.

Duodenogastric reflux

Reflux of small intestinal contents into the stomach is a physiological phenomenon. Duodenogastric reflux occurs most frequently during the last part of phase 2 of the MMC. The backwash of the alkaline material may lead to a temporary decrease of intragastric acidity and even to a rise of intragastric pH above 7. During the following phase 3, powerful antral contractions will clear the alkaline fluid from the stomach and restore the acidic pH. After resection of the distal stomach and after pyloroplasty, duodenogastric reflux is increased. It is thought that the effectiveness of distal gastric resection in peptic ulcer disease was partly due to the reduction in intragastric acidity caused by enhanced enterogastric reflux.

GASTRIC PERCEPTION

In recent years, we have become more aware of the fact that the stomach not only secretes and contracts, but also perceives what is going on. In order to do this, the gastric wall contains receptors of various types, most of which have been incompletely identified. Gastric secretion, motility and emptying are continuously adjusted on the basis of information gathered by the gastric wall receptors. Under normal circumstances this information is not consciously perceived by the individual.

GASTROESOPHAGEAL REFLUX

Reflux of gastric contents into the esophagus is a physiological phenomenon. In healthy subjects up to 50 reflux episodes may occur in a 24-h period and up to 5–6% of the time esophageal pH may be below 4. Healthy individuals do not perceive their physiological reflux at all or only rarely and it does not lead to esophagitis.

The most important structure in the prevention of gastro-esophageal reflux is the lower esophageal sphincter (LES). The crural diaphragm augments the LES, in particular during inspiration. It has been shown that the majority of episodes of gastro-esophageal reflux occurring in healthy subjects takes place during spontaneous relaxations of the LES. These transient ('inappropriate') relaxations are not induced by swallowing, but occur without identifiable evoking event. The rate of occurrence of spontaneous relaxations increases upon distension of the proximal stomach. These relaxations also provide the opportunity for gas to escape from the stomach through belching.

DISORDERED GASTRIC FUNCTION AND SYMPTOMS

Abnormal secretion

Abnormalities of the secretory function of the stomach include increased secretion (hyperchlorhydria) and decreased secretion (hypochlorhydria or achlorhydria). There is no evidence, however, that either moderately increased or decreased secretion in itself produces dyspeptic symptoms. Gastric acid secretion and intragastric pH have been found to be in the normal range in functional dyspepsia (Collen & Loebenberg 1989, Bechi et al 1992).

Inhibition of gastric secretion does not lead to a significant decrease in symptoms in patients with functional dyspepsia (Bates et al 1989). The latter observation indicates that functional dyspepsia is unlikely to represent a mild form of peptic ulcer disease.

Disordered motility and emptying

There is ample evidence that abnormal gastric motility and emptying can lead to dyspeptic symptoms. Many studies have shown that 30–50% of patients with functional dyspepsia have delayed gastric emptying, in particular for solid food (Waldron et al 1991). In fact, in all studies that compared groups of healthy controls with groups of patients with functional dyspepsia, a statistically significant decrease in the rate of gastric emptying was found. Furthermore, in patients with functional dyspepsia treatment with prokinetic drugs, such as metoclopramide, domperidone and cisapride, has been shown to be significantly more effective than placebo. There is also evidence that delayed gastric emptying plays a role in the pathogenesis of symptoms in systemic diseases that affect the stomach, such as diabetes mellitus, scleroderma and the pseudoobstruction syndromes.

The possible causes of delayed gastric emptying are summarized in Table 10.2.

In diabetes, the prevalence of gastric emptying disorders is particularly high. In some studies up to 80% of diabetics, with or without autonomic neuropathy, were found to have abnormal

Table 10.2 Causes of delayed gastric emptying

Idiopathic
    Functional dyspepsia
    Irritable bowel syndrome

Neurogenic
    Postvagotomy state
    Diabetic autonomic neuropathy

Myogenic
    Scleroderma
    Mixed connective tissue disease

Metabolic
    Ketoacidosis
    Hypokalemia
    Hypocalcemia
    Hypoglycemia
    Hypothyroidism

Drug induced
    Anticholinergic agents
    Tricyclic antidepressants

gastric emptying. In patients with diabetes, hyperglycemia may cause a further delay in gastric emptying (Fraser et al 1990). The clinical relevance of disordered gastric motility in diabetes reaches beyond the generation of dyspeptic symptoms. Due to the delayed delivery of food to the duodenum, the timing of meals and insulin administration may become extremely difficult. It is thought that gastric motor disorders are a major determining factor in difficult to manage, brittle diabetics.

The most important motor abnormality that underlies delayed gastric emptying in functional dyspepsia and in the systemic diseases described above is a decreased contractility of the antrum after a meal (Samsom et al 1996). In addition, impaired contractility of the proximal stomach, a widened gastric antrum and pyloric motor abnormalities have been found to play a role (Undeland et al 1996).

Apart from postprandial motor dysfunction, interdigestive motility may be disturbed, which may further add to the genesis of symptoms. When the MMC is absent or lacks an antral component, indigestible solids may remain in the stomach for days. In the extreme case, this may lead to formation of a bezoar.

Apart from delayed gastric emptying, accelerated emptying may also cause symptoms. A too rapid delivery of gastric contents to the small intestine causes fullness, nausea and vomiting. These symptoms may be indistinguishable from those caused by delayed gastric emptying. The classic symptoms of dumping (tachycardia, pallor, sweating, faintness, hunger sensation) may be absent. In some patients, emptying of liquids is accelerated and emptying of solids is delayed. This combination is most frequently seen in patients who have undergone truncal vagotomy (with or without distal gastric resection).

Many of the motor abnormalities described above may be associated with abnormal myoelectrical activity. Arrhythmias of gastric ECA (in particular, tachygastria) can be found in patients with dyspeptic symptoms (Geldof et al 1986, Kim et al 1988). Usually, these arrhythmias are accompanied by diminished or absent motor activity.

Duodenogastric reflux

Duodenogastric reflux of enteric contents into the stomach has been incriminated in the genesis of dyspeptic symptoms. However, little evidence for this assumption can be found. On the contrary, two recent studies have provided information that pleads against an important role for duodenogastric reflux in the pathogenesis of functional dyspepsia. Mearin and colleagues, who used a sampling technique to study duodenogastric reflux, found no significant increase in gastric bile acid concentration and no significant correlation between symptom scores and duodenogastric reflux (Mearin et al 1995a). Likewise, fasting duodenogastric reflux was found to be normal in patients with functional dyspepsia and not to be correlated with symptom severity (Bost et al 1990).

Abnormal gastric perception

In recent years, it has become clear that in a subgroup of patients with dyspepsia, symptoms develop from an altered visceral perception rather than from abnormal gastric motility or secretion (Mearin et al 1991, Mearin & Malagelada 1992). The mechanisms through which such a hypersensitivity of the stomach is brought about are still conjectural. Among the possibilities are a decreased threshold of receptors in the stomach wall, an altered conduction of afferent information or a lowered threshold for perception at the level of the central nervous system. The abnormal visceroperception found in dyspeptic patients may be site specific, e.g. an increased perception of gastric distension has been found not to be associated with an enhanced sensitivity to duodenal distension. As in the irritable bowel syndrome, the increased visceroperception in functional dyspepsia is not associated with an increased perception of somatic stimuli.

The causes of increased visceroperception are probably heterogeneous. One of the putative causes is inflammation, either posttraumatic or infective. Mediators involved in the inflammatory process, such as histamine, bradykinin, prostaglandins, leukotrienes and platelet-activation factor (PAF), stimulate firing of afferent nerve fibers. Under normal circumstances only a small proportion of visceral afferent nerves are active, due to a relatively high threshold for stimulation. The possibility that inflammation of the gastric mucosa provoked by infection with *Helicobacter pylori* causes hypersensitivity has recently been addressed by several investigators. Their reports indicate, however, that the perception of gastric distension in patients with functional dyspepsia is not related to *H. pylori* status (Mearin et al 1995b).

Gastroesophageal reflux disease

Gastroesophageal reflux disease (GERD) can be defined as reflux that exceeds the upper limit of normal (excessive or pathological reflux) or as reflux leading to esophagitis or as reflux (either excessive or normal) that leads to symptoms. Excessive (pathological) reflux may remain asymptomatic in some individuals, but can lead to symptoms and/or to inflammation of the mucosa of the distal esophagus in others. The most characteristic symptom of GERD is heartburn, defined as a burning sensation in the chest or epigastric region, often related to the postprandial period and to maneuvers such as bending forward. A second characteristic symptom of the disease is acid regurgitation. In contrast to popular belief, even the combination of these two symptoms has only limited sensitivity and specificity for abnormal gastroesophageal reflux (Klauser et al 1990). Reflux symptoms often occur in association with dyspeptic symptoms. The term 'reflux-like dyspepsia' is often used to denote this combination of symptoms.

SPECIFICITY OF DYSPEPTIC SYMPTOMS

It has been proposed that patients with functional dyspepsia could be subdivided into a number of distinct subgroups. These subgroups are ulcer-like, reflux-like, dysmotility-like and non-specific dyspepsia (Colin-Jones et al 1988, Talley et al 1991). Some working parties proposed a fifth subgroup, labeled aerophagia. It should be noted that these classifications are mainly based on clinical impressions.

Although intuitively attractive and of interest to investigators, the classification of dyspepsia into subgroups carries some risks. If accepted too eagerly by the medical community, subgrouping of functional dyspepsia may lead to several false assumptions. The first of these is that the pattern of the dyspeptic symptoms would provide certainty as to the underlying pathophysiological mechanism(s). The second is that the symptom subgroup would be a pointer to selecting treatment in individual patients with functional dyspepsia. Recent observations have made clear that some scepticism regarding the validity of such a classification is essential. One of these observations is that about half of the patients fall into more than one of the categories (Talley et al 1993). Secondly, studies which looked into the correlation between the type of symptoms and abnormalities in gastric functions have yielded negative results. For example, Waldron et al (1991) assessed gastric acid secretion, gastric emptying rate and *H. pylori*-related gastritis in a group of patients with functional dyspepsia and found no significant correlation between the type of symptoms and any of the parameters.

GASTRIC FUNCTION TESTS

Assessment of gastric motility and emptying
(Tables 10.3, 10.4)

Gross abnormalities of gastric emptying may be detected during a routine upper gastrointestinal radiographic assessment, using a <u>barium meal</u>. More subtle abnormalities are likely to be missed. Moreover, barium meal studies involve the patient in significant exposure to radiation and do not allow the rate of gastric emptying to be assessed quantitatively. <u>Radiopaque markers</u> such as plastic spheres may be used to quantify gastric emptying of indigestible solids, but the findings are not representative of the emptying of digestible solid food. At <u>endoscopy</u> one occasionally encounters solid and/or liquid food retained in the stomach. If this happens after an adequate episode of fasting, it is evidence of significantly delayed gastric emptying. Although peristaltic contractions of the antrum can be observed endoscopically, endoscopy does not allow reliable assessment of antral motility. <u>Scintigraphy</u>, using a radiolabeled test meal and γ camera, is considered to be the gold standard for the measurement of gastric emptying. The technique can be used to measure the emptying of solids as well as liquids and, using a dual isotope technique, the two components of the meal can be studied simultaneously. Differences in composition, quantity and viscosity of the meal as well as differences in analytical technique are responsible for the fact that normal values for gastric emptying,

Table 10.3 Techniques for assessment of gastric motility

Proximal stomach
  Barostat technique
Distal stomach
  Manometry
  Ultrasound
  Impedance techniques
  Scintigraphic techniques
  Electrogastrography

Table 10.4 Techniques for assessment of gastric emptying

Radiography (barium meal or radiopaque markers)
Endoscopy
Scintigraphy
Marker dilution techniques
Absorption tests
Breath tests
Ultrasound
Impedance measurement techniques

as assessed by means of scintigraphy, differ from center to center. In the analysis of the emptying pattern of a solid meal, the lag phase should be distinguished. The postlag emptying pattern for solid meals is approximately linear, while for liquid meals an exponential pattern of emptying is usually seen.

Marker dilution techniques involving gastric intubation and repetitive sampling of gastric contents have been applied in the research setting, but have not found clinical application. Other techniques make use of the absorption kinetics of orally administered substances. The absorption of substances such as paracetamol, ethyl alcohol and glucose from the stomach is negligible and their delivery to their site of absorption in the proximal small bowel is determined largely by the rate of gastric emptying. Consequently, the concentrations of these substances can be used as an index of gastric emptying. Repeated blood samples are required.

More recently, breath tests have been developed that measure absorption without requiring repetitive blood sampling. In particular, tests employing isotopes that are not radioactive hold much promise for clinical application on a large scale. Among the tests proposed, the ^{13}C-octanoic acid breath test has been validated best (Maes et al 1994). The amount of $^{13}CO_2$ in the expired breath which reflects the absorption of octanoic acid is measured with a mass spectrometer. From the $^{13}CO_2$ excretion curves thus obtained, gastric emptying parameters are derived using mathemathical models.

Real-time ultrasound utilizes dynamic imaging of the stomach to assess gastric emptying. This can be done in two ways. Firstly, the volume of the stomach can be determined by measurement of the areas of a series of cross-sectional slices along the longitudinal axis (Gilja et al 1996). Although theoretically attractive, the technique is difficult to apply in clinical practice. A much more simple approach involves the measurement of antral diameter or cross-sectional area. The decrease in antral diameter after ingestion of a liquid meal has been found to correlate significantly with the rate of gastric emptying measured scintigraphically. However, it should be realized that this technique does not really measure gastric emptying.

Changes in the electrical impedance of the epigastric region can be used as a measure of gastric emptying. This technique can only be applied when the test meal has an electrical conductivity which is either higher or lower than that of the surrounding tissues. The most sophisticated form of impedance measurement uses a circumferential array of electrodes around the upper abdomen and construction, by means of a computer, of a tomographic slice through the epigastric region. With this technique, called 'applied potential tomography' or 'epigastric impedance tomography', a more reliable assessment of gastric emptying can be made in most cases (McClelland & Sutton 1985, Avill et al 1987). Difficulties are encountered when gastric emptying is accelerated. The technique has not yet found widespread clinical application.

The myoelectrical activity generated by the stomach can be assessed by means of electrodes positioned on the abdominal surface. Alternatively, and less suitable for clinical practice, are internal electrodes held in position by magnets or negative pressure. The technique of surface recording is also called electrogastrography (EGG) (Abell & Malagelada 1988). The amplitude of the EGG signal is increased when the distal stomach contracts, although the correlation between contraction amplitude and EGG amplitude is weak. With electrogastrography, arrhythmias of electrical activity such as tachygastrias can be detected in a large proportion of cases (Geldof et al 1986).

Antral contractions can be assessed by means of intraluminal manometry (Malagelada & Stanghellini 1985, Jebbink et al 1995). Manometry can be carried out either with perfused open-tip catheters or with a catheter with miniature pressure transducers. Manometry is unsuitable for studying the motor activity of the proximal stomach. Accurate localization of the probe relative to the antroduodenal junction is important for reliable assessment of antral and pyloric motility. For this purpose the technique of transmucosal potential difference measurement (TMPD) has been developed. This technique makes use of the fact that the potential in the lumen of the antrum is over 15 mV more negative than that in the duodenal lumen. Antroduodenal manometry can be carried out in both the fasting and the postprandial state, without limitations as to the composition of the test meal.

For the assessment of the motor activities of the proximal stomach a specialized technique is used (Azpiroz & Malagelada 1987). This so-called 'barostat technique' makes use of a flaccid air-filled bag placed in the proximal stomach. The pressure in this bag is kept at a constant level using an electronically controlled pump. When the proximal stomach relaxes, air is pumped into the bag and when the proximal stomach contracts, air is withdrawn. Intrabag volume variations are monitored and the curve thus obtained reflects variations in gastric tone.

Assessment of gastric perception

For the assessment of gastric perception the above-described barostat technique is used (Mearin et al 1991). The intragastric bag is inflated to either a preset pressure or volume. Pressure or volume are then increased stepwise or in random sequence and the sensations scored, usually on a visual-analog scale. This technique has been found valuable for research purposes, but cannot yet be considered as a diagnostic tool.

Popular function tests

Only some of the tests described above have found more or less widespread clinical application. The most important factor hampering their use for non-research purposes is probably their labor- and time-consuming nature.

The most widely used test is measurement of gastric emptying with a radioactively labeled meal. In recent years, electrogastrography has gained popularity. Thus far, the application of manometric tests has remained confined largely to specialized centers (university hospitals), but it can be expected that these tests will become more widely available in the near future.

CONCLUSIONS

Much is still unknown about the pathogenesis of dyspeptic symptoms. It has become clear that organic abnormalities can only be held responsible for the symptoms in a small subset of dyspeptic patients. The abnormalities most consistently found in functional dyspepsia are postprandial antral hypomotility, impaired gastric emptying and enhanced gastric perception. When organic causes have been excluded or are felt to be unlikely, a therapeutic trial is usually appropriate. The available evidence indicates that in most cases treatment with a prokinetic agent, with or without antiemetic properties, offers the highest chance of success. An exception to this rule prevails when symptoms of gastroesophageal reflux dominate the spectrum. In that case, an inhibitor of gastric acid secretion may be more effective.

When additional function testing is considered necessary, the most relevant test is measurement of gastric emptying, preferably with a radioactively labelled meal with both a solid and a liquid component. In selected cases, further relevant information may be obtained from gastroduodenal manometry and electrogastrography. When gastroesophageal reflux is felt to play a role, 24-h esophageal pH monitoring with assessment of the relationship between symptoms and reflux is indicated.

The many other gastric function tests that have been described should be considered research tools.

REFERENCES

Abell TL, Malagelada J-R 1988 Electrogastrography. Current assessment and future perspectives. Digestive Diseases and Sciences 33: 982–992

Avill R, Magnall YF, Bird NC et al 1987 Applied potential tomography. A new noninvasive technique for measuring gastric emptying. Gastroenterology 92: 1019–1026

Azpiroz F, Malagelada J-R 1987 Gastric tone measured by an electronic barostat in health and postsurgical gastroparesis. Gastroenterology 92: 934–943

Bates S, Sjödén P-O, Fellenius J, Nyrén O 1989 Blocked and nonblocked acid secretion and reported pain in ulcer, nonulcer dyspepsia, and normal subjects. Gastroenterology 97: 376–383

Bechi P, Dei R, Amorosi A, Marcuzzo G, Cortesini C 1992 *Helicobacter pylori* and luminal gastric pH. Relationships in nonulcer dyspepsia. Digestive Diseases and Sciences 37: 378–384

Bernersen B, Johnsen R, Straume B 1996 Non-ulcer dyspepsia and peptic ulcer: the distribution in a population and their relation to risk factors. Gut 38: 822–825

Bost R, Hostein, J, Valenti M et al 1990 Is there an abnormal fasting duodenogastric reflux in nonulcer dyspepsia? Digestive Diseases and Sciences 35: 193–199

Colin-Jones DG, Bloom B, Bodemar G, Crean G, Freston J, Gugler R 1988 Management of dyspepsia: report of a working party. Lancet i: 576–579

Collen MJ, Loebenberg MJ 1989 Basal gastric acid secretion in nonulcer dyspepsia with or without duodenitis. Digestive Diseases and Sciences 34: 246–250

Fraser RJ, Horowitz M, Maddox AF, Harding PE, Chatterton BE, Dent J 1990 Hyperglycaemia slows gastric emptying in Type 1 (insulin-dependent) diabetes mellitus. Diabetologica 33: 675–680

Geldof H, van der Schee EJ, van Blankenstein M, Grashuis JL 1986 Electrogastrographic study of gastric myoelectrical activity in patients with unexplained nausea and vomiting. Gut 27: 799–808

Gilja OH, Hausken T, Wilhelmsen I, Berstad A 1996 Impaired accommodation of proximal stomach to a meal in functional dyspepsia. Digestive Diseases and Sciences 41: 689–696

Jebbink RJA, vanBerge-Henegouwen GP, Akkermans LMA, Smout AJPM 1995 Antroduodenal manometry: 24-hour ambulatory monitoring versus short-term stationary manometry in patients with functional dyspepsia. European Journal of Gastroenterology and Hepatology 7: 109–116

Kim CH, Zinsmeister AR, Malagelada J-R 1988 Effect of gastric dysrhythmias on postcibal motor activity of the stomach. Digestive Diseases and Sciences 33: 193–199

Klauser AG, Schindlbeck NE, Müller-Lissner SA 1990 Symptoms in gastro-oesophageal reflux disease. Lancet 335: 205–208

McClelland GR, Sutton JA 1985 Epigastric impedance: a non-invasive method for the assessment of gastric emptying and motility. Gut 26: 607–614

Maes BD, Ghoose YF, Rutgeerts PJ, Hiele MI, Geypens B, Vantrappen G 1994 Octanoic acid breath test to measure gastric emptying rate of solids. Digestive Diseases and Sciences 39 (suppl. 12): 104S–106S

Malagelada J-R, Stanghellini V 1985 Manometric evaluation of functional upper gut symptoms. Gastroenterology 88: 1223–1231

Mearin F, Malagelada J-R 1992 Upper gut and perception in functional dyspepsia. European Journal of Gastroenterology and Hepatology 4: 615–621

Mearin F, Cucala M, Azpiroz F, Malagelada J-R 1991 The origin of symptoms on the brain–gut axis in functional dyspepsia. Gastroenterology 101: 999–1006

Mearin F, de Ribot X, Balboa A, Antolin M, Varas MJ, Malagelada J-R 1995a Duodenogastric bile reflux and gastrointestinal motility in pathogenesis of functional dyspepsia. Digestive Diseases and Sciences 40: 1703–1709

Mearin F, de Ribot X, Balboa A et al 1995b Does *Helicobacter pylori* infection increase gastric sensitivity in functional dyspepsla? Gut 37: 47–51

Samsom M, Jebbink RJA, Akkermans LMA, vanBerge-Henegouwen GP, Smout AJPM 1996 Abnormalities of antroduodenal motility in type I diabetes. Diabetes Care 19: 21–27

Talley NJ, Colin-Jones D, Koch KL, Koch M, Nyren O, Stanghellini V 1991 Functional dyspepsia: a classification with guidelines for diagnosis and management. Gastroenterology International 4: 145–160

Talley NJ, Weaver AL, Tesmer DL, Zinsmeister AR 1993 Lack of discriminant value of dyspepsia subgroups in patients referred for upper endoscopy. Gastroenterology 105: 1378–1386

Undeland KA, Hausken T, Svebak S, Aanderud S, Berstad A 1996 Wide gastric antrum and low vagal tone in patients with diabetes mellitus type I compared to patients with functional dyspepsia and healthy individuals. Digestive Diseases and Sciences 41: 9–16

Waldron W, Cullen PT, Kumar P et al 1991 Evidence of hypomotility in non-ulcer dyspepsia: a prospective multifactorial study. Gut 32: 246–251

The stomach: clinical management

J-R Malagelada

GENERAL STRATEGY

Clinicians caring for a patient with a presumed disorder of gastric function face an immediate problem: there is no consensus on the definition, diagnostic algorithm or management strategy for such a condition. Thus, most physicians base their care on a symptom-oriented, empiric approach to therapy. They may not be far from the mark! In this chapter, however, I will attempt to direct and organize clinical thought into the most efficient routes for logical management.

The key concept is that functional symptoms are thought to arise from the upper gastrointestinal tract without a demonstrable organic cause (Colin-Jones et al 1988, Barbara et al 1989). I use the term 'upper gastrointestinal' rather than 'gastric' because, in most patients, it is impossible on the basis of symptoms alone to ascertain whether the stomach, the upper small bowel or both are dysfunctional.

The correct logic to follow must be pragmatic:

1. establish whether symptoms are consistent with a functional disorder and attempt to group the symptoms into recognizable 'syndromes or complexes';
2. exclude organic diseases that pose a significant risk to the patient or that are amenable to specific therapy;
3. pay attention to individual patient requirements (and/or demands);
4. always aim at achieving symptom relief;
5. maintain vigilant follow-up to manage relapses (likely) and to reaffirm diagnosis (startling surprises may pop up occasionally!).

Thus, symptom complexes presenting with typical features of a functional disorder occasionally develop more dramatic features of organic disease. The physician needs to be aware of such

215

possible eventualities though, in referral practice, it is more common to encounter the reverse; mainly, functional disease that is being managed as organic disease. Many unfortunate patients have received unnecessary surgical procedures, parenteral nutrition or drug therapy.

SYMPTOMS AND SYNDROMES

Common complaints in functional upper gastrointestinal disorders

Upper abdominal pain, nausea and vomiting are the cardinal symptoms of patients with functional upper gastrointestinal disorders. Often, there is also an array of accompanying complaints that sometimes coalesce into a rather colorful clinical picture. Let's review first the characteristics of the major symptoms.

Upper abdominal pain tends to be localized in the epigastrium, but it may extend into the periumbilical area or either the left or right upper abdominal quadrant. However, when the pain is exclusively localized in one of the hypochondria we tend to categorize it as a variety of irritable bowel syndrome (the so-called 'hepatic flexure' or 'splenic flexure' syndromes), rather than ascribe it to a gastric origin. Back radiation of the pain should alert one to organicity, although this may not always be the case since back radiation may sometimes occur in functional patients as well.

The pain may present at any time of the day. Some patients develop it only after meals or report that it is exacerbated by meals. Others may complain of pain early in the morning, with an empty stomach. Eating may relieve the pain, similarly to patients with peptic ulcer, but this is far less common. Nocturnal awakening with pain, long regarded as a sign of organicity, is indeed relatively rare in functional patients. However, when there is associated restlessness and insomnia the patient may be spontaneously waking up and then feeling the pain. In your interview, be subtle enough to make the distinction.

The *character of the pain* is extremely variable. Some patients describe it as a sharp, lancing sensation, whereas others report a more vague, pressure-like discomfort. There is often a coincidence between the pain and a sensation of abdominal distension, reported as bloating. In some patients the two become associated to the point that the patient describes it as painful abdominal distension.

There is considerable association (and overlap) among various functional syndromes, particularly between functional dyspepsia and irritable bowel (Talley & Phillips 1988). By convention, patients whose pain is predominantly referred to the lower abdomen and associated with bowel movement disturbances are included in the irritable bowel syndrome group. Those whose pain is predominantly referred to the upper abdomen without significant alteration in bowel rhythm are categorized as functional dyspepsia. However, in some patients it may be difficult to correctly allocate a particular clinical picture to one or the other.

Nausea and vomiting are two other cardinal features of functional upper gastrointestinal disorders. Nausea is common and may represent the only symptom, the predominant symptom or just one of the symptoms. It may occur with an empty stomach, as for instance early in the morning, or develop in response to ingestion of food or beverages. Nausea may also present in conjunction with vomiting and/or retching. Pain and nausea often occur together and add up to a very uncomfortable feeling. When vomiting is also part of the picture, some patients describe it as worsening the pain and others as alleviating the pain. In the latter instance particularly, the clinician should enquire whether the patient is actually inducing vomiting by stimulation of the pharynx to obtain quick relief by evacuating gastric contents.

There are other symptoms that by themselves rarely constitute a picture severe enough to warrant consultation with a physician, but that quite frequently accompany the main symptoms described above. These include, first, early satiety (a feeling of overfilled stomach during or shortly after eating) or what the patients describe as postprandial fullness or 'prolonged digestion', meaning the subjective feeling of food remaining in the stomach for many hours after meals. These sensations derive from a combination of epigastric bloating, satiety and regurgitation or 'tasting' of the previously ingested food.

Rumination, the regurgitation of partially digested food that is either reswallowed or expectorated, can be considered as within the spectrum of functional gastric disorders. The symptoms are always postprandial, not nocturnal or during recumbency, and should be distinguishable from reflux, but this is not always easy (O'Brien et al 1995).

Another common symptom is belching that sometimes occurs as an isolated manifestation, the so-called compulsive belching syndrome, or in combination with other symptoms. Pyrosis and regurgitation are in themselves rather typical symptoms of gastroesophageal reflux disease (GERD) and, when predominant, they should incline the clinician towards a possible GERD diagnosis. However, these symptoms may also accompany other manifestations characteristic of a functional gastrointestinal disorder.

The <u>duration of the symptomatology</u> is important. The diagnosis of functional disorder is supported by a long clinical course, although no specific limits can be set. Most clinical trials nowadays require a minimum duration of symptoms of 3 months with a minimum frequency of 25–30% of symptomatic days (Talley et al 1994). The latter requirement should, nevertheless, be flexible. Many patients are asymptomatic for relatively long periods of time and then relapse.

Syndromes

Functional disorders are symptom-based diagnoses, usually established by an exclusionary approach, that is, by ascertaining the absence of a specific structural defect or lesion that could explain the symptomatology.

Among clinicians, there are two current trends. First, a tendency to seek patterns or combinations of symptoms that could be used to label subgroups of patients with similar manifestations. Second, to match symptoms and physiological abnormalities detected by special tests, including measurement of the gastric emptying rate, contractile activity or visceral perception of distension. This latter process is aimed at establishing a diagnosis of functional disorder based on its pathogenesis. Unfortunately, the distinction between functional patients with and without detectable physiological abnormalities is often ambiguous because it depends on the tests applied, which are highly variable in their sensitivity and specificity (Waldron et al 1991).

Functional dyspepsia

This is the paradigm of functional upper gut disorders. Most define functional dyspepsia as variations of the concept: symptoms without demonstrable organic cause thought to arise from the upper gastrointestinal tract. Evolving from this general concept, Colin-Jones et al in 1988 and others subsequently attempted to subgroup patients with functional dyspepsia into three clinical varieties.

Reflux-like dyspepsia. In these patients, heartburn and other symptoms consistent with gastroesophageal reflux present in association with other symptoms more typical of dyspepsia such as epigastric pain, fullness, early satiety, etc. This subgroup of dyspepsia is more likely than others to respond to antisecretory agents, probably because gastroesophageal reflux does indeed play some pathogenetic role (Pfeiffer et al 1992).

Ulcer-like dyspepsia. The key symptom in this subgroup of patients is epigastric pain, hence the eponym ulcer-like dyspepsia. Some patients in this category may indeed incorporate other elements of acid peptic disease detectable by endoscopy such as duodenitis, prepyloric erosions, etc., but this is not a consistent feature. The question is whether these patients represent partially developed or atypical forms of peptic ulcer disease. It may be so. However, doubts also arise because response rates to antisecretory agents are not very different from those observed in the majority of functional dyspepsia patients. Furthermore, eradication of *Helicobacter pylori* infection, when present, has not been uniformly successful (see later).

Dysmotility-like dyspepsia. Symptoms in this subgroup of patients are attributed to impaired gastric emptying, inappropriate postcibal gastric distension and perhaps also to duodenal dysmotility. The chief symptoms are early satiety, epigastric fullness and upper abdominal bloating. The degree of discomfort may range from unpleasantness to frank pain. These upper abdominal symptoms tend to occur postprandially and are often associated with other symptoms that merge with the irritable bowel syndrome, such as generalized abdominal bloating and flatulence, particularly after large meals rich in carbohydrates and fat.

The three subgroups of dyspepsia described above are, in practice, difficult to separate from each other. Moreover, investigators performing clinical studies and pharmacological trials often had to resort to allotting patients to one or another subcategory and accepting large overlaps or blending them into a large, non-specific group not exactly fulfilling the criteria for any of the three subcategories. On the other hand, these subgroups may be helpful as clinical descriptors and their use among clinicians is fairly widespread.

Management-relevant physiology. Taking cases of dyspepsia individually, there is poor correlation between clinical data and physiological data. Even when the symptomatology suggests a certain physiological disturbance, subsequent investigations may not confirm it. For instance, delayed gastric emptying and/or gastric contractile abnormalities are not a uniform feature of patients with dysmotility-like dyspepsia (Greydanus et al 1991,

Waldron et al 1991). Worse still, in some patients fulfilling clinical criteria for functional dyspepsia, extensive application of up-to-date physiological tests may fail to show any detectable abnormality. The corollary is that pharmacological agents specifically designed to act on a physiological function (antisecretors, prokinetics, etc.) are usually prescribed on an empirical basis, by reference to the symptomatology, rather than based on a particular physiological derangement.

In contrast to peptic ulcer disease, there is no apparent correlation between infection with *Helicobacter pylori* and functional dyspepsia or altered functions such as delayed gastric emptying or increased perception of gastric balloon distension (Tucci et al 1992). Some studies have claimed improvement of dyspeptic symptoms after successful *Helicobacter* eradication with appropriate antibiotics. It is acknowledged that eradication may be indicated for other reasons (i.e. some believe all positive patients should be treated for prophylaxis) but it is doubtful, at this point, that eradication of the organism is an effective therapeutic measure to achieve symptomatic relief.

Since it follows from the above comments that there are no current diagnostic or physiological tests to predict the efficacy of a pharmacological agent in functional dyspepsia, it follows that assessment of the therapeutic response is also based on symptoms. Thus, if a given patient shows evidence of delayed gastric emptying before treatment with a prokinetic drug and then normalizes, the test has confirmed the pharmacological response but a symptomatic response does not necessarily follow and vice versa. When large groups of patients rather than individual cases are evaluated, however, relations between physiological responses and symptomatic responses become more apparent, at least for certain prokinetic and hypoalgesic agents.

The variability of the clinical course in functional dyspepsia is notorious. Over time, the clinical manifestations assume two principal forms: temporal variability and circumstantial variability. The first indicates that symptoms rarely persist unchanged in intensity, or even character, for long periods of time. They may vary from day to day, week to week or month to month. Circumstantial variability means that symptoms are very much affected by environmental and personal events. It is probably in this context that stress and other psychological factors influence the symptomatology of functional dyspepsia. In other words, the patient may feel better or worse about their condition depending on mood and related factors. These external influences may also explain the high placebo response often observed on clinical drug trials that may reach 60%. A variable placebo response may also relate to other factors such as the attention bestowed by clinical investigators on patients enrolled in the trial.

Idiopathic gastroparesis

Gastroparesis is a medical term that clinicians sometimes apply with different meanings. The term 'gastroparesis' implies impaired gastric motility resulting in gastric stasis. The diagnosis may be made by a radiologist or endoscopist observing abnormal retention of food particles in the stomach or by a clinician who obtains a clinical history consistent with gastric stasis, for instance vomiting of food ingested many hours previously. However, patients with a severe delay in gastric emptying may be asymptomatic and, conversely, patients with symptoms such as postprandial nausea, fullness or regurgitation, that would be consistent with gastric food retention, may show normal emptying rates when tested (Corinaldesi et al 1987). It follows that the diagnosis of gastroparesis is on much firmer grounds when the patient presents both a suggestive clinical picture and objective evidence of dysmotility and stasis. The diagnosis of gastroparesis, like all conditions deemed functional, presupposes the absence of a specific mechanical, ulcerative, neoplastic or inflammatory lesion that could be held responsible for the clinical picture. The possibility that idiopathic gastroparesis is caused by a viral illness has some epidemiological support but, unless direct proof of a viral etiology is obtained, it should not be labelled as such (Kebede et al 1987, Oh & Kim 1990).

Clinical presentation. Most symptomatic patients with gastroparesis complain of chronic nausea, epigastric discomfort and recurrent vomiting. The epigastric discomfort is usually perceived as fullness or pressure, sometimes as frank pain. Typically, although not exclusively, symptoms are induced or exacerbated by ingestion of food, especially solid meals. In severe cases there may be water and electrolyte disturbances, weight loss and other adverse nutritional sequelae.

Differential diagnosis. Gastroparesis, as a clinical entity, must be differentiated from other gut disorders, chiefly functional dyspepsia, pseudoobstruction and the irritable bowel syndrome. Differentiation from functional dyspepsia is the most difficult and ambiguous, because the symptoms may be very similar. In dyspepsia, the clinical picture is generally milder and the recurrent vomiting, nutritional problems and disabling character of gastroparesis are usually absent. On the other hand, significant gastric stasis may be asymptomatic, particularly in diabetics and patients with prior gastric surgery.

Pseudoobstruction patients usually appear more seriously ill and incapacitated. There are recurrent episodes of acute abdominal pain and distension with failure to pass flatus that mimics small bowel mechanical obstruction (Christensen et al 1990). Nausea and vomiting are common in pseudoobstruction, as is also the case in gastroparesis, but in the former, these manifestations tend to be overshadowed by the abdominal distension and intestinal manifestations.

Nevertheless, the separation of pseudoobstruction, gastroparesis and functional dyspepsia is not always easy, especially when complicated by drug therapy. Caution is needed before the decision is made to embark upon dramatic therapy such as parenteral nutrition or abdominal surgery for presumed pseudoobstruction.

Irritable bowel syndrome encompasses patients whose main distinctive features, quite unlike gastroparesis, are an alteration in bowel habit pattern and lower abdominal pain, often relieved or aggravated by defecation. Thus, it is usually possible to distinguish, on purely clinical grounds, gastroparesis from irritable bowel syndrome. However, overlaps obviously do exist and it has been estimated that about one third of patients with dyspepsia may also present with features of irritable bowel syndrome (Talley et al 1990). Unfortunately, many clinicians apply the irritable bowel syndrome label too broadly, to all kinds of unexplained digestive complaints.

Idiopathic gastroparesis must also be differentiated from the secondary forms due to specific diseases or conditions (Malagelada & Camilleri 1995). The main secondary categories are diabetic gastroparesis, postsurgical gastroparesis or gastroparesis associated with visceral myopathies. Symptoms may be identical and the distinction between secondary and idiopathic gastroparesis is made largely on the basis of a predisposing factor or disease being absent in the latter.

RISK AND COST-ADJUSTED MANAGEMENT OF FUNCTIONAL UPPER GUT SYNDROMES

Exploring the background

Functional disorders are so variable in their manifestations, their impact on well-being and the motivations of patients seeking a physician consultation that management approaches cannot be standardized. Several studies have shown that among the general population there are many individuals who acknowledge, when specifically questioned, that they experience occasional symptoms indistinguishable in character from those manifested by patients seen by physicians for functional dyspepsia (Harrison Morris 1989, Talley et al 1992). It appears that many of these persons choose to ignore their abdominal symptoms or accept them as normal and do not request medical consultation.

Therefore, in the management planning of a patient with functional symptoms the physician must include not only an analysis of the patient's symptomatology but also of the reasons for consulting. Moreover, before undertaking any investigations, risk and cost–benefit outcome should be considered. To help analyze these questions properly I will review separately issues that relate to the type of patient under assessment, the qualifications of the physician and the level of uncertainty that both patient and physician are prepared to accept.

Patient characteristics and motivations

Symptoms of dyspepsia are very common and non-specific. On the basis of anamnesis and physical examination, it is not always possible to guess whether the patient's dyspeptic symptoms are due to an underlying serious illness or represent a functional disorder. In the former instance, be it neoplasm or ulcer, a delay in diagnosis could have potentially adverse consequences for the patient whereas, in the latter, the time factor is less significant.

To differentiate secondary from essential or functional dyspepsia we begin with the patient characteristics that may help the process. Age and sex have useful statistical connotations (Williams et al 1988). Patients aged 45 years or less have a much lower probability of harboring an occult malignancy (the most feared risk of inaccurate and delayed diagnosis) than older individuals. Sex is of some relevance, since functional disorders are more common in women than in men. Symptomatic males are, therefore, more likely to suffer from an organic disorder than are symptomatic females, although admittedly the reliability of this particular point when considering an individual case is small.

Experienced physicians appropriately place great emphasis on ancillary clinical data, including constitutional signs, background illnesses, family history and so forth. Patient personality and the manner in which he or she describes the symptoms are also useful clues. Colorful descriptions are a likely sign of functional rather than organic disorder. A functional diagnosis is also favored if the patient reports many concomitant symptoms unrelated to the gut, such as lower back pain, chronic headaches, atypical urinary disturbances and so forth. Moreover, it has been reported that these non-gut complaints reflect personality traits that would induce patients to request medical advice for the same symptoms that other individuals would otherwise manage themselves.

Attitudes manifested by the patient or by accompanying relatives or friends may also be significant, because they may tip the physician about the underlying level of concern or about whether the patient is expecting immediate investigation. Hysterical or hypochondriac personalities are unlikely to be satisfied by simple reassurance or treatment without prior investigation. This may be even more likely when the patient, as happens commonly nowadays, arrives at the clinic well informed about new advances and assorted marvels of medical technology. These 'knowledgeable' patients with upper abdominal complaints tend to expect to be referred for diagnostic work-up including, at the very least, upper gastrointestinal endoscopy. Cancerophobia is a rather widespread trait among patients seeking medical consultation and, if these patients are denied what they assume would be a reasonable search for a potential tumor, they may become dissatisfied, build resentment (that in turn diminishes the likelihood of therapeutic success) or seek alternatives. These attitudes vary in degree, depending on background, culture and socioeconomic status, but it is generally useful to explore the expectations of the patient and the entourage during the initial interview, before a management plan is outlined.

Physician qualifications

Patients with dyspeptic symptoms may consult physicians with varying degrees of training, specialization and experience depending on preference, referral channels and health plan organization in a particular country or system. Generally speaking, most patients consult first with general practitioners, but many gain direct or secondary access to internists, gastroenterologists, surgeons or even psychiatrists. Physician qualifications and the attendant access to medical technology become relevant factors to what happens next. Dyspeptic patients seen by a general practitioner, in many countries the standard point of entry for ambulatory patients into the medical system, are more likely to be managed by an empirical approach. Conversely, dyspeptic patients seen initially by gastroenterologists, who have ready access to endoscopy and other advanced medical technologies, are more likely to be investigated in some depth soon after the first visit. This tendency is reinforced by the fact that most specialists have been educated to establish a diagnosis based on fact, before they initiate treatment.

Acceptance of uncertainty

Ultimately, the decision whether to observe, to treat the patient empirically or to investigate a case with advanced diagnostic methods depends on what level of uncertainty both patient and physician are prepared to accept. As we indicated earlier, on the patient's part, attitude towards the problem may be determined by personality, cultural background and pressures of different kinds arising from family, friends or working environment. Some patients will be content with physician reassurance after an initial brief interview and physical exam and willingly submit to a period of observation or a short therapeutic trial. By contrast, other patients offered the same approach may well be disappointed and even contest the decision to skip a thorough investigation of their medical problem, because they are unwilling to accept a tentative diagnosis. From a practical standpoint, the greater the patient's concern, the more carefully the physician must avoid trivializing the complaints and skipping diagnostic investigations.

Physicians' preconceived ideas and medical–cultural background also have a profound influence in the decision process. Few physicians will fail to proceed immediately with diagnostic investigations, such as endoscopy, in the presence of 'alarm symptoms' including significant weight loss, back pain, pallor, a palpable mass, jaundice and the like. Delaying procedures in the face of such indicators carries a significant risk of overlooking a serious evolving lesion. On the other hand, since diagnostic procedures increase the discomfort and cost to the patient (or third payer), physicians increasingly and appropriately refrain from applying them automatically. The degree of confidence that physicians have in their clinical judgement, the fear of legal implications and the willingness to take time to properly explain options to the patient all help determine whether to investigate immediately or not.

The diagnostic investigation circuit

The key objectives of diagnostic tests are to establish first, whether there is a recognizable lesion in the upper gastrointestinal tract and second, whether the patient has a disease outside the digestive tract that could be responsible for the abdominal complaints. Since, as pointed out previously, the management process has to be individualized, I will outline the most appropriate sequence of diagnostic investigations as a step-by-step process.

Upper gastrointestinal endoscopy is the usual starting procedure, other than a simple blood screen (Kagevi et al 1989, Johnsen et al 1991). Endoscopy will usually identify neoplastic, ulcerative or inflammatory lesions that may be responsible for the patient's symptoms. However, we should keep in mind two important endoscopy-negative conditions: gastroesophageal reflux disease without esophagitis and small bowel obstructive lesions beyond the reach of conventional upper endoscopy. If clinical concern about missing these conditions arises, the issue must be pursued further. Diagnosis of reflux may require an empiric trial with a proton pump inhibitor or an esophageal pH-monitoring test. Obstructive lesions may be identified by means of a small bowel barium series or CT scan. Ultrasonography, although often performed, has a surprisingly low yield in the absence of symptoms or blood test results suggestive of biliopancreatic disease (Nyrén et al 1987).

Assuming that the abovementioned procedures are negative and the physician continues to suspect an organic condition, the possibility of systemic disease with secondary gastrointestinal manifestations should be investigated. Before doing so, however, it is important to scrutinize the patient's list of current and recent medications and, if not done already, obtain a full blood screening for relatively common metabolic and hormonal disturbances (hyperglycemia, hypercalcemia, hypokalemia, hypothyroidism). Relevant systemic diseases to keep in mind at this stage include: diabetes mellitus with visceral neuropathy (uncommonly it may occur in mild, non-insulin-dependent diabetes), collagen vascular disease, such as scleroderma or mixed connective tissue disease, and neurological disorders including brainstem lesions, dysautonomia of various sorts and amyloidosis. All these conditions may be potentially associated with symptomatic upper gut dysmotility (Malagelada et al 1986). Demonstrating the presence of one of these conditions may or may not allow effective or curative therapy, since most have no known cure. However, establishing the correct diagnosis invariably helps focus and target management, so that emphasis can be placed on the disease rather than on its gastrointestinal repercussions.

If endoscopy discloses the presence of lesions related to acid peptic disease, such as duodenal or gastric ulceration or esophagitis, management must be directed towards the use of antisecretory drugs and, in the case of peptic ulcer disease, eradication of *Helicobacter pylori*. In contrast to past practices, there is no need to routinely perform an indepth physiologic investigation of individual patients with gastric analysis or gastrin studies. However, an apparent drawback of the fast 'treatment first' approach for acid peptic disorders is that it may lead to underdiagnosis of relatively rare, though important conditions, such as gastrinoma, antral G-cell hyperplasia or postsurgical sequelae (incomplete vagotomy or retained antrum syndrome). Of these, missing an early gastrinoma (about half are malignant) has the greatest adverse consequences for the patient. Gastrinomas, prior to metastasizing, have about one chance in three of cure, if identified and surgically excised. This applies particularly to patients with the sporadic, non-MEN-I (multiple endocrine adenomatosis) form of the disease. Special attention should therefore be paid to patients with dyspeptic symptoms who present associated diarrhea, large gastric folds or severe erosive duodenitis extending beyond the apex of the bulb. The serum gastrin level should be determined in such patients and, if found to be elevated, it should be followed with an appropriate gastrin challenge test (usually a secretin provocative test).

A primary motility disorder should be considered when there is no structural lesion at endoscopy and the other conditions listed above have been satisfactorily excluded. Clues pointing towards upper gut dysmotility may sometimes appear, for instance, when the radiologist reports delayed emptying of a barium meal or when the endoscopist observes retained food; such findings are uncommon except in advanced disease. Motility disorders are frequently diagnosed by excluding all other possibilities, but it is much better to document the disturbance by special tests such as manometry or radioscintigraphy. As a practical approach, the rule of using simple exclusion in patients with mild, non-incapacitating symptoms without nutritional compromise and performing specialized investigations in patients with more severe or recurrent problems seems logical.

Measurement of gastric emptying of a meal by radioscintigraphy is a useful test. It is most sensitive when it includes quantification of the rate of gastric evacuation of both liquid and solid components of the meal. According to most published series, delayed gastric emptying of solids is detected in approximately half of patients with mild dyspepsia. The proportion of

positive tests increases in patients with more severe manifestations but, generally speaking, there is poor correlation between
symptoms and the degree of gastric emptying abnormality
(Corinaldesi et al 1987, Davis et al 1988, Waldron et al 1991).
Ultrasonography may also be used to measure gastric emptying
non-invasively, but only liquid emptying can be quantitated,
with the consequent loss of sensitivity.

Gastrointestinal manometry, both fasting and postprandial, is
another useful test for investigating a potential motility disturbance (Malagelada et al 1986). Its sensitivity in mild cases of dyspepsia is approximately equal to that of gastric scintigraphy, that
is, about half of patients will show antral hypomotility after
ingestion of solid food. However, the real usefulness of manometry is its ability to record simultaneously gastric and intestinal
phasic pressure activity patterns, providing useful clues as to the
nature of the motor disorder. Pressure activity that is of normal
amplitude but uncoordinated (neurogenic pattern) suggests disturbed innervation, whereas weak but well-coordinated activity
(myogenic pattern) is more typical of smooth muscle disease.
There is also another fairly characteristic manometric pattern that
suggests distal mechanical small bowel obstruction. These distinctions are naturally lost with end-stage disease and bowel
atony. In any case, the information may be helpful in establishing
the correct diagnosis and in outlining a viable management plan.

In special cases, investigations may be extended to evaluate
biliary dyskinesia by motility and imaging studies of the
biliopancreatic area. Additional steps may include formal psychiatric evaluation in patients with evident psychopathology and,
exceptionally, tests for food tolerance if food allergy is suspected
(particularly in patients with a medical history of atopy).

THERAPY

The therapy of functional gastrointestinal disorders has several
aspects: 1) therapy as an empiric trial, as a tool to reduce investigational costs; 2) therapy of symptoms, to improve the quality of
life; 3) therapy to prevent complications that may carry significant morbidity and mortality.

The empiric therapeutic trial

Why and when to do it

Support for the concept of an empiric therapeutic trial in functional disease comes mainly from indirect evidence obtained

from drug trials performed in 'organic' disease. That is, in patients in whom a specific condition such as peptic ulcer or esophagitis has been demonstrated. Unfortunately, no consistently effective form of therapy is known for functional dyspepsia and the results of a therapeutic trial in an individual patient with functional dyspepsia may be ambiguous. If the patient becomes asymptomatic, it could be a placebo effect, and if the patient remains symptomatic, no diagnosis has been excluded.

The potential advantages of empiric drug trials in dyspeptic patients are twofold:

1. to 'cure' worrying functional dyspeptics with transient symptoms, who can then be reassured and excluded from the medical system at low cost;
2. to alleviate the symptoms of dyspepsia due to benign organic processes, such as gastritis or reflux disease.

In the latter case, however, the recurrent nature of these illnesses will likely make the results of a drug trial, even when successful, shortlived. It has been pointed out by recent studies that delaying endoscopy and other pertinent investigations may eventually turn out to be more costly than early investigation (Bytzer et al 1994).

The ideal duration of an empiric drug trial is also uncertain. On the basis of trials performed in patients with proven acid peptic disorders, a period of 2–4 weeks appears reasonable (Dobrilla et al 1989). By that time, placebo effects are likely to be waning and positive effects of the drugs should become apparent. An additional consideration is whether a second 2–4 week trial with a different drug should be conducted if the first trial fails. Currently, some physicians take this approach in their clinical practice, but the decision to repeat the trial must be carefully individualized to preclude delaying specific treatment of an evolving serious lesion that may have been overlooked.

What measures or agents to use

A therapeutic trial may not necessarily involve pharmacological agents but may be based on simple measures such as introducing dietary changes (i.e. low fat, bland or predominantly liquid meals), eliminating bad habits and potentially offending drugs, encouraging exercise, etc. If a drug trial is to be conducted, the first decision concerns the class of therapeutic agent most likely to be effective in each individual case. There are two classes of drugs to choose from – antisecretory agents and prokinetics – and a metaanalysis of drug trials supported prokinetics over H_2 blockers (Dobrilla et al 1989).

Nevertheless, some clinical clues may be useful in making the choice. Antisecretory agents may be empirically used first in functional disorders incorporating features suggesting acid peptic disease ('refluxlike dyspepsia' and 'ulcerlike dyspepsia'). Prokinetics would be best used first in patients with symptoms suggesting a motility disorder ('dysmotility-like dyspepsia'). However, there is no scientific support for making such a decision, because past studies have often been unable to correlate symptoms with specific physiological abnormalities. Sucralfate, though sometimes used as a therapeutic trial, is less popular than antisecretory agents or prokinetics and no better than these for treatment of acid peptic disorders. Whether eradication of *Helicobacter* infection in patients with positive serology or breath test would constitute a reasonable therapeutic trial cannot be affirmed yet. Early results indirectly support the approach (McCarthy et al 1995) but there are no conclusive data on the value of *Helicobacter* eradication on the symptoms of dyspepsia.

Therapy to relieve symptoms

In patients with an established diagnosis of functional upper gut disorder, successful symptomatic therapy often involves acting at three levels: against the symptom itself, against the presumed origin of the symptom and against the psychological background.

Acting against the symptom itself is easy to comprehend, difficult to achieve. Pain, in different forms, is the index symptom in many patients with a functional upper gut disorder. Visceral pain is rather impervious to conventional analgesics (non-steroidal antiinflammatory agents or paracetamol). Moreover, NSAIDs are best avoided for fear of inducing complicating gastric or intestinal mucosal lesions. Occasionally, opiates are required for the management of acute severe pain but, obviously, their addictive potential and disturbing effects on bowel motility make them unsuitable for sustained use. Thus, as specified below, pain is usually managed by the use of agents that act on the underlying visceral mechanisms of pain such as spasm, distension and hyperalgesia.

Nausea is another common symptom and it is amenable to direct pharmacological therapy by antiemetic drugs. Halogenated phenothiazine derivatives administered either orally, via suppository or parenterally may be helpful. However, many clinicians prefer to use partial dopamine (D_2) antagonists such as metoclopramide, to take advantage of their concomitant prokinetic and sedative actions. Ondansetron and granisetron are powerful 5-HT$_3$ antagonists with antiemetic properties but clinically negligible prokinetic action. Whether they have visceral analgesic properties is currently under study and their applicability to the therapy of functional syndromes still uncertain.

Postprandial fullness, burping and regurgitation have no specific drug therapy but may be helped by instructions on adoption of appropriate eating habits, decreasing the content of fats and irritating dietary ingredients and asking the patient to take small frequent portions rather than large and spaced meals.

Acting against the presumed origin of the patient symptoms is the approach most commonly adopted. As indicated above, gastric stasis and distension are thought, although by no means proven, to be the critical pathogenetic factors in functional dyspepsia and related upper gut syndromes. Acid peptic injury stimulating pain terminals is a second possibility. Given this premise, it should come as no surprise that both drugs that stimulate gastric evacuation and antisecretory agents are the most favored by practicing clinicians, as we already emphasized when discussing the empiric therapeutic trial. However, unlike the empiric therapeutic trial performed without prior investigation, there are now patients in whom gross lesions of esophagitis, ulcer or significant erosions have been already excluded, hence reducing the proportion of patients with active acid-peptic disease. For this reason, prokinetics are generally preferred to antisecretory agents in this group.

Prokinetics are agents that enhance gastric evacuation by increasing antral contractility, antroduodenal coordination, propulsive activity in the intestine or various combinations of the above. Their efficacy in the treatment of functional dyspepsia is generally supported by several trials (Dobrilla et al 1989, Talley 1991). The benzamide metoclopramide was the first agent developed specifically as a prokinetic and antiemetic. Metoclopramide incorporates both antidopaminergic D$_2$ action and 5-HT$_4$ agonist activity that facilitates release of acetylcholine in the enteric nervous system. The former appears to be responsible for central effects, including inhibition of nausea and vomiting and a mild anxiolytic action, whereas the latter is mostly responsible for the peripheral prokinetic effects. Unfortunately, the central dopamine-blocking effects may occasionally induce extrapyramidal-like effects including dystonic reactions. Domperidone, a derivative of metoclopramide, retains the antidopaminergic action but is less likely to produce central dystonic or sedative effects because it does not cross the blood–brain barrier well. Because domperidone lacks the 5-HT$_4$ agonist component that induces much of the prokinetic effect, another agent, cisapride, was subsequently developed and remains the current standard for prokinetics. Cisapride has strong 5-HT$_4$ agonist action and stimulates propulsive contractions at various levels of the gastrointestinal tract.

Patients with evidence of gastric stasis who are stabilized and able to ingest oral medication may be managed with a prokinetic such as cisapride (or one of several closely related compounds) that stimulates upper gut propulsive activity. In practice, cisapride is often prescribed by clinicians to treat functional dyspeptic symptoms, even without direct evidence of dysmotility (Van Ontrybe et al 1993). The scientific basis for this practice is questionable but derives some support from clinical trials in symptomatic patients. Cisapride is best given orally in divided doses increasing gradually from 5 up to 20 mg four times daily. Side-effects are rare but careful monitoring of heart electrical rhythm is warranted at high doses or in patients taking potentially interacting drugs. As with other prokinetics, individual responses to cisapride are somewhat variable. Therefore, lack of response to cisapride or analogous compounds may warrant a trial with an alternative agent such as metoclopramide (central effects may act adjuvantly) or domperidone (effects on dopamine receptors not activated cisapride). Erythromycin is an antibiotic that acts primarily, though not exclusively, as a motilin agonist. It is more useful in acute situations, administered parenterally as a slow bolus, than in chronic oral treatment, because of its antibiotic action, side-effects and apparent loss of efficacy over time (Richards et al 1993). Erythromycin derivatives retaining gastrokinetic effects but deprived of antibacterial activity are currently being developed.

Antisecretory agents also have a role in the therapy of functional gastrointestinal disorders. Patients with a dyspeptic syndrome incorporating elements of gastroesophageal reflux disease (who could be categorized as suffering from refluxlike dyspepsia or reflux plus dyspepsia) are the most likely candidates. Pyrosis is acknowledged to be a fairly specific symptom for gastroesophageal reflux disease and this symptom, at least, is likely to respond. Unfortunately, there are also patients whose pyrosis is unrelated to GERD, possibly due to 'irritable esophagus', and these are unlikely to improve on antisecretory drugs.

Some dyspeptic patients, even without GERD or GERD-like symptoms, appear to respond to antisecretory drugs. Several controlled trials comparing the symptomatic effect of these agents against placebo in functional dyspepsia attest to their partial efficacy, but the therapeutic mechanism remains a mystery. It has been postulated that some of these patients represent mild erosive precursors of peptic ulcer disease or, perhaps, increased sensitivity to luminal acid, but the evidence is shaky. The practical problem is also how to identify these responder patients among the large pool of dyspeptic individuals. Finally, I should point out that ranitidine, an H_2-blocking drug, appears to possess some prokinetic properties and that ranitidine derivatives combining motor effects and a weak antisecretory action are under development.

Since increased visceral sensitivity to distending stimuli is a common feature of upper gastrointestinal functional syndromes, drugs that decrease perception may be used for symptomatic relief. Octreotide is a long-acting somatostatin analog that, in the intestine, may initiate ectopic fronts of motor activity although, depending on dose, its net effects may be to accelerate or prolong transit. However, the effects on transit are a matter of current debate and, hence, the practical usefulness of octreotide as a prokinetic has been questioned. Octreotide may decrease abdominal symptoms by inhibiting afferent pathways that mediate intestinal perception. As a visceral hypoalgesic agent, it may be therapeutically useful in selected patients. Fedotozine is a new agent that acts on gut κ opioid receptors to decrease visceral sensitivity to pain, but clinical experience with this compound is still limited (Fraitag et al 1994).

Acting against the psychological background that sustains the clinical manifestations of functional gut disorders is at the same time important and tricky. There is a longstanding and widely held belief that many such patients have abnormal personality traits (anxiety, neuroticism, depression) or attitudes. Some studies support this view (Richter 1991, Haug et al 1994) but the matter cannot yet be regarded as conclusively settled. Neither is there proof that stress exacerbates the clinical manifestations of functional disease. Some evidence suggests that the way the patient deals with chronic stressors is the most significant factor (Bennett et al 1992). Patients with irritable bowel symptoms who consult a physician are more likely to suffer psychological disturbances than those who do not seek medical attention (Drossman et al 1988). The same could be true for upper gut functional type disorders. Thus, besides inherent heterogeneity or an as yet unidentified missing link, the explanation for the apparently tenuous connection between the psyche and the gut in functional disorders is that the former may have a greater influence on how the patient reacts to his symptoms than on the symptoms themselves. Drossman (1994) hypothesized that, in functional gut disorders, the predisposing factors (genetic, environmental, infection) act as independent variables influenced by psychosocial modifiers (culture, social support, life stress, psychological status and coping ability). The latter would largely determine clinical expression and outcome.

In managing functional patients, the clinician should take into account that any therapy acting on gut pathophysiology will be modulated by the influence of the psychosocial modifiers. This concept may provide a plausible explanation for the relative failure of prokinetics and other agents acting primarily on gut function. Thus, drugs that appropriately correct an abnormal function, i.e. delayed gastric emptying, may not achieve a clear symptomatic benefit in some patients because they have no influence on modifiers. Conversely, some agents, particularly those with psychopharmacologic action (anxiolytic, sedative, antiemetic), may help some patients without actually changing gut pathophysiology.

Therapy to prevent complications

Many patients with upper gut functional disorders suffer from relatively mild symptoms. Annoying as they may be, these symptoms do not interfere with normal body function and activity. By contrast, other patients are burdened by severe manifestations, potentially leading to complications that must be anticipated and prevented. Repeat emesis or even regurgitation and retching may significantly damage the esophageal mucosa. Recurrent vomiting tends to produce a severe form of esophagitis that may extend throughout the entire body of the esophagus. This form of esophagitis may be silent and sometimes reveals itself by severe bleeding. In other patients, it may cause heartburn, pain and dysphagia. It is effectively treated, and prevented, by proton pump inhibitors. Unfortunately, vomiting may sometimes reduce the practicality of oral medications, requiring initial treatment with parenteral drugs. Mallory–Weiss tears are another feared complication in recurrent vomiters. The most effective prevention is to block the emetic reflex pharmacologically and to teach the patient to refrain from retching, as much as possible.

Metabolic and nutritional disturbances often develop in recurrent vomiters. The most common electrolyte imbalance is hypochloremic alkalosis, with hypokalemia. Other patients markedly curtail their food intake because of anorexia or fear of eating. The latter traits may lead to cachexia and a clinical picture that resembles anorexia nervosa. Commercial liquid formulas offer a variety of well-balanced dietary supplements with pleasant flavors. These nutritional aids can be very helpful since, as a rule, liquid meals are better tolerated and empty from the stomach faster than do solid meals.

Some patients in pain will self-administer or demand analgesic drugs. Narcotics complicate the successful management of chronic abdominal pain and may induce severe constipation, occasionally producing a picture that resembles intestinal pseudoobstruction. Narcotic withdrawal must be attempted and the process may be facilitated by treatment with clonidine, an α_2 agonist agent that may attenuate the abdominal symptoms associated with narcotic withdrawal. Many patients also take aspirin and non-steroidal antiinflammatory drugs. These may induce not only gastric but also intestinal ulcerative lesions and generally must be withdrawn. If the patient refuses to do so, gastroduodenal protection, preferably with a proton pump inhibitor, must be prescribed although clearly the mid and lower gut mucosae remain unprotected. The prostaglandin analog misoprostol is another possibility for adjuvant protection but sometimes it induces unpleasant abdominal cramping and diarrhea.

LONG-TERM MANAGEMENT AND PROGNOSIS

Effective management of functional upper gut disorders requires establishing a long-term treatment plan. By nature, these disorders tend to be chronic and relapsing. Many patients respond initially to drug therapy and ancillary measures, but their symptoms recur upon withdrawal or sometimes even while continuing the same therapeutic measures that proved initially successful. What can be done about this?

First, educate the patient and his/her immediate family as to the nature of the disorder and preempt unrealistic expectations. Second, use the more likely initial response to build up protection against late relapse by modifying, if possible, the environment of the patient. Introduce changes in lifestyle, emphasize exercise, advise removal of stressful factors, build up psychological support. Advice to see a psychiatrist may sometimes be misinterpreted and angrily rejected by the patient. However, in the context of long-term planning the potential usefulness of psychological counseling may be better accepted. Third, be prepared to rotate therapeutic drugs to manage probable symptomatic relapses. Fourth, establish a surveillance plan because an overlooked organic condition may emerge, either because it went undetected during the early work-up or simply because of coincidence. Do not assume that every clinical manifestation of a functional patient remains exclusively 'functional'.

By sensibly following these general measures and appropriately using the available therapeutic aids, most functional patients may be successfully managed and their quality of life improved. However, do not be too disappointed if a patient suddenly turns to a colleague; they may do so for no apparent reason or because a new 'syndrome' develops. It may well be an orthopedic surgeon, a neurologist or even the psychiatrist, who was at first rebuffed.

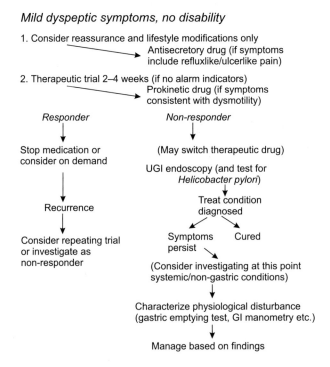

Fig. 11.1 Diagnostic algorithm for suspected functional upper gastrointestinal disorder.

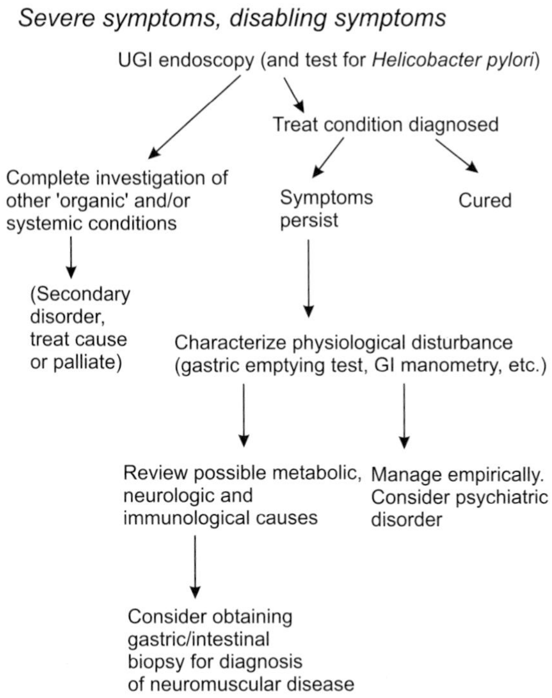

Severe symptoms, disabling symptoms

UGI endoscopy (and test for *Helicobacter pylori*)

Treat condition diagnosed

Complete investigation of
other 'organic' and/or
systemic conditions

Symptoms
persist

Cured

(Secondary
disorder,
treat cause
or palliate)

Characterize physiological disturbance
(gastric emptying test, GI manometry, etc.)

Review possible metabolic,
neurologic and
immunological causes

Manage empirically.
Consider psychiatric
disorder

Consider obtaining
gastric/intestinal
biopsy for diagnosis
of neuromuscular disease

Fig. 11.2 Diagnostic algorithm for suspected functional upper gastrointestinal
disorder.

Table 11.1 Diagnostic tests for the investigation of patients with suspected
functional upper gastrointestinal disorder

First-line tests
Screening hematology and biochemistry
Upper gastrointestinal endoscopy
Ultrasonography (only if symptoms consistent with pancreaticobiliary disease)

Second-line tests
CT scan of abdomen
24-h esophageal pH-metry
Measurement of gastric emptying (radioisotopic, ultrasonographic, other)
Gastrointestinal manometry
Expanded blood screen to look for hormonal, metabolic, immunological
disturbances, etc.

Third-line tests
Manometry of the bile ducts
Tests for food intolerance
Formal psychiatric evaluation

Table 11.2 Drugs potentially useful for the management of gastrointestinal functional type disorders

Class	Possible uses
Antisecretory agents (PPIs, H_2 blockers)	Control of symptoms
Central antiemetics (phenothiazine derivatives, 5-HT_3 antagonists, etc.)	Control of nausea/vomiting
Dual prokinetic/antiemetic (metoclopramide, clebopride)	Treatment of dyspepsia. Symptomatic control of nausea/vomiting
Peripheral dopamine antagonist (domperidone)	Treatment of dyspepsia
5-HT agonist prokinetics (cisapride, cinitapride)	Treatment of dyspepsia, gastroparesis, intestinal dysmotility
Motilides (erythromycin, macrolide derivatives)	Acute treatment of gastroparesis
Visceral hypoalgesic agents (octreotide, fedotozine, etc.)	Treatment of pain

REFERENCES

Barbara L et al 1989 Definition and investigation of dyspepsia: consensus of an international ad hoc working party. Digestive Diseases and Sciences 34: 1272–1276

Bennett EJ, Kellow JE, Cowan H et al 1992 Suppression and anger and gastric emptying in patients with functional dyspepsia. Scandinavian Journal of Gastroenterology 27: 869–874

Bytzer P, Moller Hanssen J, Schaffalitzy de Muckadell OB 1994 Empiric H_2 blocker therapy or prompt endoscopy in the management of dyspepsia. Lancet 343: 811–816

Christensen J, Dent J, Malagelada J-R, Wingate DL 1990 Pseudo-obstruction. Gastroenterology International 3(3): 107–119

Colin-Jones DG et al 1988 Management of dyspepsia: report of a working party. Lancet i: 576–579

Corinaldesi R et al 1987 Effect of chronic administration of cisapride on gastric emptying of solid meal and on dyspeptic symptoms in patients with idiopathic gastroparesis. Gut 28: 300–305

Davis RH, Clench MH, Mathias JR 1988 Effects of domperidone in patients with chronic unexplained upper gastrointestinal symptoms: a double-blind, placebo-controlled study. Digestive Diseases and Sciences 33: 1505–1511

Dobrilla G, Comberlato M, Steele A, Vallaperta B 1989 Drug treatment of functional dyspepsia. Meta analysis of randomized controlled clinical trials. Journal of Clinical Gastroenterology 11: 169–177

Drossman DA et al 1988 Psychosocial factors in the irritable bowel syndrome. Gastroenterology 95: 701–708

Drossman DA 1994 The functional gastrointestinal disorders. Holm AN (ed) Megley, USA, pp 1–24

Fraitag B, Homerin M, Hecktseiler P 1994 Double blind dose–response multicenter comparison of fedotozine and placebo in the treatment of non-ulcer dyspepsia. Digestive Diseases and Sciences 39: 1072–1077

Greydanus MB et al 1991 Neurohormonal factors in functional dyspepsia: insights on pathophysiological mechanisms. Gastroenterology 100: 1311–1318

Harrison JD, Morris DL 1989 Dyspepsia in coal miners and the general population: a comparative study. British Journal of Industrial Medicine 46: 428–429

Haug TT, Svebak S, Wilhelmsen I, Berstad A, Ursin H 1994 Psychological factors and somatic symptoms in functional dyspepsia. A comparison with duodenal ulcer and healthy controls. Journal of Psychosomatic Research 38: 281–291

Johnsen R et al 1991 Prevalences of endoscopic and histological findings in subjects with and without dyspepsia. British Medical Journal 302: 749–752

Kagevi I, Löfstedf S, Persson LG 1989 Endoscopic findings and diagnoses in unselected dyspeptic patients at a primary health care center. Scandinavian Journal of Gastroenterology 24: 145–150

Kebede D, Barthel JS, Singh A 1987 Transient gastroparesis associated with cutaneous Herpes zoster. Digestive Diseases and Sciences 32: 318–322

Malagelada J-R, Camilleri M, Stanghellini V 1986 Manometric diagnosis of gastrointestinal motility disorders. Thieme-Stratton, New York

Malagelada J-R, Camilleri M 1995 Motility disorders of the stomach. In: Hawbrich WS, Schaffner F, Berk JD (eds) Bockus Gastroenterology, 5th edn. WB Saunders, Philadelphia, pp 615–634

McCarthy C, Patchett S, Collins RM et al 1995 Long term prospective study of *Helicobacter pylori* in non ulcer dyspepsia. Digestive Diseases and Sciences 40: 114–119

Nyrén O et al 1987 The 'epigastric distress syndrome': a possible disease entity identified by history and endoscopy in patients with nonulcer dyspepsia. Journal of Clinical Gastroenterology 9: 303–309

O'Brien MD, Bruce BK, Camilleri M 1995 The rumination syndrome, etc. Gastroenterology 108: 1024–1029

Oh JJ, Kim CH 1990 Gastroparesis after a presumed viral illness: clinical and laboratory features and natural history. Mayo Clinic Proceedings 65: 636–642

Pfeiffer A et al 1992 Gastric emptying, esophageal 24-hour pH and gastric potential difference in non-ulcer dyspepsia. Gastroenterology and Clinical Biology 16: 395–400

Richards RD, Davenport K, McCallum RW 1993 The treatment of idiopathic and diabetic gastroparesis with acute intravenous and chronic erithranycin. American Journal of Gastroenterology 88: 203–207

Richter JE 1991 Stress and psychologic and environmental factors in functional dyspepsia. Scandinavian Journal of Gastroenterology 182: 40–46

Talley NJ 1991 Drug treatment of functional dyspepsia. Scandinavian Journal of Gastroenterology 26 (suppl. 182): 47–60

Talley NJ, Phillips SF 1988 Non-ulcer dyspepsia: potential causes and pathophysiology. Annals of Internal Medicine 108: 865–879

Talley NJ et al 1990 Diagnostic value of the Manning criteria in irritable bowel syndrome. Gut 31: 77–81

Talley NJ et al 1992 Dyspepsia and Dyspepsia subgroups: a population-based study. Gastroenterology 102: 1259–1268

Talley NJ et al 1994 Functional gastroduodenal disorders. Ed Drossman, DA. Little, Brown, Boston

Tucci A et al 1992 *Helicobacter pylori* infection and gastric function in patients with chronic idiopathic dyspepsia. Gastroenterology 103: 768–774

Van Ontrybe M, deNutte N, van Eaghem P et al 1993 Efficacy of cisapride in functional dyspepsia resistant to domperidone or metoclopramide: a double blind, placebo controlled study. Scandinavian Journal of Gastroenterology 28 (suppl. 195): 47–53

Waldron B et al 1991 Evidence for hypomotility in non-ulcer dyspepsia: a prospective multifactorial study. Gut 32: 246–251

Williams B et al 1988 Do young patients with dyspepsia need investigation? Lancet ii: 1349–1351

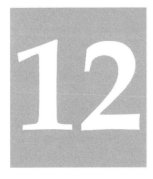

Clinical physiology of the small bowel

E Husebye

INTRODUCTION

Patients with symptoms suggesting small or large bowel involvement, for which the physician cannot identify any specific pathology, account for more than 50% of all patients with gastrointestinal complaints and about 25% of those referred to a gastroenterologist (Switz 1976). The estimated prevalence in the general population amounts to 22% (Jones & Lydeard 1992); of these, less than 50% seek medical care. Those who seek medical care, possibly due to 'illness behavior' (Sandler et al 1984), have an increased incidence of psychiatric disturbance, whereas those who do not, resemble the normal population in this respect (Whitehead et al 1988). Patients with functional disorders have the same expected survival as the general population, but the quality of life is often reduced. Patients with unexplained gastrointestinal symptoms tend to be classified as suffering from the irritable bowel syndrome (IBS) unless defecation is normal, in which case they are classified as 'patients with functional dyspepsia' (Drossman et al 1990). There is no distinct division between these two populations of patients, as illustrated by the observation that, even in IBS patients, the epigastrium is a prevalent site of pain (Kang et al 1992).

Dysfunction of the small bowel may give rise to a variety of symptoms, but periumbilical pain, bloating and diarrhea are the symptoms that particularly draw attention to this bowel segment. Alterations of bowel habit that suggest an underlying motility disorder have traditionally been attributed to colorectal dysfunction. Current concepts, however, also recognize the possible contribution of small bowel dysfunction.

In this chapter, small bowel physiology and pathophysiology with particular reference to functional disorders are reviewed. Most studies have examined the possible role of altered motor activity and this will therefore be the main focus.

SYMPTOMS

Pain: parietal, visceral or referred?

Parietal (somatic) pain originates from the abdominal wall or the parietal peritoneum and is rather sharp, well localized, and lateralized, because each side of the nervous system innervates a corresponding part of the parietal peritoneum.

Somatic pain due to entrapment of somatic sensory nerve fibers in the abdominal wall can be mistaken for a functional symptom. Triggering of the pain by digital palpation at the site of entrapment and relief of pain after infiltration of local anesthetic are useful in the identification of this pain mechanism. Scars after previous abdominal surgery, adiposity, a recent major weight reduction and diabetes mellitus are predisposing factors.

Visceral pain originates from the mesentery, the visceral peritoneum or intraabdominal organs. Visceral hollow organs are mainly sensitive to stretch and tension in the gut wall and forceful muscular contractions may result in symptoms, such as abdominal colic due to mechanical obstruction. However, in patients with visceral neuropathy, even marked distension and spasm may be asymptomatic due to the impairment of visceral afferents. Because of mainly bilateral and multisegmental innervation, visceral abdominal pain is often vague without distinct origin, symmetrical and localized near the midline. Autonomic effects such as nausea, vomiting, sweating, restlessness and pallor often accompany visceral pain.

Referred pain usually originates from more intense stimuli of visceral organs. Central pathways are responsible for referral of pain to a skin area or subcutaneous structures with afferent neurons projecting through the same neural segment. Referred pain from the small bowel is sensed as a dull back pain in the midline. This type of pain occurs in about 20% of patients with functional disorders, less frequently than in organic visceral diseases (Kang et al 1992).

The origin of pain in patients with functional disorders is by definition unknown, but evidence suggests that it is visceral. Lowered thresholds for visceral pain have now been firmly established at multiple sites of the GI tract in patients with functional digestive disorders (Whitehead et al 1990). IBS patients are also more sensitive to physiological bowel motility (Kellow et al 1991) and about 50–60% of those with functional disorders perceive visceral stimuli that do not enter the consciousness of the majority of healthy subjects (Whitehead et al 1990). Alterations in visceral afferent neurons have been suggested, because threshold for sensation of somatic pain is not reduced (Cook et al 1987).

Bloating

Bloating is defined as distension of the abdomen and 10–25% of healthy people admit to bloating (Sullivan 1994). In sufferers, it is generally absent on waking but increases progressively during the day, being provoked and exaggerated by large meals and by constipation and relieved by belching, the passage of flatus or defecation. The relationship to IBS is therefore close and recent data suggest that bloating is the cardinal symptom of this syndrome. Bloating also occurs in patients with functional dyspepsia and in some patients as the sole complaint (Sullivan 1994). There is a female preponderance of the symptom, with premenstrual clustering. Bloaters do not exhibit increased amounts of abdominal gas and 'antigas' remedies are no more effective than placebo. Recent data have shown that there are expellers and non-expellers of gas and the voluntary rectal retention of gas may contribute to the symptoms by inhibiting small bowel motility (Youle & Read 1984). The origin of bloating and gas complaints is not defined, but the small and large bowels are both likely to be involved.

Diarrhea: definition, prevalence and significance

The pathogenesis of diarrhea is heterogeneous, including a number of extraintestinal conditions besides diseases of the small and large bowel. The word diarrhea originates from the Greek terms *dia rhein* which mean flow through. In the public domain, the term is used liberally and ambiguity is also encountered in professional use. In scientific usage, diarrhea means increased volume of stools, loose stools, and frequent bowel movements; loose stools have been suggested as the main feature. Diarrhea may be the result of both small and large bowel dysfunctions. When the small bowel is responsible, propulsive colonic patterns of motility are evoked by the passage of intestinal contents into the cecum in volumes that exceed the threshold for 'colonic salvage'.

Recently, a comprehensive UK study of 838 men and 1059 women showed that only 67% of men and 57% of women enjoy the conventional normal bowel habit of one or two regular daily defecations (Heaton et al 1992); 8% of men and 5% of women reported more than two daily bowel movements, whereas 4% and 11% reported more than 51 hours between bowel movements, respectively. Irregularity is more common than regularity in the general population.

In this normal population loose stools were reported by 21% of men and 18% of women, showing that caution is needed when defining a stool pattern as abnormal. Stool consistency should be recorded carefully in patients with altered bowel habits, because stool form rather than stool frequency is a marker of intestinal transit (O'Donnell et al 1990). Moreover, after adjustment for differences in diet, significantly increased stool volume is uncommon in patients with functional disorders.

In summary, patients with functional dyspepsia have, by definition, normal bowel movements, whereas those with IBS may have alterations in stool frequency and consistency, but usually not in stool volume. Where there are changes in stool volume in functional disorders, it is generally assumed that these are secondary to altered transit through the absorptive region of the bowel rather than to mucosal dysfunction; this assumption may prove to be unjustified as our understanding of the neural control of the mucosa increases, but it is consistent with existing evidence.

MOTOR PHYSIOLOGY OF THE SMALL INTESTINE

Physiological motor activity

Smooth muscle cells of the small bowel exhibit continuous fluctuations in membrane potential called slow waves (Fig. 12.1). When recorded with extracellular electrodes, the sum of slow waves from a number of neighboring cells is seen. The frequency

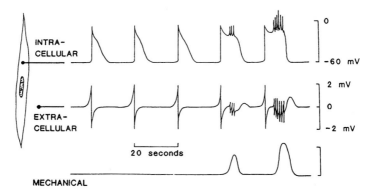

Fig. 12.1   Electric activity of gastrointestinal smooth muscle cell showing that contractions occur when spike bursts are superimposed on slow waves. The number of spikes in the burst determines the strength of a contraction. (From van Cutsem E. Thesis. University Hospital of Leuven, Belgium, 1994.)

of slow waves is about 11 per min in the proximal small bowel, decreasing stepwise to 7–8 per min in the ileum. When smooth muscle cell membrane potentials are depolarized beyond threshold by the removal of neural inhibition, by neural excitation or by excitation by hormones or locally released neuropeptides or biogenic amines, action potentials occur, leading to contraction. In extracellular recordings, spike bursts represent summated action potentials and it is when a spike burst is superimposed on a slow wave that the muscle contracts (Fig. 12.1). Thus, slow waves determine the timing of contractions and also control their rate and length of aboral propagation. Accordingly, the maximum contractile frequency in the small bowel equals the slow wave frequency, as seen during certain patterns of motility (Figs 12.2, 12.3).

Groups of contractions associated in time and aboral spread are defined as patterns of motility. These patterns are usually easy to

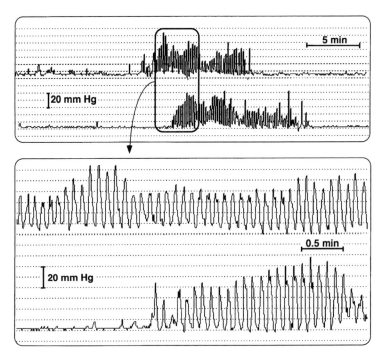

Fig. 12.2 Phase III of MMC recorded in a healthy subject during nocturnal fasting from sensors located in duodenum (upper tracing) and proximal jejunum (lower tracing). A section is expanded in the lower panel to show the regular contractile frequency of 11 per min, reflecting the underlying slow wave frequency. Phase I: the quiescent periods prior to and succeeding phase III. Absence of phase II activity is a typical feature of MMC during sleep. (Modified after Husebye et al 1991.)

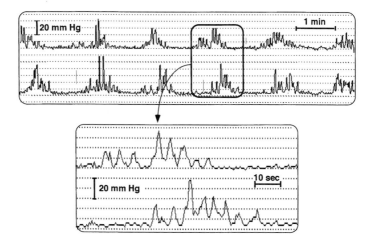

Fig. 12.3 Discrete clustered contractions (DCC) recorded from sensors located in duodenum (upper tracing) and proximal jejunum (lower tracing) during postprandial state in a healthy elderly subject. A typical sequence of minute rhythm is shown: repetitive DCC at 1–2 min intervals. The lower panel shows a blown-up section of the recording. (Modified after Husebye et al 1991.)

recognize and reflect integrated motor activity with particular functional characteristics. *Single* contractions are only defined as distinct phenomena (e.g. giant migrating contractions) if they have characteristics that are clearly different from those of normal contractions.

Patterns of motility in health

Certain patterns of motility are always present in healthy subjects if recording is performed for a sufficiently long period of time. These are the migrating motor complex (MMC) that occur during fasting and the postprandial pattern of motility that follows the intake of a nutrient meal.

The migrating motor complex (MMC)

The MMC is the most characteristic and well-studied pattern of motility. In healthy individuals it is invariably present during fasting from birth (Bisset et al 1988) to old age (Husebye & Engedal 1992). The MMC consists of three phases, of which phase III is the most distinctive and easily identified. It is a succession of regular contractions at the slow wave frequency lasting for about 5 min that migrates aborally from the proximal small bowel to terminate between the midpoint of the small bowel and the terminal ileum (Kellow et al 1986) (Fig. 12.2). Phase III occurs most frequently at the ligament of Treitz; the duodenum and antrum participate in about 85% and 60% of phase IIIs, respectively (Kellow et al 1986). The velocity of migration is 5–10 cm per min, much slower than the 1–2 cm per minute propagation velocity of the single contractions that comprise the pattern (Summers et al 1983). The generally accepted minimum duration of a succession of contractions that can be defined as phase III of the MMC is 2 min; shorter runs of contractions are considered to be 'clusters' (less than 1 min) or phase III like activities.

Phase III of the MMC recurs at average intervals of 90 to 110 min (Vantrappen et al 1977; Thompson et al, 1980; Kellow et al 1986; Husebye et al 1990). The duration of these intervals, the *MMC period*, can vary by more than 3 h in the same individual and the variance within subjects amounts to 90% of the total variance for the MMC period (Husebye et al 1990). Variance between healthy individuals is therefore difficult to distinguish. Thus, a single MMC period does not provide a valid estimate of the overall incidence of the MMC in a single subject and this has practical implications for the recording and analysis of small bowel motor activity (Husebye et al 1990). Predominant intraindividual variability also characterizes other MMC variables, except that the migration velocity of phase III is relatively specific within individuals (Husebye et al 1990).

Phase III is usually succeeded by quiescence or phase I (less than three contractions per 10 min) and then irregular contractile activity of phase II recurs before the next phase III completes the MMC cycle. During sleep, phase II is usually brief and sometimes absent (Kellow et al 1990).

The MMC pattern requires preserved enteric neuromuscular function, whereas the extrinsic nerve supply can be disconnected without abolishing the pattern; spontaneous MMC activity occurs in transplanted small bowel. Experimental evidence indicates that the normal intestinal microflora provide a substantial stimulatory drive for initiation and aboral migration of normal phase III activity (Husebye et al 1994). In addition, luminal secretions can initiate phase II activity (Smith et al 1992).

GI peptides and other cellular messengers may modulate the MMC pattern by paracrine and endocrine modes of action, but the physiological role of the different cell messengers awaits to be defined. Intravenous administration of motilin and motilin receptor agonists such as erythromycin elicit phase III of MMC in the antroduodenal region and endogenous plasma motilin is maximal during late phase II and phase III of MMC. Motilin release seems to be important for antral participation in the MMC pattern, but it is not required for the initiation or aboral migration of MMC in the small bowel. Somatostatin, serotonin and sumatriptan (5-HT 1p agonist) can also initiate phase III-like activity in the duodenum, indicating that ENS circuits with both peptidergic and serotonergic transmission are involved.

The physiological role of the MMC remains to be clearly established. Remnants of previous meals and secretions are cleared during phase III of MMC, and Code & Schlegel (1974) therefore coined the term 'gastrointestinal housekeeper'. Subsequently, the absence of MMC was demonstrated in some patients with bacterial overgrowth, suggesting a role in the control of microbial colonization in the small bowel (Vantrappen et al 1977). A close relationship between impaired MMC activity and colonization with Gram-negative bacilli was recently reported in patients with small bowel radiation injury (Husebye et al 1995).

Absent or abnormal MMC activity has been reported in patients with enteric neuromuscular disorders and in patients with extrinsic neuropathies (Stanghellini et al 1987; Anuras 1992). Moreover, the presence of duodenojejunal MMCs predicts a successful outcome of jejunal tube feeding (Di Lorenzo et al 1995) in children with chronic idiopathic intestinal pseudoobstruction. The MMC thus emerges as a marker of the integrity of enteric function. Complete absence of MMCs is, particularly during prolonged recording, a reliable indicator of severe enteric dysfunction (Hyman et al 1993; Husebye et al 1995; Di Lorenzo et al 1995), but this is an uncommon finding even in patients with known enteric neuromuscular disease. Abnormal MMC activity (Stanghellini et al 1987) and reduced intensity of MMC (Husebye et al 1995) are more sensitive indicators of enteric dysfunction.

Postprandial pattern

Food intake induces irregular contractile activity in the small bowel soon after a meal and postprandial state is defined as the elapsed time between the start of the meal intake and the return of phase III. The first postprandial phase III usually arises in the mid-jejunum when 15–80% of the meal is still in the small bowel (Read et al 1984). The duration of the postprandial state depends mainly on the caloric content of the meal (Ouyang et al 1989; Soffer & Adrian 1992) and has been reported to be 177 min, 359 min and 411 min in the proximal small bowel of healthy adults after meals of 630 kJ, 1260 kJ and 2520 kJ respectively (Ouyang et al 1989).

Meal intake immediately initiates irregular contractile activity in the entire small bowel, a response that involves vagal output and hormonal and paracrine effects. Continuing MMC activity after meal intake during experimental vagal cooling demonstrates the significance of parasympathetic control (Hall et al 1986). Truncal vagotomy is often followed by severe digestive symptoms and by a premature return of the MMC pattern after a meal (Thompson et al 1982). When nutrients are administered directly into the jejunum there is predominantly a local postprandial response, because omission of the cephalic, gastric and duodenal phases of meal stimulation reduces meal-induced vagal and hormonal responses.

Ileal motility

The ileum exhibits the patterns of motility outlined above, but there are some important differences compared with the proximal small bowel (Kruis et al 1985). The MMC pattern occurs less frequently, whereas bursts of contractions predominate (Kellow et al 1986). The distinction between fed and fasting motility is also less clear, because the remnants of a meal may remain in the ileum for several hours after the return of MMCs in the proximal small bowel (Read et al 1984). Of particular interest are prolonged propagated contractions, a highly propulsive motility pattern confined to the distal ileum, that clears refluxed cecal contents (Kruis et al 1985). Short chain fatty acids elicit this pattern of motility (Kamath et al 1987).

The ileum is involved in the reflex control of both upper gut motility and transit through the ileocecal junction and this regulatory function is reflected in greater impairment of digestion and absorption after ileal compared with jejunal resection (Quigley 1993).

Patterns seen in health and disease

Certain patterns of motility are occasionally seen in healthy individuals and have been reported to occur more frequently in certain disease states. The physiological significance of these patterns is still unclear.

Discrete clustered contractions (DCC)

DCC are composed of 3–10 contractions at the slow wave frequency (Summers et al 1983) (Fig. 12.3). They usually start in the proximal small bowel and propagate aborally at a rate similar to the individual contractions that comprise the pattern (1–2 cm per s; Fig. 12.3). DCC usually propagate for less than 30–40 cm (Kellow et al 1986) and MMC and DCC are thus distinguished by both the rate and extent of aboral propagation (Figs. 12.2, 12.3).

DCC are occasionally seen in young healthy adults during phase II of the MMC (Summers et al 1983; Kellow et al 1986; Ouyang et al 1989; Husebye & Engedal, 1992) and postprandially (Summers et al 1983; Camilleri 1989; Ouyang et al 1989). In old age, this pattern of motility becomes prevalent after meals. DCC were found in 67% of healthy elderly subjects after a mixed meal and 'minute rhythm', a pattern of repetitive DCC at 1–2 min intervals (Fig. 12.3), was seen during the postprandial period in 53% (Husebye & Engedal 1992).

The mechanism for the initiation of DCC is unknown. A similar pattern occurs in patients with partial mechanical obstruction (Summers et al 1983), suggesting that increased resistance to flow may be a trigger mechanism. An isosmotic, non-caloric solution infused into the proximal small bowel at a rate of 20 ml per min initiated DCC after 30 min (Steadman & Kerlin 1994). Reduced flexibility of connective tissue compartments of the bowel wall during aging may increase resistance to flow by reducing compliance. The presence of DCC in healthy individuals emphasizes that this pattern can be a normal response to physiological stimuli and different types of nutrients may determine its postprandial incidence.

Isolated bursts of contractions

Isolated or stationary bursts are defined as runs of contractions at high regular or irregular frequency, that are confined to a limited segment of the bowel (Stanghellini et al 1987; Husebye et al 1995). Stationary bursts may impede flow temporarily and give rise to distension and abdominal pain due to a temporary functional stenosis (Malagelada & Stanghellini 1985). Bursts are frequently seen in primary and secondary motility disorders and are considered a neuropathic feature, because of their presence in patients with autonomic neuropathy (Stanghellini et al 1987; Camilleri & Fealey 1990). The longer the duration of a burst, the more likely that it indicates an abnormality (Stanghellini et al 1987; Husebye et al 1995).

Giant migrating contractions (GMC)

GMC are contractions of prolonged duration amounting to 15–20 sec and of high amplitude (> 30 mmHg). GMC propagate over long distances and are highly propulsive, squeezing the contents out of the bowel either orally or aborally, depending on the direction they propagate. GMC with oral spread are usually called retrograde GMC and this pattern, which empties intestinal contents into the stomach, precedes spontaneous – but not self-induced – vomiting. Aboral and retrograde GMC empty bowel contents rapidly into the cecum and the stomach respectively, suggesting that they defend the gut by removing potentially harmful toxic and infectious agents.

Reflex control of bowel motility

The intrinsic nerve plexuses of the gut wall are known collectively as the enteric nervous system (ENS). The ENS is the only compartment of the nervous system outside the central nervous system (CNS) that exhibits independent reflex activity, which is why it is considered to have brain-like functions as 'the little brain in the gut' (Wood 1984). Neural control of gut motility is the combined effect of local enteric reflexes, intestinointestinal inhibitory reflexes, reflexes initiated beyond the small bowel (e.g. peritoneum, rectum, etc.) and perturbation and reflexes involving the CNS.

The peristaltic reflex results in contraction oral to and relaxation aboral to an appropriate intraluminal stimulus. This reflex also involves coordination between the circular and longitudinal muscle layer and, since it persists in extrinsically denervated bowel, is a function of the enteric nervous system. Distension of small bowel segments inhibits adjacent segments; sympathetic fibers projecting through prevertebral ganglia mediate these inhibitory intestinointestinal reflexes and extensive distension can paralyze the entire bowel through these neural pathways. Reflex inhibition of proximal small bowel motility by rectal distension (Youle & Read 1984) demonstrates modulation by a distant segment in the GI tract.

Two physiological mechanisms illustrate the functional interdependence of different regions of the small bowel. The arrival of nutrients into proximal small bowel stimulates propulsive ileal motility that serves to empty the ileum (Read et al 1985; Trotman & Price 1986) and the consequent cecal filling may evoke high-amplitude propagated contractions in the colon. Conversely, the ileum is more sensitive than jejunum to luminal stimuli and the ileal infusion of lipids inhibits both gastric emptying and motility of proximal small bowel more than infusion into jejunum (Spiller et al 1984): this mechanism is known as 'the ileal brake'.

Modulation by CNS

Conscious and unconscious brain activity can modulate small bowel motility and meal intake, stress and sleep are associated with CNS modulations of bowel motility.

Stress and small bowel motility

The effects of stress on gastrointestinal function are part of universal experience, but controlled studies are required to demonstrate regional effects. Controlled studies of the effects of stress in laboratory settings utilize two different categories of stressor: mental stress, usually in the form of problem solving or antagonistic interrogation, and somatic stress, usually as painful stimuli. These two types of stress are mediated through different pathways and may have dissimilar effects. Published studies of small bowel motility during stress are difficult to interpret because of the variety of stressors and protocols that have been used. It has been clearly shown that mental stress reduces the recurrence rate of phase III of MMC (McRae et al 1982; Valori et al 1986; Holtmann & Enck 1989), but conflicting results have been reported for the influence of stress on phase II activity. Increased phase II activity seems to be the prevailing response to the experimental stressors most commonly used (Kumar & Wingate 1985; Valori et al 1986).

Sleep and small bowel motility

Reduced CNS arousal during sleep is associated with a marked increase of phase I of MMC at the expense of phase II (Kumar et al 1990). Less prominent features of sleep modulation include a slightly shorter MMC period and slower aboral migration of phase III (Kumar et al 1986). By acute reversal of the sleep cycle Kumar et al (1990) showed that it is wakefulness rather than diurnal phase that is responsible for this modulation. The MMC and rapid eye movement (REM) sleep cycles are physiological renewal processes with a similar periodicity, but they do not coincide (Kumar et al 1990); it seems that the ENS – the gut brain – operates independently of the CNS in this respect. Recent data, however, have indicated an association between REM sleep and phase III of MMC.

The early return of MMCs after a meal taken shortly before sleep compared with an earlier meal cycle (Kumar et al 1989) has been interpreted as showing that the reduced vagal influence during sleep allows MMC to recur in spite of continuing local stimulation by nutrients; in that study, markedly increased phase II activity was seen during subsequent nocturnal MMCs. Postprandial GI peptide release seems to be similar during day and night (Soffer et al 1997), indicating that sleep modulation of fed and fasting small bowel motility is neurally rather than humorally mediated.

Sleep data show that CNS modulation is of particular importance for initiation of phase II activity. Hence, the MMC pattern as recorded during sleep reflects more selectively the enteric component of the MMC, whereas diurnal recordings during fasting also include modulation by the CNS.

SMALL BOWEL TRANSIT AND FLOW

Aboral transport in the small bowel occurs by intermittent, rapid flow pulses moving boluses of chyme in a manner resembling objects on a conveyer belt. This peristaltic type of flow differs from the continuous hydrostatic flow of the blood circulation. In the GI tract countless small pumps, coupled in series along the bowel, accomplish the movements. Peristaltic contractions are propulsive; segmenting contractions, which are transient and non-propagated, serve to separate the luminal contents into discrete boluses.

Qualitative information regarding transit has been obtained with combined manometry and radiology (Vantrappen et al 1977). During phase I, transport is limited. During phase II both segmenting and peristaltic contractions are seen and in late phase II, peristaltic contractions predominate. The peristaltic contractions of phase III remove the remnants of a meal and secretions during fasting (Read et al 1984) and seem to act as a barrier to reflux (Vantrappen et al 1977). During the postprandial state a different pattern of transit is observed. After nutrients enter the small bowel, transit is at first rapid and chyme is spread along the bowel; it then slows down during digestion (Johansson & Ekelund 1976), which favors absorption by increasing contact time with the absorptive surface.

Quantitative information regarding flow obtained using a perfusion/aspiration technique (Kerlin et al 1982) showed that during fasting about 50% of flow occurs in relation to the progression of phase III of MMC, with phase II accounting for about 30–40% . Fasting flow rates fluctuated between 0 and 1.5 ml/min. Postprandial flow rate ranged from 1 ml/min to peaks of 7 ml/min that recurred at intervals of 1.5 to 2 h.

Recently, electrical impedance has been used to detect liquid boluses passing multiple pairs of tube-mounted electrodes (Nguyen et al 1995). This technique demonstrated bolus transport events over short distances in the absence of lumen-occlusive contractions, suggesting that hydrostatic as well as pulsatile flow mechanics operate in the small bowel.

SECRETION AND ABSORPTION

Secretion and absorption fluctuate in synchrony with the MMC pattern during fasting. Bile and pancreatic secretion peak towards the end of phase II, as does net intestinal chloride secretion (Vantrappen et al 1979; Sjovall et al 1990). Similar fluctuations are found for absorption, which peaks during phase I (Sjovall et al 1990). These observations emphasize the integrated control of enteric functions by ENS.

Interestingly, pancreatic enzyme secretion continues to cycle during the postprandial period (Holtmann et al 1996), as does intestinal flow (Kerlin et al 1982). Although the MMC pattern appears to be interrupted by a meal, the precise relationship between postprandial motility and the MMC is not fully understood and the postprandial motility response was recently shown to depend on the phase of MMC in which the meal was taken (Medhus et al 1995). The ENS program that generates coordinated cyclic variations of enteric functions during fasting may continue during the postprandial period, but, in manometric recordings, is concealed by the heterogeneity of food-stimulated contractions.

METHODS FOR THE STUDY OF SMALL BOWEL PHYSIOLOGY

Motor activity

Manometry remains the 'gold standard' for clinical testing, because phasic contractions are generally lumen occlusive in the small bowel and can be reliably detected by intraluminal pressure measurements. Transit tests are more convenient, but they are time consuming and do not provide the same detailed and direct information about the timing and location of events.

Small bowel manometry

Most data on small bowel motility disorders have been obtained using stationary techniques with external transducers and water-perfused tubes (Anuras 1992; Camilleri 1993b), and abnormal patterns of motility detected with this technique have been described (Stanghellini et al 1987). The replacement of perfused tube systems with electronic intraluminal pressure sensors, initially radiotelemetry (Thompson et al 1980) and subsequently miniature strain gauge transducers with data acquisition in digital solid-state memory devices (Husebye et al 1990; Lindberg et al 1990), has enabled ambulatory recording over prolonged periods. At the same time, computer technology has simplified the processing of data recorded during stationary and ambulatory manometry; computer analysis is not only labor saving but decreases bias and errors in interpretation (Benson et al 1993).

Intraluminal pressure sensors detect changes in intraabdominal pressure due to gross body movements, including coughing and Valsalva maneuvers; these pressure changes are greater than the pressures generated by the gut smooth muscle. Because they are unwanted and tend to obscure patterns of gut motility, they are commonly described as 'artefacts', although they are all too real.

Technique

Pressure sensors For recognition of the motility patterns of upper small bowel, at least three recording sites 15 cm apart are recommended, with one recording site at the ligament of Treitz. This recording site should be used to determine the features of the MMC, as phase III occurs most frequently at this level (Kellow et al 1986) and the location is anatomically defined. The configuration of the sensors in the recording catheter otherwise depends on the purpose of the study; the MMC is optimally detected with recording sites about 15 cm apart, whereas the spatial spread of single contractions is best defined in the proximal jejunum by a recording segment of 10 cm with recording sites 2–2.5 cm apart. In water-perfused systems, eight recording sites are often used, but simultaneous recordings from 21 sites have been reported. In ambulatory manometry, six sensors are at present the technical compromise, but this may change with advances in technology.

Limitations of stationary techniques Patients are restricted to the immediate vicinity of the recording equipment, which for practical purposes precludes long-term and nocturnal recordings. Perfused tubes are wider in diameter, and therefore less comfortable, than the thin flexible catheters used in ambulatory manometry. In addition, the volume of water delivered by perfusion may contribute to luminal stimulation if multiple channels are used and in particular if the duration of recording is extended.

Limitations of ambulatory techniques   A high ratio of artefacts to contractions because of body movements during ambulant recording hampers recognition of contractile events during diurnal phase II and postprandial motility, because irregular contractions are particularly difficult to distinguish from artefacts; during normal sleep, this is less of a problem. The catheters used for ambulatory studies are expensive and fragile and their running costs are still high. Incorporation of more than six sensors in a catheter increases the fragility of the system and the risk of sensor failure. Ambulant techniques are unreliable for antropyloric manometry because of the difficulty of maintaining sensors in position over long periods of time in the terminal antrum and pylorus, where contractions are lumen occlusive.

Stationary short-term or ambulatory long-term manometry?

The answer to this question depends upon whether the examination is being performed to (i) test the integrity of enteric neuromuscular function, (ii) assess the effect of CNS perturbation through extrinsic neural and humoral pathways or (iii) test the motor response to food.

Testing the integrity of enteric neuromuscular function   When the aim of the study is to detect enteric dysfunction, nocturnal manometry is advantageous, because CNS perturbation is at a minimum during the night and the ENS program is dominant (Kumar et al 1990). Abnormal increases in the frequency of contractions are more easily detected during nocturnal fasting, when motor quiescence (phase I) normally predominates. It has been shown that a normal nocturnal MMC pattern is a reliable indicator of normal intestinal microflora, whereas an impaired MMC pattern is associated with Gram-negative colonization (Husebye et al 1995).

Because of the intrinsic variability of the MMC, prolonged recordings during fasting are required to detect and quantify MMCs reliably (Thompson et al 1980; Husebye et al 1990; Husebye et al 1995). If recording is restricted to 3–4 h during diurnal fasting, MMCs may not be detected at all, even in some healthy subjects. Prolonged and therefore ambulant manometry is thus advantageous in this context.

During ambulatory manometry, the timing and content of the evening meal should be adjusted to avoid interference between postprandial and fasting motility during nocturnal recording. A caloric content of at least 1500 kJ is sufficient to initiate a consistent postprandial response in man (Ouyang et al 1989; Soffer & Adrian 1992). After a mixed meal of 1700 kJ at 6 p.m., a typical nocturnal MMC pattern was observed during the night (Husebye et al 1990) and the meal was well tolerated by most patients with severe dysfunction (Husebye et al 1995). When a slightly larger meal of 2200 kJ was administered between 6 and 7 p.m., phase II dominated the first nocturnal MMC cycle (Kumar et al 1989). A meal eaten 15 min before going to bed resulted in persistent phase II activity during most nocturnal MMC cycles (Kumar et al 1989). Thus, a meal containing between 1500 and 2000 kJ can be administered not later than 7 p.m. without interfering significantly with the nocturnal MMC pattern.

Testing CNS perturbation of enteric neuromuscular function Predominant cluster activity in IBS patients (Kellow & Phillips 1987), alterations in MMC pattern due to stress (Valori et al 1986) and alterations in MMC patterns in subgroups of IBS patients are confined to the waking state. Diurnal recording is therefore needed to study these features. Because the restrictions imposed by immobility are, per se, stressful, ambulant manometry may be preferable to stationary manometry. In the detailed assessment of contraction patterns, particular attention should be paid to stimulation by luminal perfusion, nutrients and beverages and to the effect of age.

Testing the motor response to food Meals are normally eaten in the waking state; postprandial motility should also be recorded during wakefulness, because vagally and hormonally mediated brain–gut interactions contribute significantly to this pattern of motility. A semirecumbent or comfortable sitting position after a meal helps to reduce body movement artefacts; these are particularly difficult to distinguish from contractions during postprandial motility and stationary manometry has advantages here. This does not inevitably dictate a perfused tube system; subjects intubated with an ambulant system can be required to sit quietly after a meal.

Postprandial motility is quantified by contractile frequency and amplitude or by a motility index combining the two for defined time periods (Camilleri et al 1985). Propagation analysis of single contractions is more complicated and has not yet been validated for clinical use. Motility should be recorded for at least 2 h after meal intake to judge whether a significant response is elicited.

Intestinal manometry: summary

- Ambulatory manometry, with solid-state systems, is best suited to nocturnal recordings that allow the MMC pattern to be identified and quantified reliably. This approach seems to be superior for detecting enteric dysmotility.
- Postprandial motility should be recorded during the day with the subject at rest; stationary recording is appropriate. Either water-perfused or solid-state systems can be used, but the former allows more sensing points and is superior in the detection of antral and pyloric motor activity.
- The effects of CNS perturbation on small bowel motility require observation during diurnal fasting; ambulant systems are probably less stressful.
- Opinions on appropriate methods and protocols are convergent, but standardization has not yet been achieved as has already happened with the study of the esophagus.

Transit

Scintigraphy remains the standard for small bowel transit studies, but the hydrogen breath test is also useful for studies of physiology and specific problems in clinical pathophysiology.

Scintigraphy

The problem with measuring small bowel transit using scintigraphy is that 'regions of interest' within the small bowel cannot be clearly identified for the quantification of transit from serial images. The stomach and cecum can be clearly identified and this has led to the use of subtraction techniques; the time taken for small bowel transit is inferred from the interval between the meal leaving the stomach and arriving in the cecum. Single and dual isotope techniques have been used (Malagelada et al 1984), with labeling of the liquid and solid phase by ^{99m}technetium ^{111} or ^{113}indium, or ^{67}gallium. The time taken for small bowel transit has usually been estimated as the difference between the half-emptying time of the stomach and the half-filling time of the cecum. A more accurate approach, however, is to use the technique of deconvoluting the profiles for gastric emptying and colonic filling to obtain a spectrum of transit times and then to calculate the mean value; with this technique, there is no discrimination between transit of liquids and solids. Transit times range from 1.5 to 6 h in healthy subjects after a mixed meal (Malagelada et al 1984). This reflects the limitations in clinical use; only marked acceleration or delay can be detected, which is usually found only in patients with volume diarrhea or intestinal pseudoobstruction.

The hydrogen breath test

The measurement of breath hydrogen to detect a rise in colonic hydrogen production from ingested non-absorbable carbohydrates is, in principle, an attractive proposition because it is non-invasive and detects the transit of a quasiphysiological substance. But, in practice, studies of small bowel transit time have demonstrated great variability both within and between individuals. When the hydrogen breath test was performed under fasting conditions, using 10 ml lactulose, the coefficient of variation amounted to 18%. Di Lorenzo et al (1991) have recently shown that variations under fasting conditions are partly accounted for by the phase of MMC at the time that the test solution is administered.

With a lactose-containing meal the coefficient of variation is reduced to 4% (Staniforth & Rose 1989), but scintigraphic studies have revealed a substantial intraindividual variability for small bowel transit after meals, with a correlation coefficient of 0.43 only, for tests on different days (Argenyi et al 1995). This difference between the hydrogen breath test and scintigraphy may simply reflect that the former measures arrival of the head of the carbohydrate load in the cecum, whereas the latter is perhaps more related to the transit of the bulk of the meal.

The problem with the breath hydrogen test is its dependence on (a) the absence of small bowel bacterial overgrowth and (b) the presence of hydrogen-producing bacteria in the colon; even in healthy subjects, the latter condition is not invariably met. The hydrogen breath test is not reliable in the presence of bacterial overgrowth, which may be a factor in functional disorders, and a large discrepancy in calculated transit between normal scintigraphy and an early hydrogen peak may indicate bacterial overgrowth.

Limitations of transit studies

In theory, transit should be the most clinically relevant of all functional measurements, since it is probably disordered transit that is the clinically important consequence of functional disorders. But there is a lack of clarity about what is being measured in transit studies that remains to be resolved. Arguments about whether it is the transit of the 'head of the meal' or the 'bulk of the meal' ignore the inconvenient fact that most of the luminal contents of the small bowel are absorbed during transit and never reach the ileum. The existing techniques document the arrival of material in the cecum, but it is not possible to extrapolate the fate of non-absorbed solutes or solids with the kinetics of transit of absorbable substances through the different regions of the small bowel.

Absorption and secretion

Clinical tests for absorption and secretion have been validated for various organic gastrointestinal diseases, such as malabsorption, but they do not provide useful information in the diagnosis and evaluation of functional disorders and will not be described here. There is one exception to this, which is the measurement of total stool output. In IBS, measurement of stool output can help to resolve the occasional confusion between frequent – but often barely productive and sometimes unproductive – calls to stool and true diarrhea.

EVIDENCE FOR SMALL BOWEL DYSMOTILITY IN FUNCTIONAL DISORDERS

The early concept of IBS as a motility disorder of the gut focused primarily on the colon. Subsequently, it became apparent that small bowel function may be altered in IBS patients and the idea of a more global GI motility disorder emerged (Horowitz & Farrar 1962). Evidence for alterations in patterns of motility and transit of small bowel in patients with functional dyspepsia and IBS accumulates but controversy remains.

Functional dyspepsia

The evidence for motility disturbances in the small bowel in functional dyspepsia is conflicting; this is almost certainly due to differing criteria for patient selection and different study protocols.

For example, about 30% of the patients included by Kerlin (1989) and Stanghellini et al (1992) also fulfilled the criteria for IBS. Malagelada et al (1985) also included patients with organic diseases. Labo et al (1990) and Jebbink et al (1995) studied only patients with delayed gastric emptying, whereas Bassotti et al (1990) excluded such patients. In the studies where absence of MMCs was reported (Labo et al 1990; Bassotti et al 1990; Stanghellini et al 1992) the recording period often varied among patients and was usually too short to establish the finding as abnormal (Husebye et al 1990; Camilleri 1993a). The differences between groups, however, indicate that MMC abnormalities occur in some patients with functional dyspepsia. Absence of MMCs was most frequent in the study of Labo et al (1990) where delayed gastric emptying was the diagnostic criterion. The postprandial motility response is usually normal in patients with functional dyspepsia, but some non-specific changes have been reported (Kerlin 1989; Bassotti et al 1990; Stanghellini et al 1992; Jebbink et al 1995). Normal patterns of motility are preserved in the majority of patients with functional dyspepsia. Impaired MMC activity in some patients indicates that enteric dysmotility may contribute to the problem by interfering with gastric emptying (Waldron et al 1991). Overall, the presence of abnormal contraction patterns has not been established in functional dyspepsia.

Sleep disturbances in functional dyspepsia were studied by David et al (1994) using questionnaires and the prevalence in patients was 90% compared with 10% in controls. This was accompanied by increased nocturnal phase II activity and reduced phase III activity, indicating increased perturbation of small bowel motility during sleep in functional dyspepsia, possibly due to altered sleep states. Combined manometry and polysomnography is required to confirm this hypothesis.

Irritable bowel syndrome

Small bowel motor functions in IBS patients have been studied by manometry and by transit tests. The data are conflicting; this is attributable to variations in methodology and protocols and also to differing bias in patient selection. In particular, the assumption that 'diarrhea-predominant' and 'constipation-predominant' patients are suffering from the same disorder is open to question, as is the undoubted overlap between 'constipation-predominant' IBS and simple constipation. Although all patients that have been studied are said to have satisfied the current criteria for the diagnosis of IBS, patient samples have differed. Kellow et al (1990, 1991, 1992, Kellow & Phillips 1987) had equal numbers from the two IBS subsets, whereas Gorard et al (1994, 1995) and Schmidt et al (1996) studied only 'diarrhea-predominant' IBS.

Manometry

Patients with diarrhea-predominant IBS have a higher frequency of MMCs than patients with constipation predominance, but all are within the normal population distribution. This was demonstrated in all three studies addressing the issue. In two studies (Kellow et al, 1990, Kellow & Phillips 1987), a reduced MMC period in the diarrhoea-predominant subgroup contributed to the difference, whereas prolonged MMC period in the constipated group was detected in the third study (Kellow et al 1992). In contrast, the studies by Gorard et al (1994, 1995) and Schmidt et al (1996), limited to diarrhea-predominant IBS patients, showed similar MMC periodicity for patients and controls alike. The study by Schmidt et al (1996) is of particular interest because of the sample size of 35 IBS patients and 50 controls. The balance of the evidence suggests that MMC periodicity in IBS, and in IBS subsets, is within the normal range.

There is evidence (Kellow et al 1990) for a shorter postprandial period in IBS patients, and an increased motility index after a meal has been demonstrated for both subgroups of IBS (Kellow et al 1988). This effect was most pronounced in the ileum and for diarrhea-predominant patients (Kellow et al 1988), in whom a higher percentage of aborally propagated contractions postprandially has also been reported by Schmidt et al (1996).

An increased prevalence of discrete clustered contractions (DCC) in IBS patients compared with controls has been reported in four published studies; three other studies did not find such a difference. None of these studies can be regarded as conclusive and the discrepant findings are attributable to differences in patient selection, study protocols and data analysis. The question remains to be conclusively resolved, but the balance of evidence – if only because of the greater number of patients studied in whom excess DCC have been reported – suggests that DCC *do* occur more frequently in IBS.

Cann et al (1983a) studied 61 IBS patients and 53 healthy volunteers and found that small bowel transit time was significantly reduced (79%) in patients with diarrhea and significantly prolonged (129%) in patients with constipation-predominant IBS. Patients with pain and bloating exhibited transit rates similar to the constipated patients. The hydrogen breath test has limitations (Read et al 1985), but the use of a solid meal containing baked beans and of careful criteria to define the arrival of the meal in cecum (Cann et al 1983a) avoided some of these pitfalls. Scintigraphy demonstrated accelerated small bowel transit in diarrhea-predominant IBS patients (Jian et al 1984), as did the breath test in another study (Gorard et al 1994). But, although differences between the subgroups were highly statistically significant in the study of Cann et al (1983a), all patients had transit times within the range of healthy controls. The alterations in transit rate are thus modest and cannot be used clinically for the diagnosis of IBS; this is a typical finding in motility studies in IBS patients.

Focusing on the ileum, scintigraphy quantifying ileocecal movement of chyme showed that 10 patients with IBS and bloating had delayed emptying of the ileum when compared with eight healthy controls (Trotman & Price 1986). The almost entire separation of the data for the study groups was surprising and might indicate that more precise targeting was useful. A recent study, however, produced contrary data; scintigraphically determined ileocecal transit of an isotope from a delayed-release capsule during fasting was more rapid in 20 IBS patients, including 16 with constipation-predominant IBS and bloating, than in controls (Hutchinson et al 1995). Although the alterations in transit fall within the normal range, rapid ileocecal transit may contribute to the pathogenesis of diarrhea in a subset of IBS patients.

A relationship between transit and stress (Cann et al 1983b) underlines the close connections between CNS and ENS in regulation of small bowel motility. If, as asserted by Whitehead et al (1988), the prevalence of psychiatric disturbances is increased in this population, CNS modulation may be involved in the pathogenesis of symptoms in IBS by interfering with small bowel motility. Evidence for exaggerated response to stress was provided by Kumar & Wingate (1985), who showed that IBS patients were more prone to suppression of phase III activity during stress than were healthy controls and patients with inflammatory bowel disease. Evidence for an exaggerated small bowel motility response in IBS patients has also been provided for other challenges including cholecystokinin octapeptide, a high fatty meal and ileal distension (Kellow et al 1988). In this context, it is perhaps relevant that all the small bowel motility and transit changes that have been reported in IBS have been in the waking state; in IBS, abnormal small bowel motor function has only been documented during CNS arousal.

SIGNIFICANCE OF DYSMOTILITY IN FUNCTIONAL DISORDERS

Functional dyspepsia

The majority of studies over the years report no significant differences of small bowel motility in patients with functional dyspepsia. Within this population, however, there are some patients with abnormal essential patterns of motility (MMC and postprandial pattern) and increased prevalence of clustered contractions. These changes may result from altered CNS modulation or from enteric dysfunction. Moreover, they may contribute to the delay of gastric emptying and small bowel transit seen in about 40% (Labo et al 1990; Jebbink et al 1995) and 60% (Waldron et al 1991) of patients with functional dyspepsia. However, the clinical relevance of this possible association is dubious because mild to moderate delays of gastric emptying and small bowel transit do not necessarily provoke symptoms.

Irritable bowel syndrome

Overall, no consistent relationship has been established between motility patterns and symptoms in IBS patients with functional dyspepsia or IBS. In single patients, however, coincidence has been observed. Kellow et al (1991) carefully addressed the perception of physiological small bowel motility; the transit of phase III of the MMC through the duodenum gave rise to abdominal sensations in some healthy controls, but more frequently and intensively in IBS patients. Kumar & Wingate (1985) showed a relationship between clustered contractions and symptoms in IBS. Despite these studies, it would be foolish to conclude that the proximal small bowel is the origin of the symptoms of the irritable bowel; the cardinal symptom of IBS is, after all, disturbed defecation. A more reasonable conclusion is that IBS is a panenteric disorder.

CONCLUSION

In recent years, there have been considerable advances in our understanding of small bowel physiology. In particular, there is now a reasonably clear picture of the enteric motor events that are controlled by the enteric nervous system and the way in which these are modulated by the central nervous system and there are clearly inferences to be drawn about the relationship between perturbations of these two nervous systems and the manifestations of functional bowel disorders. But there is at present insufficient evidence to translate these hypotheses into precise descriptions of pathophysiology and the technologies and protocols that might allow this knowledge to be used for the diagnosis and management of functional disorders still lack precision. There is, however, much promise for the not so distant future.

REFERENCES

Anuras S 1992 Motility disorders of the gastrointestinal tract. Raven Press, New York

Argenyi EE, Soffer EE, Madsen MT, Berbaum KS, Walkner WO 1995 Scintigraphic evaluation of small bowel transit in healthy subjects: inter- and intrasubject variability. American Journal of Gastroenterology 90: 938–942

Bassotti G, Pelli M A, Morelli A 1990 Duodenojejunal motor activity in patients with chronic dyspeptic symptoms. Journal of Clinical Gastroenterology 12: 17–21

Benson MJ, Castillo FD, Wingate DL, Demetrakopoulos J, Spyrou NM 1993 The computer as referee in the analysis of human small bowel motility. American Journal of Physiology 264: G645–G654

Bisset WM, Wat JB, Rivers RPA, Milla PJ 1988 Ontogeny of fasting small intestinal motor activity in the human infant. Gut 33: 1331–1337

Camilleri M 1989 Jejunal manometry in distal subacute mechanical obstruction: significance of prolonged simultaneous contractions. Gut 30: 468–475

Camilleri M 1993a Study of human gastroduodenojejunal motility. Digestive Diseases and Sciences 38: 785–794

Camilleri M 1993b Perfused tube manometry. In: Kumar D, Wingate D L (eds) An illustrated guide to gastrointestinal motility. Churchill Livingstone, Edinburgh, pp 183–199

Camilleri M, Fealey RD 1990 Idiopathic autonomic denervation in eight patients presenting with functional gastrointestinal disease. Digestive Diseases and Sciences 35: 609–616

Camilleri M, Malagelada JR, Stanghellini V, Fealey RD, Sheps SG 1985 Gastrointestinal motility disturbancies in patients with orthostatic hypotension. Gastroenterology 88: 1852–1859

Cann PA, Read NW, Brown C, Hobson N, Holdsworth CD 1983a Irritable bowel syndrome: relationship of disorders in the transit of a single solid meal to symptom patterns. Gut 24: 405–411

Cann P A, Read NW, Cammack J et al 1983b Psychological stress and the passage of a standard meal through the stomach and the small intestine in man. Gut 24: 236–240

Code CF, Schlegel JF 1974 The gastrointestinal housekeeper. Motor correlates of the interdigestive myoelectric complex of the dog. Proceedings from the Fourth International Symposium on Gastro-Intestinal Motility. Mitchell Press Ltd, Vancouver, pp 631–634

Cook IJ, van Eeden A, Collins SM 1987 Patients with irritable bowel syndrome have greater pain tolerance than normal subjects. Gastroenterology 93: 727–733

David D, Mertz H, Fefer L et al 1994 Sleep and duodenal motor activity in patients with severe non-ulcer dyspepsia. Gut 35: 916–925

Di Lorenzo C, Dooley CP, Valenzula JE 1991 Role of fasting gastrointestinal motility in the variability of gastrointestinal transit time assessed by hydrogen breath test. Gut 32: 1127–1130

Di Lorenzo C, Flores AF, Buie T, Hyman PE 1995 Intestinal motility and jejunal feeding in children with chronic intestinal pseudo-obstruction. Gastroenterology 108: 1379–1385

Drossman DA, Thompson WG, Talley NJ, Funch-Jensen P, Janssens J, Whitehead W E 1990 Identification of sub-groups of functional gastrointestinal disorders. Gastroenterology 3: 159–172

Gorard DA, Libby GW, Farthing MJG 1994 Ambulatory small intestinal motility in 'diarrhoea' predominant irritable bowel syndrome. Gut 35: 203–210

Gorard DA, Libby GW, Farthing MJG 1995 Effect of a tricyclic antidepressant on small intestinal motility in health and diarrhea-predominant irritable bowel syndrome. Digestive Diseases and Sciences 40: 86–95

Hall KE, El-Sharkawy TY, Diamant N E 1986 Vagal control of canine postprandial upper gastrointestinal motility. American Journal of Physiology 250: G501–G510

Heaton KW, Radvan J, Cripps H, Mountford RA, Braddon FEM, Hughes AO 1992 Defecation frequency and timing, and stool form in the general population: a prospective study. Gut 33: 818–824

Holtmann G, Enck P 1989 Differential effects of acute mental stress on gastric acid, pancreatic enzyme secretion and gastroduodenal motility. Digestive Diseases and Sciences 34: 1701–1707

Holtmann G, Kelly DG, DiMagno EP 1996 Nutrients and cyclic interdigestive pancreatic enzyme secretion in humans. Gut 38: 920–924

Horowitz L, Farrar JT 1962 Intraluminal small intestinal pressures in normal patients and in patients with functional gastrointestinal disorders. Gastroenterology 42(4): 455–464

Husebye E, Engedal K 1992 The patterns of motility are maintained in the human small intestine throughout the process of aging. Scandinavian Journal of Gastroenterology 27: 397–404

Husebye E, Sklar V, Aalen OO, Osnes M 1990 Digital ambulatory manometry of the small intestine in healthy adults: Estimates of the variation within and between individuals and statistical management of incomplete MMC periods. Digestive Diseases and Sciences 35: 1057–1065

Husebye E, Hellstrom PM, Midtvedt T 1994 The intestinal microflora stimulates myoelectric activity of rat small intestine by promoting cyclic initiation and aboral propagation of the migrating myoelectric complex. Digestive Diseases and Sciences 39: 946–956

Husebye E, Skar V, Haverstad T, Iversen T, Melby K 1995 Abnormal intestinal motor patterns explain enteric colonisation with Gram negative bacilli in late radiation enteropathy. Gastroenterology 109: 1078–1089

Hutchinson R, Notghi A, Smith NB, Harding LK, Kumar D 1995 Scintigraphic measurement of ileocaecal transit in irritable bowel syndrome and chronic idiopathic constipation. Gut 36: 585–589

Hyman PE, Di Lorenzo C, McAdams L, Flores AF, Tomomasa T, Garvey TQ 1993 Predicting the clinical response to cisapride in children with chronic intestinal pseudo-obstruction. American Journal of Gastroenterology 88: 832–836

Jebbink HJA, van Berge-Henegouwen GP, Bruijs PPM, Akkermans LMA, Smout AJPM 1995 Gastric myoelectrical activity and gastrointestinal motility in patients with functional dyspepsia. European Journal of Clinical Investigation 25: 429–437

Jian R, Najean Y, Bernier JJ 1984 Measurement of intestinal progression of a meal and its residues in normal subjects and patients with functional diarrhoea by a dual isotope technique. Gut 25: 728–731

Johansson C, Ekelund K 1976 Relation between body weight and the gastric and intestinal handling of an oral caloric load. Gut 17: 456–462

Jones R, Lydeard S 1992 Irritable bowel syndrome in the general population. British Medical Journal 304: 87–90

Kamath PS, Hoepfner MT, Phillips S F 1987 Short chain fatty acids stimulate motility of the canine ileum. American Journal of Physiology 253: G427–G433

Kang JY, Tay HH, Guan R 1992 Chronic upper abdominal pain: site and radiation in various structural and functional disorders and the effect of various foods. Gut 33: 743–748

Kellow JE, Phillips S 1987 Altered small bowel motility in irritable bowel syndrome is correlated with symptoms. Gastroenterology 92: 1885–1893

Kellow JE, Borody S, Phillips S, Tucker RL, Haddad AC 1986 Human interdigestive motility: variations in patterns from esophagus to colon. Gastroenterology 98: 1208–1218

Kellow JE, Phillips S, Miller LJ, Zinsmeister AR 1988 Dysmotility of the small intestine in irritable bowel syndrome. Gut 29: 1236–1243

Kellow JE, Gill RC, Wingate DL 1990 Prolonged ambulant recordings of small bowel motility demonstrate abnormalities in the irritable bowel syndrome. Gastroenterology 98: 1208–1218

Kellow JE, Eckersley GM, Jones MP 1991 Enhanced perception of physiological intestinal motility in the irritable bowel syndrome. Gastroenterology 101: 1621–1627

Kellow JE, Eckersley FGM, Jones M 1992 Enteric and central contribution to intestinal dysmotility in irritable bowel syndrome. Digestive Diseases and Sciences 37 168–174

Kerlin P 1989 Postprandial antral hypomotility in patients with idiopathic nausea and vomiting. Gut 30: 54–59

Kerlin P, Zinsmeister A, Phillips S 1982 Relationship of motility to flow of contents in the human small intestine. Gastroenterology 82: 701–706

Kruis W, Azpiroz F, Phillips S 1985 Contractile patterns and transit of fluid in canine terminal ileum. American Journal of Physiology 249: G264–G270

Kumar D, Wingate DL 1985 The irritable bowel syndrome: a paroxysmal motor disorder. Lancet ii: 973–977

Kumar D, Wingate DL, Ruckebusch Y 1986 Circadian variation in the propagation velocity of the migrating motor complex. Gastroenterology 91: 926–930

Kumar D, Soffer EE, Wingate DL, Britto J, Das Gupta A, Mridha K 1989 Modulation of the duration of human postprandial motor activity by sleep. American Journal of Physiology 256: G851–G855

Kumar D, Idzikowski C, Wingate DL, Soffer EE, Thompson P, Siderfin C 1990 Relationship between enteric migrating motor complex and the sleep cycle. American Journal of Physiology 259: G983–G990

Labo G, Bortolotti M, Vezzadini P, Bonora G 1990 Interdigestive gastroduodenal motility and serum motilin levels in patients with idiopathic delay in gastric emptying. Gastroenterology 90: 20–26

Lindberg G, Iwarzon M, Stal P, Seensalu R 1990 Digital ambulatory monitoring of small-bowel motility. Scandinavian Journal of Gastroenterology 25: 216–224

Malagelada JR, Stanghellini V 1985 Manometric evaluation of functional upper gut symptoms. Gastroenterology 88: 1223–1231

Malagelada J-R, Robertson JS, Brown ML et al 1984 Intestinal transit of solid and liquid components of a meal in health. Gastroenterology 87: 1255–1263

McRae S, Younger K, Thompson DG, Wingate DL 1982 Sustained mental stress alters human jejunal motor activity. Gut 23: 404–409

Medhus A, Sandstad O, Bredesen J, Husebye E 1995 The migrating motor complex modulates intestinal motility response and rate of gastric emptying of caloric meals. Neurogastroenterology and Motility 7: 1–9

Nguyen HN, Silny J, Wyller S, Marschall HU, Rau G, Matern S 1995 Chyme transport patterns in human duodenum, determined by multiple intraluminal impedancometry. American Journal of Physiology 268: G700–G708

O'Donnell LJD, Virjee J, Heaton KW 1990 Detection of pseudodiarrhea by simple clinical assessment of intestinal transit rate. British Medical Journal 300: 439–440

Ouyang A, Sunshine AG, Reynolds JC 1989 Caloric content of a meal affects duration but not contractile pattern of duodenal motility in man. Digestive Diseases and Sciences 34: 528–536

Quigley EMM 1993 The effects of resection, restorative procedures and transplantation on intestinal motility. In: Kumar D, Wingate DL (eds) An illustrated guide to gastrointestinal motility. Churchill Livingstone, Edinburgh, pp 691–716

Read NW, Al-Janabi MN, Edwards CA, Barber DC 1984 Relationship between postprandial motor activity in the human small intestine and the gastrointestinal transit of food. Gastroenterology 86: 721–727

Read NW, Al-Janabi MN, Bates TE et al 1985 Interpretation of the breath hydrogen profile obtained after ingesting a solid meal containing unabsorbable carbohydrate. Gut 26: 834–842

Sandler RS, Drossman DA, Nathan HP, McKee DC 1984 Symptom complaints
    and health care seeking behavior in subjects with bowel dysfunction.
    Gastroenterology 87: 314–318
Schmidt T, Hackelsberger N, Widmer R, Meisel C, Pfeiffer A, Kaess H 1996
    Ambulatory 24–hours jejunal motility in diarrhea-
    predominant irritable bowel syndrome. Scandinavian Journal of
    Gastroenterology 31: 581–589
Sjovall H, Hagman I, Abrahamsson H 1990 Relationship between interdigestive
    duodenal motility and fluid transport in humans. American Journal of
    Physiology 259: G348–G354
Smith D, Waldron B, Campbell FC 1992 Response of migrating motor complex
    to variation of fasting intraluminal content. American Journal of Physiology
    263: G533–G537
Soffer EE, Adrian TE 1992 The effect of meal composition and sham feeding on
    duodenojejunal motility in humans. Digestive Diseases and Sciences 37:
    1009–1014
Soffer EE, Summers RW 1993 Ambulant manometry. In: Kumar D, Wingate DL
    (eds) An illustrated guide to gastrointestinal motility. Churchill Livingstone,
    Edinburgh, pp 200–210
Soffer EE, Adrian TE, Launspach J, Zimmerman B 1997 Meal induced secretion
    of gastrointestinal regulatory peptides is not affected by sleep.
    Neurogastroenterology and Motility 9: 1–3
Spiller RC, Trotman IF, Higgins BE et al 1984 The ileal brake – inhibition of
    jejunal motility after ileal fat perfusion in man. Gut 25: 365–374
Stanghellini V, Camilleri M, Malagelada JR 1987 Chronic idiopathic intestinal
    pseudo-obstruction: clinical and intestinal manometric findings. Gut 28: 5–12
Stanghellini V, Ghidini C, Maccarini MR, Paparo GF, Corinaldesi R, Barbara L
    1992 Fasting and postprandial gastrointestinal motility in ulcer and non-ulcer
    dyspepsia. Gut 33: 184–190
Staniforth DH, Rose D 1989 Statistical analysis of the lactulose/breath hydrogen
    test in the measurement of orocecal transit: its variability and predictive value
    in assessing drug action. Gut 30: 171–175
Steadman C, Kerlin P 1994 Response of the human intestine to high volume
    infusion. Gut 35: 641–645
Sullivan S N 1994 Functional abdominal bloating. Journal of Clinical
    Gastroenterology 19: 23–27
Summers R W, Anuras S, Green J 1983 Jejunal manometry patterns in health,
    partial intestinal obstruction, and pseudoobstruction. Gastroenterology 85:
    1290–1300
Switz DM 1976 What the gastroenterologist does all day. A survey of a state
    society's practice. Gastroenterology 70: 1048–1050
Thompson DG, Wingate DL, Archer L, Benson MJ, Green WJ, Hardy RJ 1980
    Normal patterns of human upper small bowel motor activity recorded by
    prolonged radiotelemetry. Gut 21: 500–506
Thompson DG, Ritchie HD, Wingate DL 1982 Pattern of small intestine motility
    in duodenal ulcer patients before and after vagotomy. Gut 23: 517–523
Trotman I F, Price CC 1986 Bloated irritable bowel syndrome defined by
    dynamic 99mTc brain scan. Lancet ii: 364–366
Valori RM, Kumar D, Wingate DL 1986 Effect of different types of stress and of
    'prokinetic' drugs on the control of the fasting motor complex in humans.
    Gastroenterology 90: 1890–1900
Vantrappen G, Janssens J, Hellemans J, Ghoos Y 1977 The interdigestive motor
    complex of normal subjects and patients with bacterial overgrowth of the
    small intestine. Journal of Clinical Investigation 59: 1158–1166
Vantrappen G, Peeters TL, Janssens J 1979 The secretory component of the
    interdigestive migrating motor complex in man. Scandinavian Journal of
    Gastroenterology 14: 663–667
Waldron B, Cullen PT, Kumar P et al 1991 Evidence for hypomotility in non-

ulcer dyspepsia: a prospective multifactorial study. Gut 32: 246–251

Whitehead WE, Bosmajian L, Zonderman AB, Costa PT jr, Schuster MM 1988 Symptoms of psychologic distress associated with irritable bowel syndrome: comparison of community and medical clinic samples. Gastroenterology 95: 709–714

Whitehead WE, Holtkotter B, Enck P et al 1990 Tolerance for rectosigmoid distension in irritable bowel syndrome. Gastroenterology 98: 1187–1192

Wood JD 1984 Enteric neurophysiology. American Journal of Physiology 247: G585–G598

Youle MS, Read NW 1984 Effect of painless rectal distension on the gastrointestinal transit of a solid meal. Digestive Diseases and Sciences 29: 902–906

Colon and anorectum: constipation, urgency, pain syndromes. Clinical physiology

IJ Cook

INTRODUCTION

The functions of the colon include prolonged storage of excreta by retarding aborad flow; facilitation of water, electrolyte and short chain fatty acid absorption; and effective voluntary evacuation when convenient and acceptable. Prior to defecation there is a central awareness of the need to defecate and if circumstances are appropriate, colonic evacuation is achieved by a combination of colonic and rectoanal reflexes. In the interim there is periodic to and fro motion together with short stepwise movements of colonic content which result in a slow, net aborad movement of content.

A range of symptoms, by virtue of their site and relationship to stooling habit, are attributed to colonic dysfunction. Constipation is clearly a 'colonic' symptom. Rectal urgency is a rectal symptom but in some instances may be due to deranged function proximal to the rectum resulting in rapid rectal filling. Less clearcut symptoms, such as pain, bloating, flatulence and 'gas', need not be ascribed to colonic dysfunction. Furthermore, IBS is likely to be a mixed disorder involving visceral hypersensitivity, enhanced intestino-intestinal reflexes and dysmotility, not only of the colon but of many regions of the gut.

This chapter will concentrate on the colon and will review the available data implicating sensorimotor dysfunction in the pathogenesis of common, functional 'colonic' symptoms. The reader will be aware that much of our knowledge of such mechanisms is incomplete. Hence, current opinion on pathophysiology of these syndromes remains largely speculative.

MEASUREMENT TECHNIQUES

Mass movements of colonic content were first identified radiologically at the turn of the century. Thirty years ago important observations relating pressure and flow were made using time-lapse cinefluoroscopy and combined manometry in the distal colon (Ritchie et al 1962). However, the utility of radiology as a means of studying colonic movements and transit has been limited by the hazards of radiation. Less invasive techniques are now available for the measurement of human colonic motility including transit studies, intraluminal manometry, myoelectrical recordings and measurement of colonic wall tone. The anorectum, due to its accessibility, has been studied more extensively using methods such as defecography, anorectal manometry and electromyography.

Measurement of colonic transit

Radiopaque marker studies

Marker studies actually measure total gut transit time, but because the colon residence time comprises the major proportion of total transit, it is accepted as a suitable estimate of colonic transit. Transit was first measured by tracking progress of ingested radiopaque markers of various shapes either given on one day or on three consecutive days followed by abdominal X-rays on specific days. This technique was further simplified necessitating only a single abdominal X-ray, thereby further limiting radiation exposure (Metcalf et al 1987).

Colonic scintigraphy

This technique delivers a low radiation dose to the patient and permits capture of unlimited numbers of images without additional radiation exposure. Technetium and indium are the most commonly used isotopes with half-lives of 6 h and 3 days respectively. A standard dose of ^{99m}Tc bound to a non-absorbed vehicle (DTPA) yields an effective total body dose equivalent to that received from a plain abdominal X-ray. Initial studies utilized a long nasoenteric tube to instil the isotope directly into the cecum as a single bolus (Krevsky et al 1986). Because the distal ileum empties periodically, not continuously (Camilleri et al 1989), simpler techniques utilizing oral administration of isotope have now been validated, further simplifying the test.

The colon can be divided into up to seven regions of interest and time–activity curves for each and the entire colon are calculated to determine regional emptying times. The progress of the geometric center of the isotope column can also be tracked against time (Krevsky et al 1986). The high resolution of this method also enables detection of individual movements as well as luminal capacitance and wall motion. More recently, a combination of scintigraphy and manometry is providing insight into the determinants of colonic propulsion.

Which test for colonic transit – radiopaque markers or scintigraphy?

The marker transit study remains a simple, inexpensive, non-invasive and very useful screening test in clinical practice but lacks the necessary resolution and temporal precision for detecting regional dysfunction demanded of research studies. Net aboral motion of colonic content is slow while component movements are a complex mix of brief antegrade and retrograde movements over short distances with infrequent sporadic mass movements over long distances (Cook et al 1990, Picon et al 1992).

Unlimited images are obtainable with scintigraphy which means discrete motor events are not likely to be missed and the technique is well suited to capture the minute-to-minute movements required for research studies. Scintigraphy also yields a precise measure of transit in any desired region of interest. It is more sensitive than a marker study in detecting accelerated transit in disorders such as IBS but this is not a clinically relevant application at present. Scintigraphy can be measured during stimulation of the colon by colonic prokinetic agents or irritants known to induce propulsive motor patterns. This approach may in the future identify regional colonic denervation. The author believes scintigraphy is a superior technique but the decision to use it instead of a marker study in the clinical setting will depend upon local availability of expertise and resources.

Colonic manometry

Recording techniques

The human colon imposes substantial technical demands in the measurement of motility in that it is a large and relatively inaccessible organ containing semisolid and solid fecal matter. These properties pose difficulties in the placement of recording catheters per rectum. Initial manometric recordings were localized to the rectosigmoid (Connell 1962, Ritchie et al 1962), but because of marked regional variations in type and quantity of motor patterns, rectosigmoid recordings are not at all representative of the whole colon (Cook et al 1990). Propulsive motor patterns and movements are infrequent and demonstrate both regional and diurnal variations. These considerations have lead to the advent of techniques capable of recording motor patterns along the entire colonic length for prolonged periods (Bassotti & Gaburri 1988).

Three types of manometric device have been widely used. Two of these have been adapted to ambulatory recordings: the radiotelemetry capsule and tube-mounted strain gauges (Soffer et al 1989). Perfusion manometry has been used for static recordings with catheters being placed per rectum after prior bowel preparation (Bassotti & Gaburri 1988, Furukawa et al 1994). While the radio pill can be used under truly physiological conditions, its major limitation is that it can only record from one site at any one time, making determination of migratory pressure patterns impossible. Miniaturized solid-state catheters, incorporating three transducers, have been passed transnasally into an unprepared colon in fully ambulant subjects (Soffer et al 1989). The major current limitation of solid-state ambulatory, colonic manometry is its high cost, catheter fragility and inability to record from the large number of closely spaced recording sites.

Long perfused catheters with multiple side holes can now be positioned, with the aid of a colonoscope, into the proximal colon (Bassotti & Gaburri 1988, Furukawa et al 1994). The major disadvantage of colonoscopic placement is the need for prior bowel preparation although the effect of bowel cleansing on some motor patterns may not be as great as was once believed (Lemann et al 1995). Emerging nasocolonic intubation techniques represent a promising advance in overcoming such obstacles (Lemann et al 1995) (Fig. 13.1). New miniaturized, extruded, Silastic catheters, incorporating a weighted balloon tip to assist passage, can be passed transnasally to the rectum in healthy subjects in 24–30 h. These catheters are soft, well tolerated for long periods and miniaturization has dramatically reduced the perfusion rate required for faithful recordings of colonic motor patterns (Omari et al 1994). The major advantage of perfusion manometry is that up to 16 closely spaced recording sites have now been achieved which has markedly improved the spatial resolution of motor patterns (Fig. 13.2).

Classification of colonic motor patterns

The apparent lack of propagating motor patterns in early manometric studies confined to the rectosigmoid (Connell 1962) made meaningful classification and analysis of human colonic motor

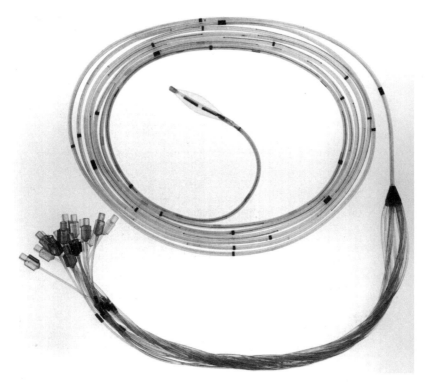

Fig. 13.1   Miniaturized, Silastic, multiport, perfused colonic manometry catheter (Dentsleeve, Bowden, Sth Australia). The 4.5 m long catheter has a diameter of 4 mm, enabling it to be passed nasoenterically. The weighted balloon tip facilitates passage through the small bowel and colon. With this catheter, recordings can be made at 16 colonic sites from the cecum to the rectum for 24 h.

patterns difficult. Activity was quantified by calculating the area under the pressure curve, yielding a 'motility index'. Prolonged multipoint myoelectrical and manometric recordings throughout the colon have identified more predictable, albeit infrequent, propulsive motor patterns (Bassotti & Gaburri 1988, Cook et al 1990). Two broad categories of motor pattern can be identified: propagating and non-propagating (Fig. 13.2).

Non-propagating activity

The predominant motor pattern throughout the human colon is non-propagating activity. It was termed 'segmenting activity' on the basis of radiological appearances and, at least in the distal colon, has been thought to retard rather than promote flow (Connell 1962). Non-propagating activity displays considerable

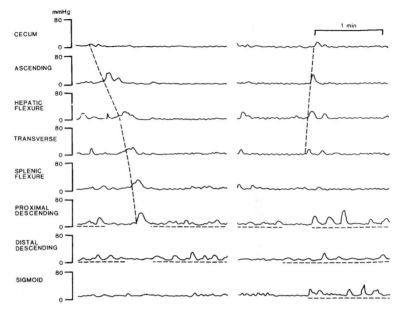

Fig. 13.2 Manometric tracing with recording sites spaced at 10 cm intervals from the cecum to the sigmoid colon in a healthy volunteer showing the major types of pressure patterns including non-propagating and antegrade and retrograde propagating pressure waves. The most prevalent pressure pattern is non-propagating, phasic on tonic pressure activity (underscored by dashed lines).

regional variation with the proportion of time occupied by it increasing with distance from the cecum (Cook et al 1990). Non-propagating activity increases after a meal (Cook et al 1990), decreases at night and increases sharply on early morning waking before breakfast, suggesting a modulatory influence from the CNS (Bassotti & Gaburri 1988, Furukawa et al 1994).

Propagating Activity

The distribution of propagating sequences (PSs) is the reverse of that seen for non-propagating activity in that PSs are more prevalent in the proximal colon and most originate in the cecum (Cook et al 1990) (Fig. 13.3). PSs can propagate antegradely or, less commonly, retrogradely. Antegrade PSs occur roughly every 30 min while retrograde PSs occur on average every 2 h. The distance propagated by PSs is regionally dependent. The average distance travelled by a PS originating in the cecum is twice that of a PS originating in the descending colon and only 4% of all PSs reach the rectum. The majority of these waves cease to propagate

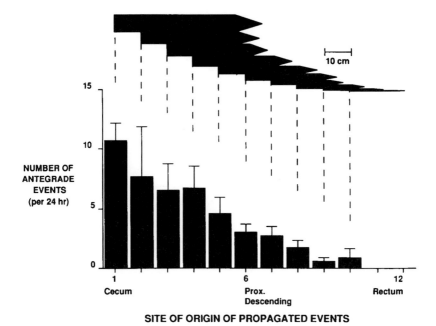

Fig. 13.3 Distribution and distance propagated by antegradely propagating pressure waves according to their site of origin in the healthy human colon. The bottom panel plots the number of propagating pressure waves that originate in each colonic region. The top panel shows the mean distance of antegrade propagation of waves. Note that propagating sequences originate more frequently in the proximal colon and, in most instances, do not propagate beyond the splenic flexure.

at the splenic flexure or proximal descending colon. PSs virtually disappear during sleep and are stimulated immediately with spontaneous or induced nocturnal arousal and following early morning waking (Furukawa et al 1994) (Fig. 13.4). Hence, central nervous system input is an important modulator of colonic PSs. Meals can induce PSs (Bassotti & Gaburri 1988) but the effect of eating on PSs is not as predictable as it is on non-propagating activity (Hammer & Phillips 1993).

PSs of high amplitude, sometimes called high amplitude propagating contractions (HAPCs), are propagating contractions of higher amplitude that can propagate along the entire length of the colon. There is no universal definition for a HAPC. Depending on the length and segment of colon studied, the distance between recording sites, the duration of study and the actual definition of 'high', the frequency of HAPCs varies from 4/day (Bassotti & Gaburri 1988) to 10/day (Cook et al 1990). The site of origin of HAPCs, distance propagated and their velocity are all similar to those of propagating sequences.

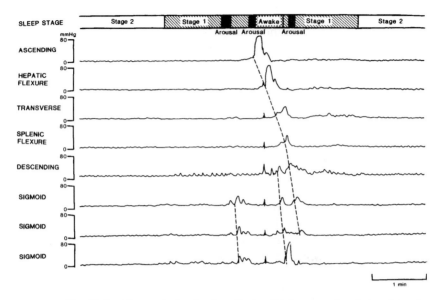

Fig. 13.4 Manometry tracing from the healthy human colon during sleep. A nocturnal arousal is defined as lightening of sleep level which need not necessarily be associated with actual waking. This example demonstrates an arousal-induced event propagating from proximal to distal sigmoid colon followed by another arousal-induced event propagating from ascending colon to sigmoid. A brief period of waking followed the second arousal. (Reproduced with permission from Furukawa et al 1994.)

Evaluation of rectoanal function

Defecography

Defecography involves video fluoroscopic recording of rectal evacuation of 120 ml of barium paste while the patient 'defecates' on a radiopaque commode. Its major strength is that it permits visualization of the rectum and pelvic floor during the expulsion phase. The major drawback is that it is not strictly a test of normal defecation, but rather the voluntary evacuation of contrast which may or may not be associated with the desire to defecate (Shorvon et al 1989). The investigation can more appropriately be considered a test of rectal emptying (evacuation proctography) and rectal and pelvic floor mechanics. Appropriate measurements and their interpretation are covered below.

Anorectal manometry

This technique utilizes a multilumen perfused or solid-state pressure-sensitive recording catheter incorporating a distending rectal balloon. The balloon permits testing of rectal sensory perception and the rectoanal inhibitory reflex in response to distension. Resting and squeeze pressures developed by the rectoanal sphincter are also measured but are not particularly useful in the diagnosis of constipation. These pressures are generally normal unless straining and excessive pelvic floor descent have caused pudendal nerve damage, in which case resting and squeeze pressures will be reduced. Sensory threshold, defecation urge and maximum tolerable volume are measured in response to incremental rectal distension. Alterations in rectal sensory perception indicate a disturbance of rectal afferent neural innervation.

Ambulatory anorectal manometry is of limited usefulness at present due to technical constraints but the technique is attractive and has promise in the determination of mechanisms of obstructed defecation and of incontinence, particularly if confined to sleep. This method permits prolonged recordings in the home environment under physiological conditions which are not always achievable with simulated defecation under observation in the laboratory. It also records infrequent motor events such as sampling reflexes (see below).

NORMAL PATTERNS OF COLONIC FILLING, STORAGE, TRANSIT AND EXCRETION

Colonic filling

A specialized muscle zone at the ileocolonic junction (ICJ), assisted by the closely approximated ileocecal ligament, is likely to regulate colonic filling and prevent coloileal reflux (Quigley et al 1985). In addition, a low-pressure tonic sphincter zone, with frequent superimposed phasic contractions, is demonstrable in humans (Cook et al 1995). In the fasted state cecal filling is slow and erratic and chyme is retained in the distal ileum for prolonged periods. Most of the transfer of ileal chyme to the cecum in humans occurs within 90 min of a meal, in a pulsatile fashion as a series of large boluses (Camilleri et al 1989). The motor correlates of ileocolonic transfer in the fed state are probably ileal propagating sequences synchronized with inhibition of phasic contractions within the ICJ. The ICJ contracts vigorously in response to cecal distension consistent with its role in preventing ileal contamination by colonic content.

Proximal colonic storage and emptying

In 1902, on the basis of radiological observations, Cannon proposed that the proximal colon is the site of storage and mixing while the distal colon acted as a conduit during the expulsion phase. Subsequent marker studies found no difference in dwell time for markers in middle, proximal and distal colon (Metcalf et al 1987) while scintigraphic transit studies on a liquid diet suggested a prolonged dwell time in the transverse colon (Krevsky et al 1986). However, storage patterns of the unprepared human colon, on a mixed diet, suggest that both particulate matter and liquids are stored primarily in both ascending and transverse colon and unlike the stomach and ileum, the right colon does not seem to discriminate between solids and liquids which empty at the same rate (Hammer & Phillips 1993).

Proximal colonic emptying correlates inversely with the diameter or capacitance of the right colon which is dependent upon colonic wall tone (Spiller et al 1986). Chemical stimulants can reduce proximal colonic capacitance and increase the rate of emptying, probably by increasing ascending colonic wall tone and stimulating propagating sequences (Spiller et al 1986). The observation that an isotonic fluid infusion stimulates proximal colonic emptying suggests distension may be a factor in the genesis of propulsive motor patterns (Hammer & Phillips 1993), although fluid infusion into the proximal canine colon need not induce propagating sequences. Hence, changes in wall tone, with or without superimposed non-propagating activity, could mediate this response in the absence of propagating activity.

Relationship of colonic motor patterns and flow

Mass movements of colonic content along the greater length of the colon were first recognized radiologically (Cannon 1902) and the motor correlate of the mass movement is the HAPC (Bassotti & Gaburri 1988). However, the majority of discrete movements of colonic content are less obvious, occurring in a stepwise manner over short distances, either to and fro or aborad in direction (Cook et al 1990, Picon et al 1992). Retrograde movements in humans have also been identified, as have retrogradely propagating sequences (Spiller et al 1986, Cook et al 1990).

Our current understanding of the relationship between PSs, stepwise transport and defecation remains incomplete. Studies combining scintigraphy and manometry in the left colon found a gradient in averaged motility indices in adjacent regions between which net isotope movement was observed. Isotopic movements are infrequent, motor events are frequently localized and the nature of pressure profiles varies markedly from moment to moment (Cook et al 1990, Picon et al 1992). Therefore, determination of the precise motor correlates of flow demands simultaneous and continuous flow measurements together with closely spaced multipoint pressure recordings. Such studies indicate that roughly 25% of all discrete movements are associated with PSs (over distances of 10–40 cm); roughly 50% are related to non-propagated motor patterns (over shorter distances <20 cm); and 25% of movements could not be linked directly to any identifiable pressure event (Cook et al 1990). The amplitude, velocity of propagation and colonic region also determine whether a PS is propulsive or not. For example, propulsive contractions traversing the greater length of the colon frequently lose their propulsive function in the descending colon where these events frequently transform into a synchronous contraction.

Defecation

Rectoanal function during defecation

A series of propagating sequences sweep across the colon, propelling contents into the rectum. Rectal filling stimulates rectal and probably anal sensory receptors which are important to defecation as they relay the sensation of distension to consciousness and mediate rectal reflexes including internal anal sphincter relaxation. These events initiate the urge to defecate and if the time and place are appropriate, the individual permits the subsequent combination of colonic contractions and pelvic reflexes to culminate in defecation. The necessary pelvic floor muscular actions are coordinated by brainstem centers and mediated by pelvic nerves. Defecation is augmented by voluntary straining by the diaphragm and abdominal musculature which aid in pushing the rectal contents further into the proximal anal canal. With straining, the levator muscles contract, the external anal sphincter relaxes and stool is expelled under the assistance of continuing colorectal propulsive activity. Once initiated, the expulsion of stool can continue without abdominal strain, its passage achieved entirely by the propulsive action of colonic peristalsis.

Is defecation a rectal or colonic function or both?

Defecation was traditionally conceptualized as a rectoanal function. Radiopaque marker studies and scintigraphic recordings made immediately prior to and during actual defecation have shown propulsive activity originating in the proximal colon which is capable of emptying the greater proportion of the entire colonic content in a single defecation act (Lubowski et al 1995) (Fig. 13.5). Conversely, the rectum can easily expel a balloon without the aid of HAPCs (Karaus & Sarna 1987) and local rectal pressures, together with abdominal strain, can at least empty the rectum in the absence of demonstrable colonic propagating sequences (Cook, unpublished observations).

How do HAPCs relate to defecation?

HAPCs are frequently associated with the urge to defecate or with actual defecation (Bassotti & Gaburri 1988) and these events are the motor equivalent of the radiologically observed mass movement. HAPCs are also responsible for major shifts in colonic content that do not necessarily culminate in defecation (Spiller et al 1986, Cook et al 1990). It is not currently known precisely how important HAPCs are to defecation. For example, an ambulatory manometric study in healthy individuals reported that only one of 10 bowel movements was associated with HAPCs (Soffer et al 1989) and defecation is possible in dogs in the absence of these contractions (Karaus & Sarna 1987).

PATHOPHYSIOLOGY OF FUNCTIONAL COLONIC DISORDERS

Constipation

Classification of constipation

Healthy bowel habits vary widely among individuals with a normal stool frequency ranging from three motions per day to three per week. Hence, the term 'constipation' means different things to different people. Furthermore, the correlation between reported symptoms and objective measures of transit is poor with approximately half the patients seeking help for constipation having normal colonic transit.

The complaint of constipation therefore can represent a disorder of: transit; rectal evacuation; perception of rectal sensations; or of the individual's expectations of their own bowel. Subclassification of constipation into either slow-transit constipation or obstructed defecation is based on symptomatic differences backed up by demonstrable differences in the mechanics of defecation between the two types. Many constipated patients do have

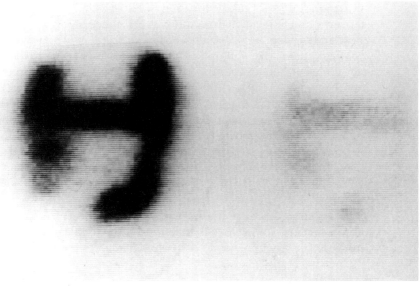

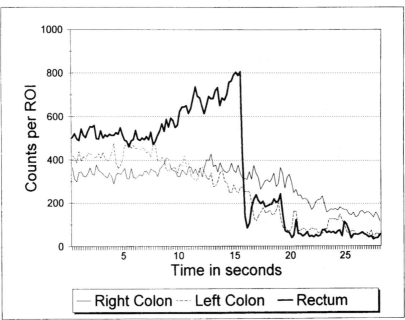

Fig. 13.5 Dynamic scintiscans of a healthy human colon during defecation. (a) Anterior images before (left) and immediately after (right) defecation demonstrating emptying of virtually the entire colon. (b) Isotope counts during defecation in the three regions of interest (ROI). Note early emptying of the left colon coincident with rectal filling followed by rapid rectal emptying together with continued emptying of the proximal and distal colon. (Reproduced with permission from Lubowski et al 1995.)

an abnormality of rectal expulsion, as demonstrated by slower and incomplete rectal evacuation of a simulated stool. Typically, these individuals are unable to evacuate rectal contents despite frequent, ineffective attempts, in the context of the urge to defecate, with marked straining and frequently aided by self-digitation. Conversely, those with slow-transit constipation rarely have a normal defecation urge combined with very infrequent defecation. Such a distinction can be a useful guide to therapy and seems to have prognostic value (Wald 1986). However, such a distinction does have some limitations in that there is considerable overlap in the nature of dysfunction in each of these groups. For example, patients with slow-transit constipation can have normal or abnormal rectal evacuation while those with obstructed defecation can have normal or abnormal colonic transit. It is also possible in some cases that abnormal proximal colonic function is secondary to a distal obstructive phenomenon.

Mechanisms of slow-transit constipation

Diffuse slow colonic transit is logically the consequence of inadequate propulsive motor patterns, due to either defective efferent neuronal function or desensitization of sensory nerves mediating colocolonic reflexes. In some cases at least, the possibility exists that hypermotility might cause constipation. For example, a paradoxical relationship has been reported whereby sigmoid-segmenting activity is increased in constipation and reduced in diarrheal states and that opiates, capable of inducing constipation, induced a similar increase in rectosigmoid motility (Connell 1962). Hence, segmenting sigmoid hyperactivity, together with the haustral pattern of the distal colon, might retard forward fecal flow.

Slow-transit constipation – colonic hypomotility. Migrating myoelectrical spike bursts are less prevalent in the fasted state and demonstrate an attenuated fed response in patients with constipation. In the prepared bowel mid and distal colonic HAPC frequency was reduced in constipated patients and absent in 30% who demonstrated a blunted response to a meal (Bassotti et al 1988). Patients in that study reported decreased defecatory urge in association with HAPCs, highlighting the importance of rectal sensation in the overall integration of defecation.

The relative contribution of deficient HAPCs to abnormal colonic transit remains unclear because meal-stimulated movement of isotope is preserved in at least 50% of individuals who lack HAPCs (Bazzocchi et al 1990); HAPCs are not deficient or absent in all patients with constipation and the neural apparatus necessary for generation of HAPCs is intact in many patients with severe slow-transit constipation. These observations suggest first-ly that other, less readily identifiable motor patterns must influ-ence colonic movements and secondly, that extrinsic or intrinsic factors capable of modulating the propulsive characteristics of propagating contractions are likely to contribute to the pathogen-esis of constipation.

Rectal sensory disorder. Fifty percent of patients with idio-pathic constipation have high rectal thresholds to the sensation of urgency induced by rectal balloon distension and this abnormal-ity is more prevalent in those with slow-transit constipation. The internal sphincter periodically and transiently relaxes, presum-ably to permit the anal canal sensors to 'sample' rectal content, thereby facilitating selective passage of flatus when appropriate. Ambulatory anorectal pressure monitoring has shown this sampling reflex to be less frequent in patients with slow-transit constipation. These observations suggest that, in some types of slow-transit constipation, sensory dysfunction and desensitiza-tion of local reflexes might lead to absence of the normal rectal stimulus to defecation upon entry of stool into the rectum, there-by delaying overall colonic transit.

Mechanisms of obstructed defecation

Obstructed defecation can result either from defective rectal sen-sory function (either attenuated or enhanced rectal perception) or from ineffective expulsion. Expulsion may be defective due to impedance to outflow which can be caused by failure of sphinc-ter relaxation (anismus) or mechanical factors such as non-pro-lapsing hemorrhoids or to rectal prolapse or intussusception. The rectal expulsive forces can also be dissipated, thereby interfering with evacuation in the context of ballooning of rectum due to rectocele or increased perineal descent.

Attenuated rectal sensitivity. Sixty-eight percent of severely constipated children and adult women have impaired rectal sen-sitivity to balloon distension. Impaired sensory neural transmis-sion could influence defecation by hindering central perception of the need to defecate or by interrupting anorectal and colo-colonic reflexes. This hypothesis is supported by the finding of impaired external anal sphincter relaxation (anismus) and inappropriate contraction of the puborectalis in some patients with obstructed defecation (Preston & Lennard-Jones 1985). However, the concept of anismus is controversial and these findings may simply reflect the individual's reticence to voluntarily relax the external sphincter while under observation. Not all individuals with obstructed defecation demonstrate anismus and even normal volunteers can demonstrate it. Patients with anismus generally have an empty rectum; the EMG finding of anismus correlates poorly with the ability to evacuate the rectum proctographically. Furthermore, surgical sphincter myotomy is ineffective treatment in individuals who demonstrate this abnormality and the presence of anismus does not adversely affect the outcome following colectomy and ileorectal anastomosis.

Enhanced rectal sensitivity. Ambulatory monitoring techniques have been used to record the correlation between rectal 'sampling' events (spontaneous rises in rectal pressure coincident with internal anal sphincter relaxation) in patients with constipation and controls. This technique showed that perception of rectal sampling events is enhanced in patients with obstructed defecation compared to both normals and patients with slow-transit constipation. A subgroup of individuals with constipation-predominant IBS have both heightened rectal perception and enhanced rectal motor responses to distension (Prior et al 1990). These findings support the concept that patients with obstructed defecation have early and too frequent central perception of anorectal events, resulting in frequent but ineffectual attempts at defecation, the passage of small stools, urgency and straining.

Rectal urgency

One disease or many?

Urgency can be induced by either precipitous rectal filling or heightened perception of rectal stimuli. The defecatory urge, if premature, results in attempted defecation of lesser rectal stool volumes and consequently unproductive straining may result. Using simulated stools of various sizes, it has been shown that smaller stool pellets require higher pressures and more prolonged straining for expulsion. Hence, individuals with an 'irritable rectum' repeatedly strain in response to small rectal volumes and have great difficulty expeling small fecal pellets.

Rapid rectal filling occurs in response to enhanced propulsive activity in the proximal or distal colon. For example, postprandial propagating sequences, which are more prevalent in patients with functional diarrhea, are likely to induce more rapid rectal filling, causing rectal urgency. Proximal colonic emptying and transit have been shown to influence the rate of stool delivery to the rectum and stool frequency in patients with IBS (Vassallo et al 1992). Sigmoid hypomotility may paradoxically cause rectal urgency by impairing the retarding effect of sigmoid-segmenting activity, leading to precipitous rectal filling and urgency (Connell 1962).

Are rectocolonic reflexes upregulated?

Using tests of rectal perception, Read & Sun (1991) have identified a subgroup of individuals with the 'irritable rectum'. Rectal sensitivity to balloon distension is enhanced in 30% of patients with constipation-predominant IBS. Importantly, this subgroup of constipated subjects with a rectal sensitivity have enhanced rectal motor responses to distension and, unlike constipated patients without rectal sensitivity, experience a frequent desire to defecate, rectal urgency and straining with the passage of small fecal pellets (Prior et al 1990). Rectal sensitivity can be enhanced by a number of extrinsic and intrinsic factors implicated in IBS such as stress, sleep deprivation, bile acids and prior hysterectomy.

Irritable bowel syndrome (IBS)

The pathogenesis of IBS is not clearly understood. The available evidence would indicate the existence of a number of different and frequently coexistent pathogenetic mechanisms to account for the range of clinical features seen in this heterogeneous disorder.

Is IBS a behavioral disorder?

The finding of an increased prevalence of psychopathology and of life stress events in patients with IBS (Ford et al 1987) lead to the hypothesis that IBS might be a psychosomatic disorder, as did the finding of a beneficial effect in some patients following psychotherapy. However, there is no personality profile specific for IBS. Indeed, IBS symptoms are common in the community but only a minority of individuals with these symptoms seek medical advice for them (Drossman et al 1988). What makes some present to the clinic while others do not? When the frequency and severity of psychosocial dysfunction were examined in these two groups of sufferers, higher levels of behavioral abnormalities were found in those presenting to the clinic compared to non-presenters (Drossman et al 1988, Smith et al 1990). Comparable levels of psychopathology are found in IBS and Crohn's disease (Cook et al 1987) and other painful, gastrointestinal diseases with identifiable structural abnormalities and symptoms similar to those of IBS. Notwithstanding the strong *association* with psychosocial dysfunction, these data strongly suggest that IBS is not *caused* by psychopathology. Rather, psychosocial factors are likely to determine exactly who will present to the clinic with their symptoms rather than who will get symptoms in the first place.

Is IBS a colonic motility disorder?

There is no intestinal motor pattern yet identified that is specific for IBS, nor has there been a consistent demonstration of increased colonic motility in the basal state. Exaggerated colonic motor responses have been identified in response to colonic stimuli such as distension, food, CCK and bile acids (Rogers et al 1989). Food commonly induces symptoms in IBS and a meal produced a prolonged myoelectrical response in one study. An exaggerated rectosigmoid motor response to a meal was found in the unprepared colon (Rogers et al 1989), but this has not been a consistent finding in the prepared colon. An exaggerated rectal contractile response to balloon distension is a consistent finding among several studies which suggests that upregulation of colocolonic reflexes might be implicated in IBS (Whitehead et al 1980). In these studies showing a reduced threshold for rectal sensation, the finding of a poor correlation between the magnitude of the rectal motor response and the perceived sense of rectal urgency indicates that the motor response is not necessary for the generation of symptoms. These findings also suggest that the afferent, not the efferent, limb of the rectorectal reflex is likely to be upregulated in IBS.

In the small bowel certain normal motor patterns, such as discrete clustered contractions, are more prevalent in (but not unique to) patients with IBS and, in some instances, these patterns correlate with symptoms (see Chapter 9). Such a correlation between spontaneous contractile patterns and symptoms is lacking in the colon of the IBS patient suggesting that colonic distension, rather than contraction, might explain symptoms in some. For example, the onset of postprandial pain and bloating coincides with the arrival of a carbohydrate meal in the cecum in IBS (Cann et al 1983). Migrating distal ileal propagating sequences associated with a phasic cecal pressure response have been shown to be associated with pain in IBS patients. These two observations are consistent with the notion that, at least in some IBS patients, uncontrolled postprandial colonic filling might cause a sense of bloating or pain from distension, with or without a reflex contractile response.

Notwithstanding the above, there are data militating against abnormal colonic motility underlying IBS. Perhaps the most compeling is the poor response of symptoms to smooth muscle relaxants such as calcium channel blockers in therapeutic trials. There has been no consistent demonstration of increased basal motility in IBS. One carefully conducted study failed to confirm quantitative differences in myoelectrical activity from controls in the basal state, in response to a meal or to cholinergic stimulation (Latimer et al 1981) and at least one study has shown sigmoid motility to be diminished compared to controls.

Is IBS a disorder of visceral pain perception?

The vast majority of afferent traffic from the gut is dedicated to the regulation of intestinal motor and secretory responses and never reaches our consciousness. Whether a visceral event is centrally perceived or not and whether it is pleasant (e.g. postprandial satiety) or noxious (e.g. postprandial nausea and pain) depend on the magnitude of the stimulus and on how the gut mechanoreceptor response threshold to that stimulus has been 'tuned'. Such a left shift in the stimulus–response curve has been consistently demonstrated as a reduced threshold to pain induced by rectal distension in patients with IBS (Ritchie 1973, Whitehead et al 1980). Ritchie also found that the rectal pressure–volume relationship in patients was comparable to controls, indicating that the response was not due to a loss of rectal compliance (Ritchie 1973). This indicates that a lower rectal wall tension is required to evoke visceral pain in IBS, suggesting that rectal mechanoreceptors have been sensitized. The exaggerated rectal motor response to distension in diarrhea-predominant IBS does not correlate with subjective pain experienced by these patients (Whitehead et al 1980). Hence, muscular contraction need not be a prerequisite for afferent discharge nor for pain. If mechanoreceptors in the intestine of patients with IBS are in fact sensitized and if an exaggerated motor response is not necessary for pain transduction, then one might expect to see symptoms associated with physiological levels of intestinal motor activity. This phenomenon remains to be demonstrated for the colon but it has been found in the small intestine of some patients with IBS.

The reduced visceral pain threshold in IBS is not due to a generalized reduction in pain threshold. Thresholds to somatic pain have been shown to be increased in IBS and the more conservative response to somatic pain demonstrated in IBS patients is comparable to somatic pain perception in patients experiencing pain due to Crohn's disease (Cook et al 1987). This discrepancy in perception of visceral and somatic pain in IBS suggests visceral afferent transduction may be upregulated somewhere distal to the point at which visceral and somatic afferents converge in the dorsal column of the spinal cord. This hypothesis has been explored by comparing rectal sensory responses to different types of distension in IBS with responses in patients with spinal lesions. That study suggested that sacral afferents are not involved but that splanchnic afferents, projecting to the thoracolumbar spinal cord, are likely to mediate visceral hyperalgesia in IBS (Lembo et al 1994).

A working model for IBS?

Can the varied hypotheses of sensitized local reflexes, visceral hyperalgesia and variable alterations in gut motor patterns all be reconciled into a unifying model of IBS? One interpretation of the available data is that the primary defect is sensitization of the gut's mechanisms of afferent transduction somewhere between the sensory terminals in the gut muscle or mucosa and the dorsal horn of the spinal cord. This in turn could account for visceral hyperalgesia as well as exaggerated motor responses which may be enhanced by upregulation of the afferent limb of the affected intestino-intestinal reflexes. At a higher level, one can postulate a regulatory influence from hormonal or descending pathways within the CNS which either facilitate or attenuate the sensitized peripheral reflex pathways. The extent of such autonomic tuning would determine the intensity of symptoms experienced. Behavioral and psychosocial factors would influence the individual's perception, interpretation and affective responses to these symptoms and ultimately determine which IBS sufferer will select him or herself from the silent majority to present to the clinic and become a 'patient'.

Proctalgia fugax

The etiology of proctalgia fugax is unknown. It is characterized by severe, intermittent rectal pain. It commonly wakes the patient from sleep, suggesting that it is not psychogenic. Spasm of the levator muscles has been proposed as a cause although there has been no consistent demonstration of anorectal motor dysfunction on dynamic testing. One manometric study suggested increased sigmoid pressures might be implicated. A recent manometric and histopathological study of a family suffering from proctalgia and constipation found a hypertrophic myopathy of the internal anal sphincter in affected members and marked ultraslow wave pressure activity in the internal anal sphincter. Importantly, that study demonstrated pain during manometry coinciding with internal anal sphincter contractions and resolution of pain following sphincter myectomy (Kamm et al 1991).

HOW SHOULD WE TEST FOR DISORDERED COLONIC FUNCTION AND HOW SHOULD WE INTERPRET RESULTS?

Which dynamic tests and in which order?

IBS is a clinical diagnosis with no pathological marker. The clinical diagnosis is supported by exclusion of other disorders which manifest similar symptoms. The vast majority of patients with IBS will not require dynamic tests. Exceptions to this would be those with prominent constipation, profound straining or urgency, rectal irritability or associated fecal incontinence.

Constipation is common and only a small minority of refractory patients will require extensive evaluation. For the purpose of this review, it is assumed that history and examination have not defined a cause for constipation and that metabolic and endocrine disorders have been excluded. Particular investigations are only valuable if we can prognosticate or treat the patient on the basis of the test findings. While marked overlap exists between the subtypes of constipation, it is useful for the clinician to classify the patient as having diffuse slow transit or obstructed defecation. Such a distinction helps establish investigational priorities and has prognostic value in those patients considered for surgery. Notwithstanding this, variable results at long-term follow-up following colectomy for intractable constipation suggest that patient selection for surgery remains an inexact science.

A combination of colonic transit measurement, evacuation proctography and anorectal physiology is widely available and most useful to the clinician faced with the patient with difficult constipation. Rarely, a single investigation provides the necessary information to dictate management. A number of investigations are usually required to yield a reasonable understanding of an individual patient's problem upon which rational therapeutic decisions can be made (Fig. 13.6).

Colonic transit measurement

In most cases of constipation, a colonic transit study is the first step in distinguishing a defecation disorder from a generalized disorder of colonic motility. Whether a radiopaque marker study or scintigraphic study is used will depend primarily on availability and cost.

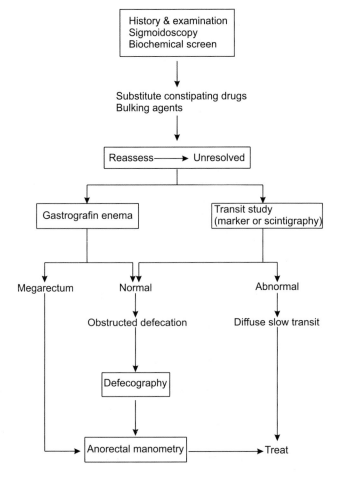

Fig. 13.6 Algorithm for the evaluation of severe constipation.

Radiopaque marker study

Using these techniques, there seems to be reasonable agreement on a mean mouth–anus transit time of 36 h, with the upper limit of normal (mean + 2 SD) being 70 h. Because of substantial inter- and intrasubject variation, only markedly prolonged delay, i.e. < 80% marker excretion within 5 days, can be considered to be unequivocally pathological.

Scintigraphic transit

Normal ranges differ among laboratories depending on the mode of isotope administration, image acquisition rate and analysis methods. From time–activity curves derived for defined colonic regions of interest, the percentage of isotope remaining within each region of interest over time is calculated and compared with normative values for the laboratory (Fig. 13.7).

Soluble contrast enema

In longstanding constipation in young adults, in whom Hirschsprung's or megacolon might be suspected, it is important to determine the caliber of the colon which is best achieved with an unprepared enema using a soluble radiocontrast such as 500 ml of Gastrografin. The bowel is not prepared because this is difficult to achieve and the empty, dilated bowel can collapse, obscuring its natural dilation. Barium should be avoided as it may lead to impaction. On the basis of systematic measurements in controls and different types of constipated patients, megarectum is defined as an anteroposterior rectosigmoid diameter greater than 6.5 cm, measured at the pelvic brim in lateral projection. Patients with idiopathic slow-transit constipation have diameters less than this. The soluble contrast enema will diagnose Hirschsprung's in the majority but distinction from a very short segment Hirschsprung's can be difficult.

The results of the above investigations will dictate further evaluation or management. If these tests are indicative of idiopathic slow transit, more aggressive therapeutic measures are appropriate. If the findings are consistent with obstructed defecation, further dynamic studies (defecography) and physiological studies (manometry) of anorectal function are indicated.

(a)

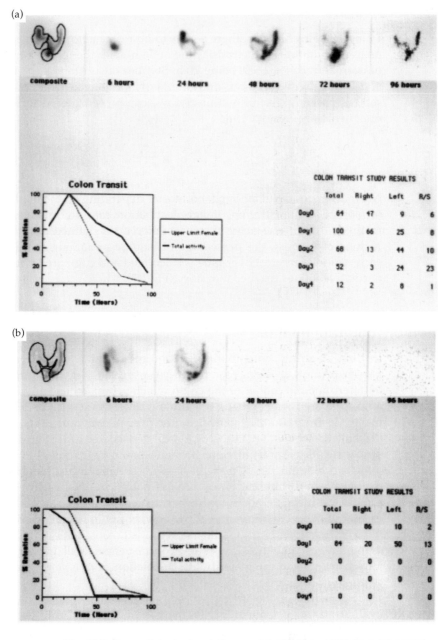

Fig. 13.7 Sequential colonic scintiscans at 6, 24, 48 and 72 h from (a) normal colon and (b) colon in a patient with diffuse slow-transit constipation. (a) Activity is present in the transverse colon by 6 h and only 3% remains in the rectosigmoid after 48 h. (b) Activity appears in the cecum at 6 h. At 24 h most activity is in the ascending and transverse colon where it remains unchanged by day 4. The time–activity curve is clearly very abnormal.

Defecography

Evacuation proctography should probably be done before anorectal manometry, unless short segment Hirschsprung's is suspected radiologically. It will identify rectal wall and pelvic floor abnormalities that may be corrected surgically and will indicate the completeness of rectal emptying which is a good predictor of outcome following surgery.

Defecography can detect increased pelvic floor descent (> 3 cm), intussusception, prolapse and rectocele. It can measure the rate of emptying and the completeness of rectal emptying. Rectocele is quite common in women who frequently use digital pressure to the posterior vaginal wall to facilitate evacuation. Surgical repair of a rectocele is more likely to be beneficial if defecography demonstrates significant barium retention following evacuation.

Anorectal manometry

Anorectal manometry is useful in the work-up of obstructed defecation, but it should also be done in cases of slow-transit constipation if surgery is contemplated because it can influence the choice of operation. For example, those with a weak sphincter and leakage on rectal loading with saline may be more suitable for an ileostomy rather than ileorectal anastomosis.

What conditions can be identified by manometry?

Short segment Hirschsprung's disease can be investigated by confirming the presence or absence of a normal rectoanal inhibitory reflex. The intramural nerves mediating this reflex are preserved in idiopathic megarectum while both are absent in Hirschsprung's. Caution is necessary in interpreting this test in the context of a markedly dilated rectum in which the balloon is sometimes unable to stretch the rectal wall sufficiently to elicit the reflex. Notwithstanding, if the reflex is present, Hirschsprung's can be confidently ruled out. Failure of external sphincter relaxation on straining (anismus) is detected manometrically or electromyographically (Preston & Lennard-Jones 1985). This is a relatively common finding in constipated patients. Its significance is controversial (see above) and it has limited relevance in guiding treatment.

Manometry can implicate other disorders in constipation including anismus, non-prolapsing hemorrhoids and solitary rectal ulcer syndrome although these problems are frequently readily apparent clinically (Read & Sun 1991). Non-prolapsing hemorrhoids can be associated with the symptom of obstructed defecation. Ultraslow waves and persisting high pressures have been demonstrated in the distal anal canal, despite internal sphincter relaxation, in response to rectal distension in these patients. This residual pressure is probably a direct mechanical effect of the hemorrhoids. Manometric findings in the solitary rectal ulcer syndrome and partial anterior rectal wall prolapse include low anal resting and squeeze pressures and internal anal sphincter tone is very low. These findings are believed to predispose to herniation of the rectal wall through a lax sphincter.

Can rectal sensory function predict outcome from treatment?

A high rectal sensory threshold may be a predictor of adverse outcome following colectomy for slow-transit constipation. Patients with an insensitive rectum have a higher chance of persisting constipation postoperatively than those operated on with normal rectal sensation (Akervall et al 1988). A subgroup of patients demonstrate an irritable rectum with heightened rectal sensitivity, exaggerated rectal contractions and sustained internal anal sphincter relaxation with rectal distension (Prior et al 1990). Similar hypersensitivity and exaggerated rectal contractions have been found in solitary rectal ulcer syndrome and rectal prolapse which probably contributes to incontinence in some of these patients. At present, there is no proven way to treat rectal sensitivity but if effective pharmacological approaches could be developed, determination of rectal sensitivity may become much more important in these syndromes.

Is colonic manometry clinically useful?

Colonic manometry, at present, does not have a defined clinical application. We have a rudimentary understanding of meaningful normal motor patterns and an even poorer understanding of disordered colonic pressure patterns. The pharmacology of colocolonic reflexes is not well understood and there are no currently available drugs known to modify colonic motility to therapeutic advantage. In the future, it is likely that motility studies will identify different subsets of slow-transit constipation or further subgroups of IBS.

REFERENCES

Akervall S, Fasth S, Nordgren S, Oresland T, Hulten L 1988 The functional results after colectomy and ileorectal anastomosis for severe constipation (Arbuthnot Lane's disease) as related to rectal sensory function. International Journal of Colorectal Diseases 3: 96–101

Bassotti G, Gaburri M 1988 Manometric investigation of high-amplitude propagated contractile activity of the human colon. American Journal of Physiology 255: G660-G664

Bassotti G, Gaburri M, Imbimbo BP et al 1988 Colonic mass movements in idiopathic chronic constipation. Gut 29: 1173–1179

Bazzocchi G, Ellis J, Villanueva-Meyer J et al 1990 Postprandial colonic transit and motor activity in chronic constipation. Gastroenterology 96: 686–693

Camilleri M, Colemont LJ, Phillips SF et al 1989 Human gastric emptying and colonic filling of solids characterized by a new method. American Journal of Physiology 257: G284-G290

Cann PA, Read NW, Hobson N, Holdsworth CD 1983 The irritable bowel syndrome (IBS) relationship of disorders in the transit of a single solid meal to symptom patterns. Gut 24: 405–411

Cannon WB 1902 The movements of the intestine studied by means of the röntgen rays. American Journal of Physiology 6: 251–277

Connell AM 1962 The motility of the pelvic colon. II. Paradoxical motility in diarrhoea and constipation. Gut 3: 342–348

Cook IJ, van Eeden A, Collins S 1987 Patients with irritable bowel syndrome have greater pain tolerance than normal subjects. Gastroenterology 93: 727–733

Cook IJ, Furukawa Y, Panagopoulos V, Collins PJ, Simula M, Dent J 1990 Correlation between intraluminal pressures and movement of contents in the healthy human colon: a combined manometric and isotope transit study. Gastroenterology 98: A338

Cook IJ, Dinning PG, Kennedy ML, de Carle DJ, Lubowski DZ 1995 Development of a new technique for measuring motor responses in the human ileocolonic junction. Neurogastroenterology and Motility 7: 252 (abstract)

Drossman DA, McKee DC, Sandler RS et al 1988 Psychosocial factors in irritable bowel syndrome. A multivariate study of patients and nonpatients with irritable bowel syndrome. Gastroenterology 95: 701–708

Ford MJ, Miller PM, Eastwood J, Eastwood MA 1987 Life events, psychiatric illness and the irritable bowel syndrome. Gut 28: 160–165

Furukawa Y, Cook IJ, Panagopoulos V, McEvoy RD, Sharp DJ, Simula M 1994 Relationship between sleep patterns and human colonic motor patterns. Gastroenterology 107: 1372–1381

Hammer J, Phillips SF 1993 Fluid loading of the human colon: effects on segmental transit and stool composition. Gastroenterology 105: 988–998

Kamm MA, Hoyle CVH, Burleigh D et al 1991 Hereditary internal anal sphincter myopathy causing proctalgia fugax and constipation. A newly identified condition. Gastroenterology 100: 805–810

Karaus M, Sarna SK 1987 Giant migrating contractions during defecation in the dog colon. Gastroenterology 92: 925–933

Krevsky B, Malmud LS, d'Ercole F, Maurer AH, Fisher RS 1986 Colonic transit scintigraphy: a physiologic approach to the quantitative measurement of colonic transit in humans. Gastroenterology 91: 1102–1112

Latimer P, Sarna S, Campbell D, Latimer M, Waterfall W, Daniel E 1981 Colonic motor and myoelectrical activity. A comparative study of normal subjects, psychoneurotic patients and patients with irritable bowel syndrome. Gastroenterology 80: 893–901

Lemann M, Flourie B, Picon L, Coffin B, Jian R, Rambaud JC 1995 Motor activity recorded in the unprepared colon of healthy humans. Gut 37: 649–653

Lembo T, Munakata J, Mertz H et al 1994 Evidence for the hypersensitivity of lumbar splanchnic afferents in irritable bowel syndrome. Gastroenterology 107: 1686–1696

Lubowski DZL, Meagher AP, Smart RC, Butler SP 1995 Extent of colonic evacuation during defaecation. International Journal of Colorectal Diseases 10: 91–93

Metcalf AM, Phillips SF, Zinsmeister AR, MacCarty RL, Beart RW, Wolff BG 1987 Simplified assessment of segmental colonic transit. Gastroenterology 92: 40–47

Omari T, Bakewell M, Fraser R, Malbort C, Davidson G, Dent J 1996 Intraluminal micromanometry: an evaluation of the dynamic performance of micro - extrusions and sleeve sensors. Neurogastroenterol Motility 8: 241–245

Picon L, Lemann M, Flourie B, Rambaud JC, Rain JD, Jian R 1992 Right and left colonic transit after eating assessed by a dual isotopic technique in healthy humans. Gastroenterology 103: 80–85

Preston DM, Lennard-Jones JE 1985 Anismus in chronic constipation. Digestive Diseases and Sciences 30: 413–418

Prior A, Maxton DF, Whorwell PJ 1990 Anorectal manometry in irritable bowel syndrome: differences between diarrhoea and constipation predominant subjects. Gut 31: 458–462

Quigley EMM, Phillips SF, Cranley B, Taylor BM, Dent J 1985 Tone of canine ileocolonic junction: topography and response to phasic contractions. American Journal of Physiology 249: G350–G357

Read NW, Sun WM 1991 Disordered anorectal motor function. In: Dent J (ed.) Practical issues in gastrointestinal motor disorders. Baillière Tindall, London, pp 479–503

Ritchie JA 1973 Pain from distension of the pelvic colon by inflating a balloon in the irritable bowel syndrome. Gut 14: 125–132

Ritchie JA, Ardran GM, Truelove SC 1962 Motor activity of the sigmoid colon of humans. A combined study by intraluminal pressure recording and cineradiography. Gastroenterology 43: 642–668

Rogers J, Henry MM, Misciewicz JJ 1989 Increased segmental activity and intraluminal pressure in the sigmoid colon of patients with the irritable bowel syndrome. Gut 30: 634–641

Shorvon PJ, McHugh S, Diamant NE, Somers SE, Stephenson GW 1989 Defecography in normal volunteers: results and implications. Gut 30: 1737–1749

Smith RC, Greenbaum DS, Vancouver JB et al 1990 Psychosocial factors are associated with health care seeking rather than diagnosis in irritable bowel syndrome. Gastroenterology 98: 293–301

Soffer EE, Scalabrini P, Wingate DL 1989 Prolonged ambulant monitoring of human colonic motility. American Journal of Physiology 257: G601–G606

Spiller RC, Brown ML, Phillips SF 1986 Decreased fluid tolerance, accelerated transit, and abnormal motility of the human colon induced by oleic acid. Gastroenterology 91: 100–107

Vassallo MJ, Camilleri M, Phillips SF, Brown ML, Chapman NJ, Thomforde GM 1992 Transit through the proximal colon influences stool weight in the irritable bowel syndrome. Gastroenterology 102: 102–108

Wald A 1986 Colonic transit and anorectal manometry in chronic idiopathic constipation. Archives of Internal Medicine 146: 1713–1716

Whitehead WE, Engel BT, Schuster MM 1980 Irritable bowel syndrome: physiological and psychological differences between diarrhoea-predominant and constipation-predominant patients. Digestive Diseases and Sciences 25: 404–413

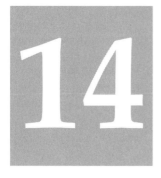

Irritable bowel syndrome: clinical management

SE Phillips, DL Wingate

INTRODUCTION

The symptom clusters thought to arise from dysfunction of the small and large intestines are usually categorized as the 'irritable bowel syndrome' (IBS). Preceding chapters describe the clinical physiology of the small and large intestines; here we address the clinical evaluation and practical management of patients whose symptoms are presumed to be the consequence of intestinal dysfunction.

Unfortunately, the diagnosis of irritable bowel syndrome is often attached to any patient with an abdominal complaint for which a structural and/or biochemical abnormality cannot be identified. Such indiscriminate designations are often based on no more than ignorance or clinical frustration, leading some to propose that IBS does not exist (Christensen 1992, 1994). While such conclusions have the virtue of intellectual rigor, they evade the reality that all doctors, and gastroenterologists in particular, must deal daily with patients who fit generally into this category (Switz 1975). Such patients present a major problem for physicians and thus a considerable burden on health-care systems; we argue here for a rational approach that, though imperfectly based on science, has the redeeming virtue of clinical value.

We propose a working definition of IBS that allows the categorization of patients into several subgroups according to their symptoms. Recognition of these symptom clusters can rationalize the management of patients who are often unhappy and frustrated by simplistic and vague explanations of their discomfort. To help understand the complaints, mechanisms of normal physiology need to be appreciated by the physician, even if the pathophysiological processes of dysfunction may remain obscure. Management of patients is easier when their concerns, fears, frustrations and expectations are explored; unfortunately, not all physicians are sympathetic to this approach and some may even expose their own frustrations in dealing with IBS patients. We argue that the key aspects of management – investigations, education and therapy – must be tailored specifically for each patient.

DEFINITION OF IRRITABLE BOWEL SYNDROME: HISTORICAL PERSPECTIVE

Fifty years ago, in a major challenge to clinical logic that still endures, Sir Thomas Lewis (1944) asserted that the process of diagnosis can be a two-edged sword; attaching a name to a compilation of symptoms and signs may seem to be useful but may be no more than intellectual rationalization. By conferring a name, diagnosticians achieve a goal, but one which 'may only be a temporary (and unstable) way-station that might, indeed, be only a cloud of ignorance'. The history of IBS bears out Lewis' logic. There is, indeed, a danger in conferring a single title on a group of related disorders – which is what IBS may be – because it deludes us into the belief that a single name implies a common pathology. We should not be the servants of definitions and names; we must acknowledge not only what we know but also what we don't know. Effective clinical management can only be based on paradigms that are generally recognized and accepted.

The syndrome of IBS was well recognized a century ago. Osler, Hurst, Bockus, Jordan, Truelove and other notables recorded their clinical experiences and pontificated on the etiology and management of this condition. Fashions change; as pointed out by Christensen (1992, 1994), it is notable that 'mucus colitis' was well described by these keen observers but is now a rare clinical presentation of IBS. The radical step of subtotal colectomy, popularized by Arbuthnot Lane (1909) for the treatment of chronic constipation ('intestinal stasis'), was also proposed for those with intermittent diarrhea (IBS). It is possible, therefore, that the clinical features of IBS may have changed; we do not see many examples of florid mucus colitis, but we recognize other symptom complexes. But although the possible reasons for this change – dietary, the use of popular purges or other drugs, environmental toxins – are interesting topics for speculation, they are not of immediate clinical relevance. More recent attempts at diagnosis deserve our attention because they reflect the current presentation of IBS.

Manning and his colleagues (1978) addressed the positive diagnosis of IBS, clearly an important component for the effective management of patients. They selected a small cohort in whom the diagnosis of IBS was agreed upon and seemingly proven by the lack of alternative diagnosis during follow-up. Using logistic regression analysis, they determined that certain symptoms were associated with the diagnosis of IBS, the key features being changes in the patterns of defecation that were associated with abdominal pain. Thus, by the late 1970s, functional disorders attributed to the mid and hind gut were characterized by pain, disorders of defecation and, less stringently, by abdominal bloating, the passage of mucus and unsatisfactory defecation.

Kruis et al (1984) took a more practical approach. They evaluated historical features, findings on physical examination and the results of simple laboratory tests as a means of separating organic from non-organic etiologies for abdominal complaints. The duration of symptoms, the lack of physical findings and the normality of certain laboratory tests were predictive of the absence of organic disease.

The 'Rome Criteria' refined the diagnostic criteria for IBS (for details, see Chapter 4 and Drossman et al 1994) using the 'Delphic' technique of consensus within a group of experts. The initial object was to establish a firm basis for clinical research, to facilitate comparative studies, but not to create restrictive clinical definitions. Building on the work of Manning, the focus remained on abdominal pain and the associated intestinal complaints (bloating, unsatisfied defecation, rectal mucus and a change of bowel pattern). The establishment of criteria by which clinical researchers can define study populations has obvious advantages for research, but restrictive definitions tend to exclude patients who nonetheless demand help. It can be argued that an overemphasis on pain and an underemphasis on the disturbances of defecation detract from the clinical value of these guidelines. In our view, IBS is not exactly what was defined by the Rome Criteria.

Our clinical bias is that IBS is best considered as a disorder of defecation, one that will usually be accompanied by abdominal pain (or discomfort) and which is often associated with fecal urgency; these are the features that most often prompt referral to gastroenterologists. Abdominal distension and bloating, unsatisfied defecation, rectal mucus and other systemic symptoms (fatigue, backache, headache, arthralgias and myalgias) are common aspects of co-morbidity that perhaps reflect the reality that IBS is a spectrum of disorders.

EPIDEMIOLOGY AND PATHOPHYSIOLOGY

What must the clinician understand for the effective management of IBS patients? Earlier chapters have addressed these areas directly but here we summarize information that we believe to be important for the clinician encountering the patient.

As discussed fully in Chapter 4 , population surveys of symptom prevalence have consistently demonstrated that 10–20% of unselected persons who respond to questionnaires experience symptoms compatible with a diagnosis of IBS, as judged by the standard criteria. The population prevalence appears to be fairly stable, with 10–20% of most cohorts losing their symptoms between successive questionnaires, to be replaced by an approximately equal number of new persons. Of those who reply positively to questions about symptoms, only about 10% seek medical care each year; over a lifetime perhaps 50% never seek care and 50% do. Thus arises the concept of *patients and non-patients* (Fig. 14.1). It is important to recognize that this concept is not unique to IBS patients; individuals with symptomatic organic disorders such as arthritis, obstructive airways disease and ischemic heart disease may not seek medical advice. These diseases can, however, be diagnosed by objective physical changes and the symptoms per se may be of lesser diagnostic significance. In contrast, IBS is a cluster of symptoms which cannot be objectively verified by a physician and thus the factors that determine whether an individual with IBS becomes a *patient* are clinically significant. In diseases with objective physical changes such as cardiovascular disease, the correction of physical deficits is a major goal of therapy but in IBS, the relief of symptoms is a paramount aim.

For example, the reasons why an individual seeks advice should be elicited; is it the severity of symptoms or an exacerbation of long-standing symptoms or perhaps the development of associated symptoms? Again, a small but definite number of

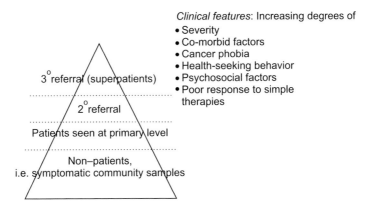

Fig. 14.1   Patients, superpatients and non-patients.

patients can be expected to lose their symptoms; is this a natural remission of postinfectious diarrhea or a normal fluctuation of symptoms or no more than the patient's awareness of discomfort? In the global perspective, however, the majority of patients have lifelong symptoms, albeit with cycles of severity. It is also possible that the psychosocial disturbances of non-patients and patients relate to their desire for medical care rather than to the intrinsic severity of the symptoms (see Chapters 5 and 6). However, 'non-patients' exhibit no more abnormalities of psychosocial behavior or care-seeking behavior than do asymptomatic controls (Whitehead et al 1988). In practical terms, patients seeking help exhibit self-selective bias and the reasons for their presentation should be sought.

In addition, an understanding of the natural history and epidemiology of IBS should alert the clinician to the 'superpatient'. These are more easily identified in the setting of secondary and tertiary referral practice, but their presence needs to be suspected early in the trail of referral. Generally, these are individuals who use mild to moderate IBS symptoms, together with an abundance of associated (often non-gastrointestinal) symptoms, to justify major alterations of lifestyle, that may include elements of secondary gain. Often prominent is the desire for the physician, rather than the patient, to be responsible for all features of the condition. The typical 'superpatient' is intolerant of all drugs, has undergone multiple, usually needless surgical procedures and has a life that revolves around the symptoms. Although these are special challenges to the subspecialist, they can be treated appropriately if recognized early.

Important practical aspects of normal pathophysiology need to be understood by clinicians. Attention to these basic principles can help elucidate some clinical dilemmas, facilitate management by the physician and suggest useful coping strategies (Table 14.1) to patients. Phenomena that need to be considered include:

1. The *gastrocolonic reflex* (Duthie 1978). Mediated by neural or humoral elements (or both), the stimulation of colorectal motility by distension of the stomach (by mixed meals, water or even a balloon!) is the presumed prompt for major symptoms such as diarrhea, urgency and fecal incontinence. Symptoms in IBS are so often aggravated by eating or drinking that many patients can be classified operationally as exhibiting an exaggerated gastrocolonic response.

2. *Visceral sensitivity*. One of the few consistent pathophysiological findings in IBS is the greater appreciation of discomfort by

patients when the gut is distended. These changes have been reported from the esophagus to the rectum (Trimble et al 1995). As described in other chapters, the underlying mechanisms are still unspecified, but the observations are so well founded experimentally that heightened visceral sensation must be accepted as an important mechanism for some symptoms.

3. *Colonic production of gas.* Digestion and absorption of foods is often incomplete in the upper gut; these concepts apply especially for carbohydrates and fats (Stephen et al 1983, Levitt et al 1987). Most adults ingest several hundred grams of carbohydrate each day and some foods contain molecules that escape digestion/absorption in the small bowel, thereby reaching the colon, where bacterial fermentation occurs. Thus, most supplemental sources of fiber consist of unabsorbable but fermentable carbohydrate; their benefits, of increasing stool volume and facilitating defecation, cannot be achieved without an increase in colonic gas production. These phenomena depend upon subtle ecological interactions among the colonic flora and available substrates. Moreover, the metabolic properties of the fecal flora are plastic, as bacterial populations can alter their metabolic properties (Florent et al 1985), so that after a few days of excessive production of gas, tolerance may develop and fiber supplements may be better tolerated.

4. *Intolerance of food.* Although food sensitivities and allergies are often claimed, they are rarely confirmed. However, digestive-absorptive capacity certainly varies among individuals and it is likely that we all have thresholds for the metabolism of starches, fruits, vegetables and other complex carbohydrates. Excessive ingestion of these materials, in a highly individualistic manner, may aggravate symptoms of IBS. Although uncommon, intake of artificially sweetened foods (sorbitol) or of fruit containing fructose can precipitate carbohydrate malabsorption, gas and diarrhea.

Table 14.1   Underlying principles of pathophysiology

Phenomenon	Description	Clinical significance
Gastrocolic 'reflex'	Stimulation of colonic motility in response to food or gastric distension	Postprandial pain Postprandial bowel movements
Visceral hypersensitivity	Exaggerated pain or discomfort with intestinal distension	IBS pain. Rectal hypersensitivity
Bacterial production of gases	Fermentation in the colon of 'unavailable carbohydrate'	Gaseousness. Intolerance of added fiber
Individual food tolerances	Excessive colonic fermentation	Diarrhea, gas
Drugs	Side-effects leading to . . .	. . . diarrhea, constipation

5. *Drugs, including caffeine and alcohol,* have demonstrable effects on gut function which, though still ill defined, may be prominent in some individuals.

6. *Mental stress.* Modulating influences of the central nervous system have been well characterized and central stimulation, most commonly aroused due to mental stress, certainly plays an important role in some persons with IBS (see Chapters 4 and 12). Levels of cerebral arousal influence autonomic function and thereby influence absorption/secretion and motor function of the gut.

Consideration of these modifying factors may clarify some clinical dilemmas, facilitate management and prompt appropriate coping strategies.

The etiology of IBS is, for the most part, an enigma; this is an additional frustration for patients who would like to know why they have been burdened with the problem. Not all, however, is obscure; it is generally accepted (although poorly documented) that IBS can be a sequel (postinfective IBS) of an acute gastroenteritis. On direct questioning, a cohort of IBS patients, estimated to be 20–25% of all patients, can date the onset of their symptoms to an acute and often severe gastroenteritis, usually traveler's diarrhea (Chaudhary & Truelove 1962). Their management does not differ from other IBS sufferers, but at least they can be reassured that they are not the victim of psychological disorders or inappropriate lifestyles; they at least have the consolation of 'an explanation'.

HIDDEN AGENDAS

Transactions between patients and physicians are relatively, perhaps deceptively, simple when they concern physical ailments and treatment outcomes that are objectively verifiable. The management of discomfort is more complex; here we list some of the 'hidden agendas' that often complicate and may even negate the open patient–physician relationship that is essential for the successful management of IBS.

Unspoken frustrations of patients

Even before seeking an initial evaluation, many patients have been advised by family, friends and paraprofessionals. Frustrations grow as the patient proceeds up the ladder, often receiving unsatisfactory answers from family physicians, internists and at the apparent ultimate court of appeal, the sub-specialist gastroenterologist! The patient's actual agenda has often not been addressed and the level of frustration increases as the ladder is ascended. Unfortunately, not all of us always recognize this sequence and the inevitable consequences of yet another unsatisfactory referral!

Questions in the minds of many patients with IBS can be summarized as:

- Will this physician tell me what is wrong with me? I have been told that there is *nothing* wrong, yet I still have the symptoms.
- Will I get the impression, once again, that 'it's all in my head'?
- Will the same uncomfortable tests be done again? With the same negative results?
- Will *this* physician also fail to diagnose the colitis (cancer?, diverticulitis?, adhesions?) that all the others have missed?
- Will *this* physician spend enough time with me to recognize that my stressful (hopeless?) life can (or cannot) be changed? Will *this* physician, if my stresses are identified, help me change my life?
- How can I control this urgent diarrhea (or constipation or pain) that is compromising my life in major ways (regardless of the cause)?

These uncertainties, worries and frustrations from prior therapeutic failures represent the broad forces that drive most consultations. Waiting to receive the patient, the physician is often unprepared psychologically and professionally to deal with a problem that may be either an extremely complicated psychosocial–physiological amalgam or a relatively simple pathophysiological phenomenon that has just not been handled effectively by prior consultants, or even a mixture of the two.

Concerns of physicians

These include the following.

- Here is another IBS patient that I will not be able to make more comfortable. The patient will only ask questions that I cannot answer.

- What has been done before? What might have been missed? Is this the patient with an occult cancer, Crohn's disease or malabsorption that I might also fail to diagnose?
- It's best just to do everything again; upper endoscopy with biopsies, colonoscopy with biopsies, small bowel X-rays, perhaps CT scans of the abdomen and a screen for malabsorption. Then I can see again and can say that we have excluded major diseases completely.
- However, it's very likely to be IBS. I have no effective treatment to offer and I will merely have another unhappy patient who will keep calling me.
- Health care is in short supply; this patient is wasting time and resources that should go to patients with more serious problems.

These background agendas can negate a consultation, but they need not be daunting. They need to be addressed openly, by selective historical inquiries and by introspection on the part of the physician. In the correct context, this can be the beginning of a positive encounter. Initial strategies of questioning might be: what is the reason for this consultation, why now and what do you expect?

Two brief anecdotes highlight these issues. When a 30-year-old, male lawyer explained that most of his siblings and his father had frequent postprandial stools and that these habits were a family joke, the next question was obvious. If he has had this symptom since adolescence (a 'non-patient') and it was now no worse, why was he now presenting (as a patient)? The answer was revealing. Recently married to a nurse, from a family with strong views on health, the patient was propelled to consultation by the wife's concern over his frequent visits to the lavatory. Indeed, house visits to the wife's family were embarrassing for the husband (and the wife), since he was unable to participate in Sunday morning breakfast discussions!

A second example is the 50-year-old woman who denied concern about organic colonic disease, saying that there was no family history of cancer. When interviewed subsequently with her husband, she admitted that she was worried about malignant disease because of colon cancer in two relatives of a slight acquaintance ('no family and no close friends with cancer!').

THE CONSULTATION

All that has been discussed above is intended to prepare the physician for the first encounter with the patient. Though effective physician–patient interactions are a necessary component for the management of all diseases, these issues are especially relevant to patients with IBS. Time spent evaluating the following points will be well repaid in patient satisfaction and some amelioration of symptoms. Rapport established over the medical and psychosocial factors prompting this consultation is likely to be helpful in future encounters. The consultant's goal should be that additional referral, and a repetition of the same sequence of events, should not be necessary.

Major complaint

Requiring the patient to identify the most important or distressing inconvenience serves two purposes. Firstly, it brings the patient face to face with the symptoms, leading to responsibility for the symptom and for the consultation. This allows the physician subsequently to direct complaints *to the patient*, not allowing responsibility to be delegated to the physician. This is a frequent source for doctor–patient frustrations. Secondly, a subset of patients with IBS will have major non-colonic (Whorwell et al 1986) or even non-intestinal complaints (Prior et al 1988) that must be attended to. Specialist gastroenterologists are often confused by, and unable or unwilling to deal adequately with, these associated complaints of headache, fatigue, menstrual disorders and myalgias. These will often be presented at great length; they must be noted but not permitted to divert attention from the major symptoms. Similarly, a past history of multiple abdominal surgical procedures can obfuscate. Some will be important. Cholecystectomy, gastric resection or vagotomy and colonic surgery are poorly tolerated by those with background symptoms of IBS; probably postvagotomy diarrhea, postcholecystectomy and postgastrectomy symptoms are more prevalent in those with underlying IBS. Intimate knowledge of the spectrum of IBS is required with reassurance of the patient that the major symptoms will be evaluated and treated.

A vital corollary is determination of the major impairment of lifestyle resulting from the symptoms. These aspects will be discussed in more detail with the specific symptom clusters but this logic, which is important to patient education, should begin early in the consultation. How do the major symptoms disturb the preferred lifestyle? Does the patient fear leaving the security of her house, and bathroom facilities, because of previous episodes of urgency incontinence? Does gaseous distension and discomfort preclude late afternoon business meetings? Is there a need to spend 3 hours in the morning, with multiple bowel movements, before the work day can commence?

What has been done before?

Careful review of previous diagnostic studies is clearly important. For most patients who reach the level of secondary referral, more diagnostic tests than are necessary have been performed. Nevertheless, the physician needs to review and discuss these critically. Are they complete, have they been performed adequately? In general, the physician should have reached a decision as to the adequacy of prior investigation before meeting the patient. The questions settle on whether or not structural investigations are adequate. Have tumors, inflammation, malabsorption syndromes been excluded satisfactorily? With most examples of IBS, these factors are easily decided ahead of time. Though it is sometimes necessary to revise one's initial judgement, it is helpful if the physician feels no need to change tactics in midstream. Whatever reassurance that can be given about *not repeating* tests will be helpful in the overall management. Direct questions as to fears about life-threatening disease need to be raised and discussed openly.

What does the patient know about IBS?

This simple but fundamental question summarizes what is perhaps most important to the patient. The central issues bothering people usually revolve around perceptions they received from others that (i) 'It's all in my head' or (ii) 'I know I don't have colitis or cancer'. However, the relevant concerns of many patients are 'Even so, I still have these symptoms; what do they indicate or presage and how am I to gain some relief?' Clarification of these issues is fundamental to adequate rapport and effective education and they will be detailed in the section on therapy. However, the declaration of this playing-field early in the consultation establishes a basis for later dialog.

What does the patient want?

Along the same lines, the patient's expectations from this consultations need to be defined. On one hand, some with IBS negate all personal responsibility for symptoms (or their ability to cope), appearing to lay all blame on the physician (who thus feels threatened); unless recognized, this is a fruitless and frustrating scenario. Others request, usually without being specific or objective (unless they are asked the appropriate questions), 'Can you help me cope better with my life?'. The physician can best help by describing the symptoms that can be treated effectively, together with those that are less easily relieved. Lack of a panacea must be faced and discussed.

COMMON CLINICAL PATTERNS

Symptom clusters help the clinician evaluate the major complaints, lead to their logical investigation and point towards a path of future management. These clusters have not always been identified and described, perhaps because their pathophysiology is still understood incompletely and, in some instances, may not even have been examined! Some with IBS will exhibit more than one of these features but, as described above, it serves clinical management well if the dominant cluster can be specified.

Diarrhea with urgency

It is very common to encounter patients with such fecal urgency that their lifestyle is greatly disturbed by this single complaint. They are often older women who may become housebound, but it can also affect younger men or women who have prolonged periods of commuting and those whose jobs take them away from ready access to toilet facilities. They may be forced to alter their habits, to the point of resigning from jobs. They may have little pain and may not qualify strictly for a Manning/Rome Criteria diagnosis of IBS yet this is the most appropriate diagnosis. When asked directly, they may notice bloating and mucousy stools, allowing the physician to feel more justified nosologically.

These symptoms are best explained by rectal sensitivity and a heightened gastrocolonic reflex, since the distress is usually greatest postprandially. The issue of fecal incontinence often enters into this scenario and some will have been referred for subspecialty care for the major indication of 'incontinence'. However, this is urgency incontinence, as contrasted to stress incontinence, if the same terms are used as are applied commonly to bladder function.

These disturbing complaints are the consequences of increased rectal sensitivity and uncontrolled rectal propulsive motility caused by stools that are unformed and therefore difficult to control. These patients are rarely incontinent of solids (a feature that suggests a primary defect of sphincter function). This degree of urgency is rare in painless postinfective or postantibiotic diarrheas but is one of the classic presentations of IBS. In women, obstetrical trauma is often raised as a contributing factor, though those with severe trauma develop incontinence soon after the injury, not later in life, as is common in IBS. Moreover, the complaint, though less common, occurs in men with no history of sphincteric trauma.

Constipation

Severe constipation that is otherwise symptomless is now thought to include two major pathophysiologies, colonic inertia and failure of evacuation (dyschezia, anismus, pelvic floor dysfunction). The constipation-predominant form of IBS is accompanied by multiple other abdominal symptoms, pain, bloating, straining and a failure of defecation to achieve full relief of the distress. The pattern of defecation is then complicated by the frequent use of laxatives, enough to achieve liquid stools, or of enemas and suppositories to facilitate evacuation. It is important to evaluate whether purging is adopted as a means of relief from multiple other symptoms (fullness, bloating, discomfort, etc.).

We propose, therefore, that a distinction be made between patients with pure constipation (due to colonic inertia or evacuatory failure) and IBS with constipation accompanied by other complaints. Thus, comparable to otherwise symptomless diarrhea, which probably should not be categorized as IBS, symptomless constipation should perhaps be distinguished from typical IBS in which the patient most often describes an alternating pattern of bowel movements.

Bloating and distension

Though sometimes attributed to disturbances of perception at the CNS level (Alvarez 1949), these are real symptoms and physical signs can be elicited. As has been documented, the abdomen distends visibly and abdominal girth increases (Maxton et al 1991). The condition is *not* due to lumbar lordosis, excessive descent of the diaphragm or an increase in intraabdominal gas (Catnach et al 1990, Maxton et al 1991). Distension is usually associated with abdominal discomfort and tenderness, not with major pain or colic. The abdominal wall may be tender, this being relieved partially by loosening of the clothes or by a bowel movement. The symptom is often mild in the mornings and becomes more severe in the afternoon and evening. The timing is therefore in contrast to that of the frequent bowel movements which characteristically are passed in the morning hours.

Chronic abdominal pain

These patients are a major challenge and we must outline our approach very clearly. For our practical purposes, IBS is a clinical condition characterized by an alteration of bowel function accompanied by abdominal pain and discomfort. Our views represent only a subtle modification of the Manning/Rome approach; however, we place more emphasis on the disturbance of bowel function and less on the aspects of pain. Chronic pain syndromes, without major disorders of defecation or any of the other features of Manning/Rome *should not* be categorized as IBS though the diagnosis of IBS is often the basis for referral. Our definitions would exclude those with pain alone as belonging to the IBS classification, though this book recognizes the overall importance of chronic pain in Chapters 5 and 6.

Those with chronic pain syndromes are extremely demanding and we do not wish to downplay their importance, *but this is not IBS*. The picture is usually clouded by the use of analgesics. It takes little extension of the spectrum of symptoms to reach the all-too-common syndrome of the 'narcotic bowel'. Opiates have major effects on the function of an otherwise normal gut; transit, manometric tracings and stooling patterns are influenced markedly. The consultant gastroenterologist needs to be alert to the pain syndrome–narcotic bowel association which can lead, if unrecognized, to inappropriate therapy. Few gastroenterologists have not encountered examples of narcotic bowel complicating chronic pain syndromes (or IBS) that have led to multiple abdominal explorations (adhesions being the usual indication) and even to diagnoses of intestinal pseudoobstruction treated with parenteral nutrition.

Associated complaints

The consultant should be cognizant of the non-intestinal symptoms expressed by many patients, though to a degree that varies widely. Chronic fatigue, fibromyalgic complaints, headache, as well as features of other functional disorders (postprandial epigastric pain and bloating, alterations of the appetite and nausea) may be major co-morbid features. Indeed, despite the apparent selectivity of Rome Criteria for functional disorders, overlap among these conditions is considerable (Agreus et al 1995).

Menstrual symptoms and irregularities and functional disorders of the urinary bladder are perhaps most common and, some would argue, are integral to a broad definition of IBS (Prior et al 1988).

Aggravation of symptoms by stress

Many patients deny relationships between their symptoms and mental or physical stress, often volunteering that symptoms are more severe when they are 'on holiday' or removed from the more obvious causes of stress. If the triggers for their symptoms are, for example, dietary, this is not surprising. Alternatively, the assumption that work is stressful while family life is not may not be justified. It is because IBS patients vary so much in these respects that the physician must inquire about the specific circumstances of social, familial or working life during which symptoms may be more severe, more inconvenient and a greater threat to the desired lifestyle.

It is important for the physician to appreciate that many GI disorders (peptic ulcer, inflammatory bowel disease, etc.) are aggravated by stress; in this respect IBS is not different. Stress management is more important in IBS because of the absence of specific therapy to attack the causal lesion. For most GI disorders, the Victorian therapies of rest and strict diet have been replaced by specific chemotherapy, but with IBS we still have to control the aggravating factors because there are no specific therapeutic options.

CLINICAL EVALUATION

Recommendations in this section must be non-specific, since they must be flexible enough to respond to the needs of individual patients and the degree to which the symptoms have been evaluated previously. Moreover, the level to which otherwise healthy young persons need to be investigated varies greatly among countries and cultures. Thus, different societies view differently the degree to which even unlikely organic diseases need to be excluded. The nature of the health system (population based or fee for service), the nature of the payer (public or private), social and cultural mores and the level of litigiousness may all have effects. In the USA, the legal climate tempts physicians to practice 'defensive medicine' in which no stone is left unturned; in other continents, this is less important. We list here only a number of the questions that need to be addressed by the examining physician.

How much reassurance is required for this patient?

Is there a family history of intestinal disease? Are there 'red flags', such as weight loss, anemia or rectal bleeding (it should be noted that bleeding in IBS is usually of the outlet type)? The expectation of the patient and the family varies widely with their social, cultural and medical sophistication.

What has been done already?

Is it necessary to repeat prior investigations? The consultant should obtain all reports, copies of radiographs and endoscopic details, evaluate the record and reach conclusions based on these data. Additional and repetitive studies are not only contraindicated, on the basis of cost and discomfort, but may disturb the stepwise progression towards a positive diagnosis; repetitious investigations may lead the patient to conclude that the physician remains uncertain of the diagnosis. The variable subjectivity of the different tests should be considered. For example, radiographic examination of the small intestine is probably more operator dependent than are examinations of the foregut or colon. If Crohn's disease of the distal small bowel is a realistic clinical possibility, then an additional examination of the small intestine may be justified.

What does the medical and global society expect?

As we have already remarked, some patients, in some societies, may be encouraged towards litigation, thus forcing local physicians into a defensive posture. Repetition of structural studies may be usual. Physicians need to be aware of the sensitivity and specificity and the positive and negative predictive values of all tests they order. These issues are never so germane as they are with IBS. An invariable formula cannot be developed, but we shall attempt to address the multiple, sometimes conflicting, factors in the algorithm.

OPTIONS FOR MANAGEMENT (Table 14.2)

We now reach a 'bottom line'. What can we do to relieve symptoms or, more importantly, to reduce the degree to which symptoms disturb the patient's desired lifestyle? Of necessity, this discussion must be a reprise; moreover, it must be flexible, with individual variations on a common theme. We do not apologize for such a philosophy and several approaches are worthy of reemphasis.

Table 14.2   Underlying principles of the patient–physician interaction

Feature	Significance or question
Prevalence of IBS	Reassurance that the patient is not unusual
Non-patients, patients, superpatients	Why is patient presenting to you, at this time?
Patient's concerns and expectations	Previous referral experiences.
	Hidden fears or other agendas. What is expected of the physician? What is patient prepared to do to help?
Physician's concerns	How much time can I devote to this patient?
What is the major life-altering symptom?	What treatment is most specific for this symptom?

Education and reassurance

Aspects that need to be taught and addressed include the following.

1. Prevalence of IBS symptoms in the general population and among those who present for medical advice.

2. Physiological education regarding the gastrocolonic response, gas production, the presence of heightened sensitivity to physiological stimuli of the gut (food, volumes of secretion, passage of stool) and the possibility that dietary excess might aggravate (but not cause) symptoms.

3. The potential role of stress in aggravating symptoms. At the same time, reassurance must be given that symptoms (certainly urgency, fecal frequency, bloating, etc.) are not 'in the head'.

4. Specific worries of each patient, fears of underlying disease and/or major concerns about the impossibilities of certain symptoms. Finally, the diagnosis of IBS can be made positively and treatment is available.

5. The lack of any pharmacological 'silver bullet' that will regularize bowel function and relieve discomfort. This must be contrasted, in a positive mode, with the strong possibility that, together, symptoms can be reduced in severity to those of an inconvenience.

6. The need *for the patient* to deal with the condition, not the physician. The point must be made that the patient must manage his/her bowel, rather than the reverse.

Drugs and diet

The chapter on pharmacology (Chapter 3) should be consulted and the classes of pharmacological agents likely to be of help need to be known, together with their limitations and side-effects.

It is tempting to exhibit therapeutic nihilism, to colleagues if not to patients, when confronting the drug treatment of IBS. In his important and timely review, Klein (1988) concluded that not a single published study offered convincing evidence of effective therapy. Major deficiencies in design, duration and power were noted in most reports. Therein may lie another dilemma; certain drugs will ameliorate certain symptoms and patient selection criteria could certainly determine the outcome of some trials. Moreover, the 50% placebo response is loud background noise.

Nevertheless, the outlook is not entirely pessimistic.

Antidiarrheals

The lesser opiates (paregoric, codeine and the newer agents diphenoxylate and loperamide) are effective and safe. The modern drugs have minimal or no central effects and patients should be encouraged to employ them on an 'as required' basis. Too many physicians are reluctant to prescribe these effective, safe drugs in adequate dosages. It should be remembered that many sufferers with IBS are quite sensitive to antidiarrheals. They may pass easily into a 'constipated' phase; they should be so informed and instructed to learn to control their symptoms by an 'as required and as anticipated' dose. Antidiarrheals prior to travel – especially traveling to work or shopping expeditions – or before a stressful meeting may greatly enhance the quality of life. Patients should also avoid large meals to reduce gastrocolonic reflexes.

Bulking agents and laxatives

In contrast to what has become the accepted, if unthinking, dogma, increased dietary or supplemental fiber has not proven to be a universal answer to IBS. This should not surprise (Francis & Whorwell 1994) since non-digestible carbohydrates increase the production of fermentative gases in the colon and, if taken in doses that are excessive, may even increase symptoms. If constipation or wild swings in the stooling pattern are a strong feature, progressively increasing amounts of fiber can be more confidently expected to help. However, the patient needs to be instructed in their proper use and potential side-effects (gas production, bloating and distension). The process should be incremental, with plateaux of response being established prior to any escalation of dosage. Duration of use and realistic expectations also must be addressed.

Muscarinic (M) blockers

The standard anticholinergics are generalized relaxants of smooth muscle, but they may be helpful in dealing with peaks of pain originating from the gut. Since they are non-specific antagonists of M receptors, they cause side-effects from their actions on the salivary glands, intrinsic muscles of the eye and the urinary bladder. Many also have central effects that cause distress. Short-acting preparations of hyoscyamine can help lessen some episodes of cramping pain. In general, we favor on-demand rather than routine use of these agents.

Centrally acting agents

Extensive but uncontrolled observations have supported the use of tricyclic antidepressants (Clouse 1994). These are often effective in small doses, amounts that would be ineffective for the treatment of major depression. Their mode of action is unclear and for some agents, muscarinic side-effects may be bothersome and may aggravate constipation.

Novel pharmacotherapies

The pragmatic theme of this chapter does not lend itself to speculation, but new specific (M3) muscarinic blockers that may have more selective actions on gastrointestinal smooth muscle are being tested. In addition, κ opiate agonists may inhibit visceral sensitivity and be useful for treating pain, as may inhibitors of the serotonin-receptors. These all await the outcome of systematic clinical trials.

SUMMARY

Overall, however, effective management of IBS depends more on the duration of effective interactions between patient and physician than upon further consultation (e.g. specific psychiatric referral) or specific pharmacotherapy. The frustration of some physicians, educated in an era of spectacular biomedical advance, in confronting IBS is only too understandable, since the management of IBS depends little, as yet, on 20th century scientific medicine. On the contrary, it remains the exemplar of an older tradition, the art of healing.

REFERENCES

Agreus L, Svardsudd K, Nyren O, Tibbling G 1995 Irritable bowel syndrome and dyspepsia in the general population: overlap and lack of stability over time. Gastroenterology 109: 671–680

Alvarez WC 1949 Hysterical type of nongaseous abdominal bloating. Archives of Internal Medicine 84: 217–245

Catnach SM, Dewsnap P, Herdman M, Libby G, Farthing MJG, Fairclough PD 1990 Abdominal bloating in the irritable bowel syndrome (IBS). Gut 31: A1171-A1172

Chaudhary NA, Truelove SC 1962 The irritable colon. Quarterly Journal of Medicine 31: 307–322

Christensen J 1992 Pathophysiology of the irritable bowel syndrome. Lancet 340: 1444–1447

Christensen J 1994 Defining the irritable bowel syndrome. Perspectives in Biology and Medicine 38: 21–35

Clouse RE 1994 Antidepressants for functional gastrointestinal syndromes. Digestive Diseases and Sciences 39: 2352–2363

Creed FH, Guthrie E 1987 Psychological factors and the irritable bowel syndrome. Gut 28: 1307–1318

Drossman DA 1994 The functional gastrointestinal disorders: Diagnosis, pathophysiology, and treatment. Little, Brown, Boston

Drossman DA, Sandler RS, McKee DC, Lovitz AJ 1982 Bowel patterns among subjects not seeking health care. Gastroenterology 83: 529–534

Duthie HL 1978 Colonic response to eating. Gastroenterology 75: 527–529

Florent C, Flourie B, Leblond A, Rautureau M, Bernier J-J, Rambaud JC 1985 Influence of chronic lactulose ingestion on the colonic metabolism of lactulose in man (an in vivo study). Journal of Clinical Investigation 75: 608–613

Flourie B, Leblond A, Florent C, Rautureau M, Bisalli A, Rambaud J-C 1988 Starch malabsorption and breath gas excretion in healthy humans consuming low and high starch diets. Gastroenterology 95: 356–363

Francis CY, Whorwell PJ 1994 Bran and irritable bowel syndrome: time for reappraisal. Lancet 344: 39–40

Klein KB 1988 Controlled treatment trials in the irritable bowel syndrome: a critique. Gastroenterology 95: 232–241

Kruis W, Thieme CH, Weinzieri M, Schussler P, Holl J, Paulus W 1984 A diagnostic score for irritable bowel syndromes: its value in the exclusion of organic disease. Gastroenterology 87: 1–7

Lane WA 1909 Chronic intestinal stasis. British Medical Journal 1: 1408–1411

Levitt MD, Hirsh P, Fetzer CA, Sheahan M, Levine AS 1987 Hydrogen excretion after ingestion of complex carbohydrates. Gastroenterology 92: 383–389

Levitt MD, Furne J, Olson S 1996 The relation of passage of gas and abdominal bloating to colonic gas production. Annals of Internal Medicine 124: 422–424

Lewis T 1944 Reflections upon reform in medical education. Lancet i: 619–621

Manning AP, Thompson WG, Heaton KW, Morris AF 1978 Towards positive diagnosis of the irritable bowel. British Medical Journal 2: 653–654

Maxton DG, Martin DF, Whorwell PJ, Godfrey M 1991 Abdominal distension in female patients with irritable bowel syndrome: exploration of possible mechanisms. Gut 32: 662–664

Moriarty KJ, Dawson AM 1982 Functional abdominal pain: further evidence that whole gut is affected. British Medical Journal 284: 1670–1672

Prior A, Wilson K, Whorwell PJ, Faragher EB 1988 Irritable bowel syndrome in the gynecological clinic. Survey of 798 new referrals. Digestive Diseases and Sciences 34: 1820–1824

Stephen AM, Haddad A, Phillips SF 1983 Passage of carbohydrate into the colon. Direct measurements in humans. Gastroenterology 85: 589–595

Swarbrick ET, Bat L, Hegarty JE, Williams CB, Dawson AM 1980 Site of pain from the irritable bowel. Lancet i: 443–446

Switz DM 1976 What the gastroenterologist does all day. Gastroenterology 70: 1048–1050

Talley NJ, Phillips SF, Bruce B, Zinsmeister AR, Wiltgen C, Melton LJ 1991 Multisystem complaints in patients with non-ulcer dyspepsia and irritable bowel syndrome. European Journal of Gastroenterology and Hepatology 3: 71–77

Thompson WG, Heaton KW 1980 Functional bowel disorders in apparently healthy people. Gastroenterology 79: 283–288

Trimble KC, Farouk R, Pryde A, Douglas S, Heading RC 1995 Heightened visceral sensation in functional gastrointestinal disease is not site-specific. Digestive Diseases and Sciences 40: 1607–1613

Whitehead WE, Bosmajian L, Zonderman AB, Costa PT, Schuster MM 1988 Symptoms of psychologic distress associated with irritable bowel syndrome. Comparison of community and medical clinic samples. Gastroenterology 95: 709–714

Whorwell PJ, Prior A, Faragher EB 1984 Hypnotherapy in irritable bowel syndrome. Lancet ii: 1232–1234

Whorwell PJ, McCallum M, Creed FH et al 1986 Non-colonic features of irritable bowel syndrome. Gut 27: 37–40

Biliary tract: symptoms in the right upper quadrant. Clinical physiology

WJ Hogan

INTRODUCTION

Pain in the region of the right upper quadrant is one of the most frequent maladies of the abdomen encountered by the practicing physician. Although right upper quadrant pain can originate from local viscera, this location is notorious for referred pain from distant sites (Magrini et al 1988). Often, the specifics of abdominal pain other than its location are poorly described by the patient and sketchily detailed by the physician. The regional location, e.g. the right upper quadrant, is the only common theme in the over-all pain descriptor. Despite knowledge about the vagaries of pain and the presence of several organ systems in this location, invari-ably the physician will initially focus on the biliary tract as the source for right quadrant pain. The gall bladder is the prime sus-pect for right upper quadrant pain. If the patient has had a chole-cystectomy, the remaining biliary tract, particularly the sphincter of Oddi, is then suspect (Dodds 1990). Therefore, a review of bili-ary-type pain would be in order at the outset of this discussion concerning right upper quadrant pain.

BILIARY PAIN

The term biliary-type pain is widely used but for the most part has lacked clear definition. Although biliary-type pain is often defined as occurring in the right upper quadrant or epigastrium, it is interesting that only 56% of gall stone patients report pain in this area. In a blind population survey, biliary pain was reported with and without gall stones at equal frequency. In a classic 30-year-old study, biliary pain was reported to be steady in quality in 98% of cases and truly colicky in only 2% of patients. In an effort to better define this distress, a panel of experts at the National Institutes of Health Consensus Conference on Laparoscopic Cholecystectomy (1993) developed the following

319

key characteristics for the criteria of right upper quadrant pain, suggesting biliary disease. The distress is:

- severe, steady right upper quadrant or epigastric pain which is gradual in onset and lasts 2–5 h;
- customarily exceeds 3 months' duration and a single episode rarely lasts more than 24 h;
- associated frequently with nausea, sweating and restlessness. The patient may walk about during periods of distress in an effort to gain relief;
- occurs predominantly after meals and at intervals of weeks to years;
- may awaken the patient, paradoxically, from sleep in the early morning hours.

The features of biliary pain are present and indistinguishable from disorders involving the gall bladder, the common bile duct or the sphincter of Oddi. For example, balloon distension of the human bile duct elicits pain in the epigastrium or right upper quadrant similar to the pain associated with cholecystitis (Doran 1967).

When structural disorders of the biliary tract cannot be identified by conventional diagnostic tests in patients who have right upper quadrant pain, suspicion of dysfunction of the gall bladder or the sphincter of Oddi is often the refuge of the frustrated physician. Dysfunction of these biliary tract components has been termed 'biliary dyskinesia' (Hogan & Geenen 1988).

BILIARY DYSKINESIA

Biliary dyskinesia is a somewhat nebulous descriptor for right upper quadrant pain assumed to be caused by motor dysfunction of the gall bladder or the sphincter of Oddi or both. The term 'biliary dyskinesia', however, has been clouded in confusion and mistrust by clinicians during the last century primarily because of the lack of a reliable test which could identify this disorder and correlate the results with subsequent positive clinical outcome. Resolution of this quandary appears to be imminent with the introduction of sophisticated techniques to evaluate the function of the gall bladder and the sphincter of Oddi such as ultrasonographic imaging, isotopic scintigraphy and ERCP manometry.

The impact of biliary dyskinesia on health resources is significant. Approximately 750 000 cholecystectomies are performed yearly;

10–20% of these patients may have persistent dyskinesia-like symptoms despite removal of the gall bladder. Additionally, the number of patients presenting to the physician with epigastric and right upper quadrant pain who have an intact gall bladder is legion.

BILIARY TRACT DYNAMICS

Biliary tract dynamics are keyed to maintain a low pressure system (Fig. 15.1). The gall bladder fills and empties (even during fasting) in concert with sphincter of Oddi contraction and relaxation. Following meal stimulation, the gall bladder empties 50% of its volume in 30 min. A recent study demonstrated that gall bladder filling begins immediately postprandially and handles

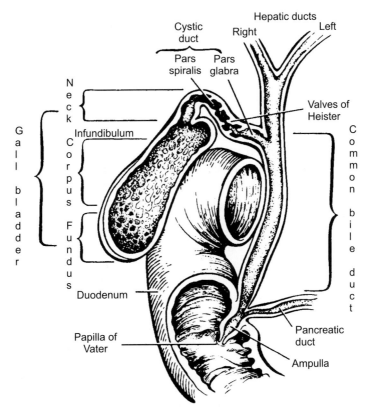

Fig. 15.1 Schema of the biliary tract structures. Biliary tract dynamics are programmed to maintain a low-pressure system. The gall bladder functions in concert with the sphincter of Oddi and the duodenal motor activity, providing a finely orchestrated 'Internet' system.

up to six times its basal volume within a period of $1\frac{1}{2}$ h (Jazrawi et al 1995). The sphincter of Oddi has an intermittent sustained basal tone with superimposed phasic contractions which are principally simultaneous in onset but demonstrate periodic antegrade propagation. These phasic waves occur at a mean frequency of four per minute along the 8–10 mm sphincter zone (Guelrud 1993).

Distension of the gall bladder is associated with relaxation of the sphincter of Oddi. In one report, intraoperative sphincter of Oddi motility studies performed during balloon distension of the gall bladder demonstrated concurrent relaxation of the sphincter of Oddi, suggesting a local reflex between the gall bladder and the sphincter of Oddi (Thune et al 1991a). It was concluded that this reflex was probably neurally mediated and injury at the time of cholecystectomy might play an important role in subsequent sphicter of Oddi (SO) dysfunction. Following the release of cholecystokinin (CCK) with meals, the gall bladder contracts and the sphincter of Oddi relaxes (Hogan 1991). In the animal model, projections of nerve cells from the duodenum to the sphincter of Oddi and the gall bladder have been demonstrated (Padbury et al 1993). Both the gall bladder and the sphincter of Oddi are closely integrated into the phase III activity front of the migrating myoelectrical complex as it sweeps from the proximal to the distal gut during the fasting state. Is it any wonder, therefore, that this finely orchestrated biliary tract 'Internet' system may be subject to dysfunctional problems over time?

GALL BLADDER DYSKINESIA

Dysfunction of the gall bladder is suspected when conventional imaging studies do not detect gall bladder stones or structural abnormalities and the source of right upper quadrant pain remains elusive to diagnosis. In the past, a number of potentially promising diagnostic studies have unsuccessfully failed to identify dysfunction of the gall bladder (Brugge et al 1986). More recently, the quantitative DISHIDA scan with concurrent CCK intravenous infusion has allowed quantitation of gall bladder emptying (Fig. 15.2). The gall bladder ejection fraction (GBEF) has been used to detect gall bladder dysfunction in patients with acalculous chronic cholecystitis (Yap et al 1991). In a randomized study validating the results of this test, a group of 87 patients with chronic right upper quadrant pain were evaluated. Twenty-six patients had an abnormal GBEF ($< 40\% \pm 3$ SD). The 26 patients were randomized to operative or conservative therapy. All 13

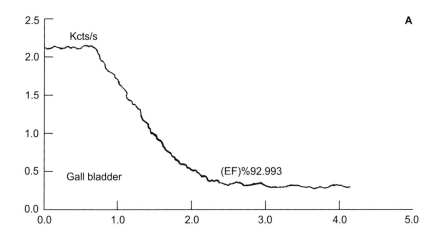

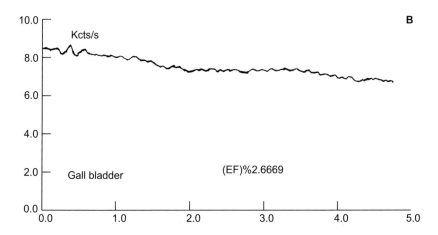

Fig. 15.2 Cholescintigraphy with CCK stimulation. The study measures gall bladder emptying by computer-generated time–activity curves in response to stimulus (CCK). Plots of changing counts over the gall bladder with time are shown here. GBEF in patient A is >90% (normal) and in patient B is <3% (abnormal). (GBEF 45 min after CCK infusion in normals >40%.)

patients with an abnormal GBEF randomized to operation had confirmed chronic cholecystitis by predetermined histologic criteria. These patients did significantly better clinically than the non-operative group of patients with an abnormal GBEF. On the other hand, the remaining 59 patients with chronic right upper quadrant pain who had a normal GBEF test showed no significant or predictable outcome difference whether they were operated or conservatively treated.

There have been a number of other studies confirming or debating the clinical usefulness of the quantitative DISHIDA scan for screening patients with suspected gall bladder dysfunction (Westlake et al 1990, Ruffolo et al 1994). However, the GBEF test currently appears to be the best discriminating test in evaluating the possibility of gall bladder dyskinesia.

SPHINCTER OF ODDI DYSKINESIA

The concept of sphincter of Oddi 'dyskinesia' originated with Dr Ruggero Oddi whose name is identified with the sphincteric muscle that entwines the confluence of the biliary and pancreatic ducts as they penetrate the duodenal wall. Over a century ago, Dr Oddi wrote, 'It is possible that the sphincteric function of the distal choledochal musculature explains some clinical problems that are still obscure . . .'. Since that time, clinicians and investigators have focused considerable energies in pursuit of an answer to this question. Subsequently, myriad techniques have been developed to study sphincter of Oddi function in humans. The majority of these techniques indirectly studied sphincteric function by measuring pressure changes within the ductal system presumably caused by alterations in resistance within the sphincter of Oddi zone. Following the introduction of diagnostic pancreaticobiliary endoscopy and radiographic visualization of the ductal systems, it was a relatively easy step to introduce a manometry catheter and directly record pressure events within the sphincteric zone.

ERCP MANOMETRY

The standard ERCP catheter is a triple-lumen polyvinyl tube with three distal open tips fashioned circumferentially at 2 mm intervals. The tube is perfused with water (0.25 ml/min) by a non-compliant pneumohydraulic pump system. (Solid-state microtransducers have been adapted for endoscopic use to measure ductal pressures within the pancreaticobiliary zone (Tanaka & Ikeda 1988). A three-lumen manometric tube which utilizes the third open tip as an aspiration port has been used when measuring the pancreatic duct portion of the sphincter of Oddi (Sherman et al 1990).)

ERCP manometry depends upon suitable and appropriate placement of the manometric catheter into the desired ductal system by a patient, talented and experienced endoscopist. Sphincter of Oddi pressure profile is obtained during station pull-through of the catheter from the duct into the duodenum (Fig. 15.3). With

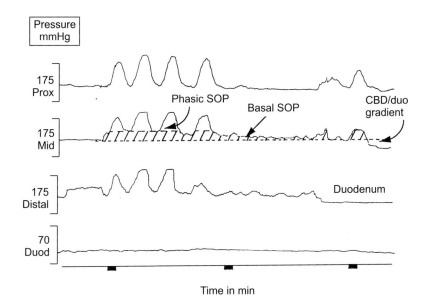

Fig. 15.3 SO pressure profile obtained during pull-through of the three recording catheter ports. The three ports (prox, mid, distal) encompass a 4 mm linear segment; pressure is denoted by the vertical bars, time by the horizontal marks. A separate catheter attached to the duodenoscope monitors pressure transients within the duodenum. Common bile duct (CBD) pressure, phasic and basal SO pressure and CBD/duodenal gradient are shown.

the manometry catheter positioned in the zone of peak basal pressure, select pharmacologic challenges can be administered while observing the response of the sphincter. The technique and the interpretation of sphincter of Oddi manometry measurements have been detailed elsewhere (Carron & Hogan 1993). A number of features of the sphincter of Oddi (SO) have been described using ERCP manometric recordings. Variations in the propagation sequencing of phasic SO waves, rapid phasic SO activity (tachyoddia) (Fig. 15.4), elevated basal SO pressure and sphincteric response to a variety of pharmacologic agents and smooth muscle relaxants have been described (Rolny & Arleback 1993, Cuer et al 1995). For example, cholecystokinin (20 ng/kg) administered intravenously immediately decreases phasic SO activity and reduces basal SO pressure in normal subjects and patients with a normally functioning sphincter of Oddi (Geenen et al 1980). Cholecystokinin has been demonstrated to cause a 'paradoxical' contraction of the sphincter of Oddi in a small subset of patients with sphincter of Oddi dysfunction (Rolny et al 1986, Evans et al 1995), mimicking the

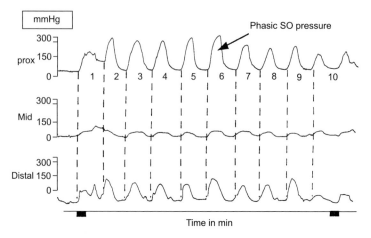

Fig. 15.4 SO tachyoddia. Three-lumen catheter recording of rapid phasic sphincter of Oddi pressure waves (numbered) at a rate of 9/min (N=4/min). While a few of the waves are propagated antegrade, the majority are simultaneous in sequence.

response that has been elicited in the denervated feline sphincter of Oddi model.

Biliary dyskinesia: manometric definition

It is difficult if not impossible sometimes to determine whether sphincter of Oddi dysfunction is caused by a structural alteration (stenosis) or a smooth muscle disorder (dyskinesia). Sphincter of Oddi manometric studies have been useful in defining these sphincter of Oddi disorders (Hogan & Geenen 1987).

Sphicter of Oddi stenosis is considered present when an elevated basal SO pressure does not respond with a decrease in resting pressure following administration of a pharmacologic smooth muscle relaxant (amyl nitrite or nitroglycerine) or cholecystokinin. On the other hand, SO dyskinesia is more likely present when an elevated basal SO pressure is rapidly diminished by smooth muscle relaxants or CCK. Phasic SO contractions that are very rapid (greater than 8/min) and sustained (tachyoddia), an increased frequency of retrograde propagation of phasic SO contractions and a paradoxical contraction response by the sphincter of Oddi to CCK are believed to represent SO dysfunction or dyskinesia (Table 15.1). Because rapid phasic SO contractions can be seen in concert with the migrating myoelectrical complexes, the significance of tachyoddia has been questioned (Torsoli et al 1986). Normally, rapid phasic SO contractions persist for several

Table 15.1 Manometric criteria for defining structural (stenosis) or functional (dyskinesia) SO disorders

Manometric criteria	SO Dysfunction	
	Stenosis	Dyskinesia
Tachyoddia	−	+
Paradoxical CCK-OP response	−	+
High basal SO pressure	+	+
Smooth muscle effect (relaxation)		
CCK-OP	−	+
Amyl nitrite	−	+
Glyceryl trinitrate		
Glucagon	−	+

− absent; + present

minutes during the duodenal expression of phase III of the MMCs and there is concurrent contractile activity recorded by a duodenal catheter. In the instances in which 'tachyoddia' has been present, the rapid contractile activity has persisted for over 5 min and there is no evidence of similar duodenal contractile activity recorded by our intraluminal catheter attached to the shaft of the duodenal scope (Helm et al 1988). The paradoxical response of the sphincter of Oddi to CCK has been duplicated by many other investigators but is a relatively infrequent occurrence and SO pressures need to be monitored carefully (Toouli et al 1982a). The duodenum normally contracts following CCK activity, but sphincteric response is recorded 5–10 s prior to any duodenal activity. An increase in retrograde propagation of phasic SO contractions has been documented in a group of patients who had choledocholithiasis (Toouli et al 1982b), but cause and effect have never been substantiated.

Biliary patient group stratification

Patients with biliary tract disorders have been classified into three groups based on their clinical presentation (Lans et al 1991) (Table 15.2). All three groups have 'biliary-type' pain, but are subsequently stratified according to the number of associated objective findings, e.g. group I has at least three objective clinical findings; group III has none. This clinical classification has been quite helpful in determining therapeutic outcomes of diagnostic studies and subsequent treatments in at least two of the three groups (I and II).

Group I patients have been shown to have dysfunction of the sphincter of Oddi mechanism in 65–80% of cases (Rolny et al 1991). A minority of these group I patients, however, have

Table 15.2 Stratification of biliary tract disorders based on clinical presentation

Group	Biliary pain	LFT Abn	CBD ↑ Diam	↑ Drain	Etiology Stenosis	Dyskinesia
I	√	√	√	√	√	
II	√		1 or 2 above		√	√
III	√		None			√

normal ERCP manometry of the sphincter of Oddi. The explanation for this finding is not fully understood, but may relate to structural alterations occurring above the zone of the sphincter. Based on this clinical classification, group I patients have routinely responded to sphincterotomy, albeit endoscopic or operative. The underlying etiology in this patient group is generally accepted to be structural alteration of the distal choledochus.

Group II patients with biliary disorders have been more critically and extensively evaluated in a prospective, randomized outcome study (Geenen et al 1989). Forty-seven patients (45 females, two males) who met the criteria for group II were extensively evaluated by conventional diagnostic and laboratory test prior to randomization to endoscopic sphincterotomy or sham

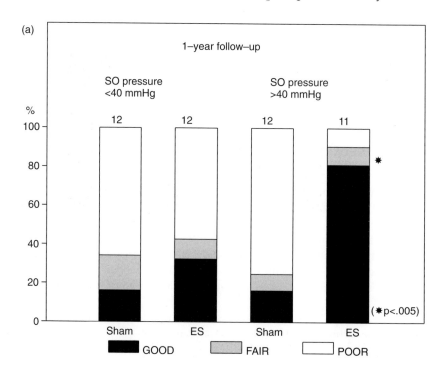

(a)

endoscopic sphincterotomy. A number of potential outcome predictors were evaluated, e.g. liver function tests, common bile duct
diameter and drainage, response to the morphine prostigmine
challenge and sphincter of Oddi manometry. At the 1-year follow-up period (Fig. 15.5a), only that group of patients who had
abnormal sphincter of Oddi pressures and endoscopic sphincterotomy were doing well. Ten of 12 patients were completely
well and one patient was much improved. These results were
based on both subjective and objective criteria. The outcomes of
patients in both sham and SO sphincterotomy groups who had
normal basal SO pressure were not significantly different from
each other at 1-year follow-up. Only the SO manometric study
results, i.e. an abnormal basal SO pressure, appeared to be predictive of positive clinical outcome. After 1 year, several of the
patients from the sham group with elevated basal SO pressure

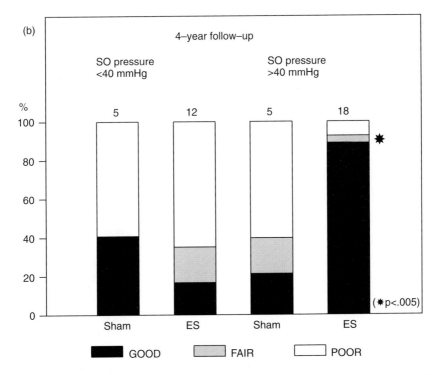

Fig. 15.5 (a) Clinical outcome of biliary type II patients at 1-year follow-up based
on their clinical and objective assessment, randomized to endoscopic
sphincterotomy (ES) or sham (good, fair or poor). (b) Several patients from the
original sham groups of 24 patients were offered endoscopic sphincterotomy at
1-year follow-up. Patient well-being based on symptomatic evaluation and
comparison was significantly better in the group with abnormal SO pressure
who had sphincterotomy.

were offered endoscopic sphincterotomy. At 4-year follow-up (Fig. 15.5b), patient well-being based on symptomatic evaluation was very good; the correlation between elevated basal SO pressure and therapeutic outcome was even stronger (17 of 19 patients were markedly improved). This study has been continued for 12 years now and these results have persisted; the patients who had abnormal basal SO pressure and endoscopic sphincterotomy have continued to do well (Kaikaus et al 1995).

Two other important clinical features were evaluated during the study of group II patients. SO manometric pressure recordings in patients obtained at study entry and at 1-year intervals showed a significant correlation for reproducibility between the two manometric recording periods. This has been verified by other investigators (Thune et al 1991). In those patients with elevated sphincter of Oddi pressures, the sensitivity and specificity of the sphincter of Oddi manometric study was 71% and 89% respectively, at the 1-year period.

Group III patients are the most difficult clinical group because the presumption of sphincter of Oddi dysfunction is based only on quality and location of pain. Results of treatment in group III patients are much less impressive (Dean et al 1991, Thune et al 1991). Calcium channel blockade medications may be useful to reduce SO pressure, but an appropriately controlled study has not been performed on patients with suspected SO dysfunction. Endoscopic sphincterotomy performed on the basis of elevated basal SO pressure in this group has demonstrated significant results in one study (Sherman et al 1991), but several other studies have not shown significant results.

The frequency of basal SO pressure elevation in a group of patients with biliary disorders stratified into the three groups has been compared in two Midwest centers where ERCP manometry is routinely performed. The results are shown in Table 15.3.

Table 15.3 Comparison of the incidence of SO dysfunction in biliary group patients from two Midwest centers

Biliary group	Indiana			Wisconsin		
	Patient (n)	Abnormal basal SOP	%	Patient (n)	Abnormal basal SOP	%
Type I	14	12	86	17	11	65
Type II	69	37	55	47	24	51
Type III	32	9	28	31	4	13

Benefits and risks

Manometric study of the sphincter of Oddi has both positive and negative features (Table 15.4). On the positive ledger, sphincter of Oddi manometry is the only diagnostic test that directly measures the motor function of the sphincter of Oddi. In addition, many clinical studies have now proven the efficacy of this test in determining SO dysfunction (Sherman et al 1992). However, on the negative side of the ledger, sphincter of Oddi manometry is an invasive procedure associated with a higher incidence of post-ERCP pancreatitis. This incidence of post-ERCP pancreatitis ranges from 10% to 20% depending on the ductal site of recording (Rolny et al 1990), i.e. the incidence of pancreatitis is much higher when SO manometric pressures are recorded from the pancreatic duct segment of the sphincter of Oddi. Manometric studies using the aspiration-type manometry catheter report a marked decrease in incidence of pancreatitis (Sherman et al 1990), but this system sacrifices a third recording port which is important when averaging SO basal pressures during catheter pull-through. Additionally, ERCP manometry is short term. Manometric studies of SO sphincteric function for 10–15 min may not be applicable to real-life events. SO manometry is also technically difficult and interpretation still varies depending on the technology, observer training and experience and the ability of the endoscopist to obtain an adequate artifact-free manometric tracing from the sphincter of Oddi zone (Gandolfi & Corazziari 1986, Smithline et al 1993).

Finally, the results of many ERCP manometry studies have not been reported according to any patient stratification. Often, there is a mixture of all three patient groups which further confuses the issue. The classification of patients into the three groups is both arbitrary and obviously overlaps real-life

---

Table 15.4 SO manometry study

Positives
Directly measures SO motor function
Proven efficacy in many clinical studies

Negatives
Invasive procedure
Short-term recording
Technically difficult
Interpretation varies
Patient mixture
ERCP pancreatitis

situations. However, it is an effort to better identify and stratify these patients so that outcome therapies on these patients can be assessed.

IMAGING TESTS AND SO DYSFUNCTION

Two types of radiologic imaging tests have been used to evaluate sphincter of Oddi dysfunction. The fatty meal ultrasonography test and a cholescintigraphy study with and without CCK-OP stimulation have received most of the interest from investigators over the last 10 years. The fatty meal ultrasonography study can be used with the gall bladder intact; cholescintigraphy studies are not useful if the gall bladder is intact or there is dilation of the common bile duct.

Fatty meal ultrasonography (FMUS) consists of an initial control measurement of the common bile duct diameter followed by repeat measurement at 45 min after the ingestion of a fatty meal consisting of lipomul (1.5 ml/lb) (Darweesh et al 1988). The rationale proposed for the fatty meal test is that in the presence of a partial common bile duct obstruction or a distal choledochal resistance factor, fat-induced increases in serum level of CCK are associated with an increased output of bile and subsequent change in the diameter of the common bile duct. In one report (Darweesh et al 1988), 44 control subjects (24 without gall bladders) were evaluated with the FMUS. The common bile duct diameter never increased more than 1 mm at 45 min. The results of the FMUS in 47 patients with suspected partial common bile duct obstruction were negative in all 28 true negative cases (specificity 100%) and were positive (CBD diameter increased by ≥ 2 mm) in 14 of 19 true positive cases (sensitivity 74%). A negative study result, therefore, eliminated the likelihood of a partial common bile duct obstruction. Additionally, FMUS correctly identified seven of eight patients with dysfunction of the sphincter of Oddi as determined at ERCP manometry.

A recent FMUS study of 31 patients with suspected SO dyskinesia (type III) compared the results to those obtained at sphincter of Oddi manometry (Dean et al 1991). A close correlation was not found between the two studies. The SO manometric study detected five patients with basal sphincter of Oddi pressures >40 mmHg. At the same time, the FMUS study was abnormal in only one of these patients but was positive in another patient with normal basal SO pressure with tachyoddia demonstrated at the time of manometric study. Nevertheless, the FMUS study is a non-invasive physiologic screening test which may be particularly useful when the patient with RUQ pain has an intact gall bladder.

The cholescintigraphy study is a computer-generated time–activity curve obtained over regions of interest, for example, the right lobe of the liver, liver hilum and the common bile duct following administration of radioisotope-labeled DISHIDA. In one well-designed study, quantitative hepatobiliary scintigraphy was performed in 56 postcholecystectomy patients (22 asymptomatic controls, 28 patients with suspected partial common bile duct obstruction and six non-jaundiced patients) (Corazziari et al 1994). Individual hepatic, hilar and common duct time–activity curves were monitored. The most sensitive indicator of a positive test was a 45-min isotope clearance time from the liver. Based on this value, the quantitative hepatobiliary scintigraphy (QHS) had a 67% sensitivity and a specificity of 85%. As previously discussed, scintigraphy cannot be used effectively with patients with significant liver disease, intact gall bladder or dilated common bile duct. However, it was suggested that the QHS test might be 'converted' to a 'biliary stress test' by the concurrent administration of cholecystokinin.

Recently, the QHS test has been performed to evaluate possible SO dysfunction in 11 asymptomatic control subjects and 19 patients with symptoms postcholecystectomy. The hepatic hilum–duodenal transit time (HHDT) was specifically evaluated in this group (Corazziari et al 1994). The HHDT values in this study show a direct correlation with manometric basal sphincter of Oddi pressure measurements. The HHDT had a 100% specificity and 83% sensitivity in diagnosing SO dysfunction when compared to the sphincter of Oddi manometric pressure measurement. Another group has developed a 'scintigraphic score' formulated around the QHS test in an attempt to improve sensitivity and specificity. A modified scintigraphic technique was developed using a 3-min infusion of CCK followed 15 min later by intravenous administration of DISHIDA. The scoring system combined both quantitative and visual criteria for interpretation of hepatobiliary scans and for the diagnosis of SO function (Sostre et al 1992). Twelve patients with suspected SO dysfunction determined by ERCP manometry and 14 patients with normal SO manometric pressures were evaluated by this combined scintigraphic scoring technique. A sensitivity and specificity of 100% was recorded by the study (Fig. 15.6). However, other groups have not had as much success duplicating these results using this modified scintigraphic technique.

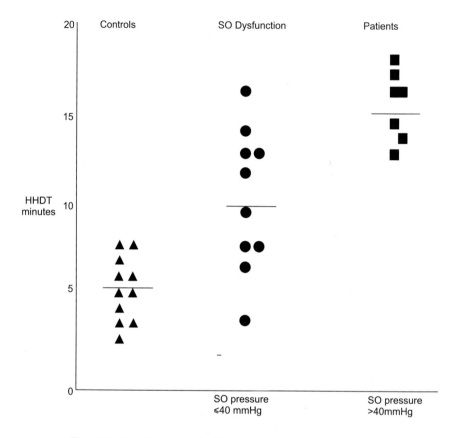

Fig. 15.6 Quantitative hepatobiliary scintigraphy study evaluating possible SO dysfunction in 11 control subjects and 19 postcholecystectomy patients. The hepatic hilum–duodenal transit time (HHDT) correlated directly with the basal SO pressure measured at ERCP manometry.

COMPARISON STUDIES 'IN THE FIELD'

The results of sphincter of Oddi manometry, fatty meal ultra-sound and quantitative scintigraphy studies were evaluated in a group of 304 patients with suspected SO dysfunction (catalono et al 1995). All patients had the three diagnostic studies and each study was scored based on the accepted standard criteria. Community-based radiologists and pancreaticobiliary endo-scopists participated in this study. However, neither the FMUS or the QHS findings appeared to be very helpful in determining sphincter of Oddi dysfunction based on comparison with SO manometry results. The FMUS showed a sensitivity of 21% and a specificity of 97%, while the QHS showed a sensitivity of 49% and a specificity of 78% when compared to SO manometric pressures.

There are obvious concerns in using the SO manometric study results as the basis for diagnostic 'truth'. Nonetheless, the study shows that there is a great discrepancy between all three tests when used in an attempt to diagnose sphincter of Oddi dysfunction. In yet another study, the results of the gall bladder ejection fraction were compared to SO manometric pressures (Ruffolo et al 1994). It was felt that distal choledochal dysfunction should impact negatively on the GBEF and, therefore, correlate with SO manometric pressure results. This apparently was not the case. The results of the two studies were in disagreement approximately 50% of the time.

DYSFUNCTION OF BOTH THE GB AND SO

There appear to be clinical situations in which either or both the gall bladder and sphincter of Oddi may be dysfunctional in patients with biliary-type pain. In one report (Pasricha et al 1993), a group of 25 patients with biliary pain and an intact gall bladder were studied with both the gall bladder ejection fraction and SO manometry. Five patients demonstrated decreased GBEF and had acalculous cholecystitis confirmed after cholecystectomy. Five patients had an increase in basal SO pressure and responded positively to endoscopic sphincterotomy. Two patients had abnormalities in both systems and they were treated with endoscopic sphincterotomy. Both patients responded. Thirteen of the initial 25 patients in this group demonstrated no abnormality whatsoever. In other reports, the finding of sphincter of Oddi manometric abnormalities in patients with intact gall bladders has also been reported at a surprisingly high incidence (Venu et al 1992, Catalano et al 1993).

The quest continues for a more accurate, readily available imaging study which can detect dysfunction in both the gall bladder and the biliary tree. Clinical outcome studies for biliary tract imaging modalities in patient groups with suspected biliary dysfunction need to be pursued. In the interim, long-term sphincter of Oddi manometric recording techniques need to be developed which are safe and tolerated by patients and findings compared to those obtained by scintigraphic studies. A non-invasive highly sensitive and specific test which identifies motor dysfunction in the pancreaticobiliary system remains an elusive goal at this time.

DIAGNOSTIC ALGORITHMS

An algorithm for screening patients with suspected SO dysfunction who may or may not have an intact gall bladder has been developed using imaging tests and SO manometric study (Fig. 15.7). Recognizing the imperfections of all the current diagnostic tests in evaluating the patient with possible biliary dyskinesia, nevertheless, this is a working approach to the clinical evaluation of patients who are suspected of having this problem.

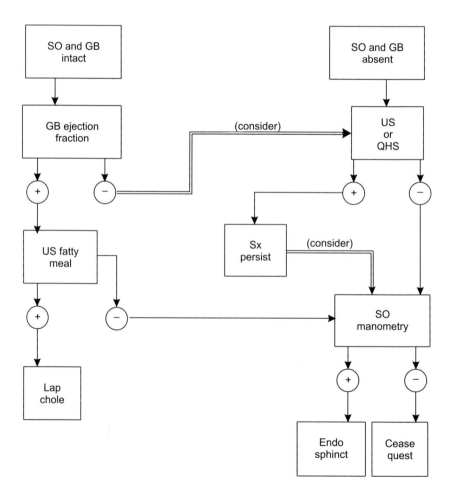

Fig. 15.7 A practical approach to the diagnosis and management of biliary dyskinesia.

CONCLUSIONS

The role of ERCP manometry, ultrasonography and radioisotope imaging in the clinical screening of patients with suspected biliary dyskinesia has been reviewed. Gall bladder ejection fraction is currently the single modality which may be helpful in determining motor dysfunction of the gall bladder. ERCP manometry is the only direct measurement of SO motor function and it has proven efficacy in select clinical situations which has been substantiated by long-term patient outcome studies. Quantitative scintigraphy with CCK stimulation may be a positive adjunct to screening patients who have suspected SO dysfunction after cholecystectomy. A fatty meal ultrasound study may be a useful screening test when the gall bladder is intact. Further refinement and redefinition of these diagnostic studies and this cosmopolitan clinical group with complaints of right upper quadrant pain remains a challenge for future investigators.

REFERENCES

Brugge WR, Brand DL, Atkins HL et al 1986 Gallbladder dyskinesia in chronic acalculous cholecystitis. Digestive Diseases and Sciences 31: 461–467

Carron DA, Hogan WJ 1993 Gallbladder and biliary tract. In: Schuster M (ed) Atlas of gastrointestinal motility: in health and disease. Williams and Wilkins, Baltimore, pp 250–267

Catalano MF, Sivak MV, Falk GW et al 1993 Sphincter of Oddi dysfunction in patients with intact gallbladder: therapeutic effect of endoscopic sphincterotomy. Gastrointestinal Endoscopy 39: 311

Catalano MF, Geenen JE, Pruessing et al 1995 Comparison of Oddi manometry (SOM), fatty meal ultrasound and hepatobiliary scintigraphy in the diagnosis of Oddi dysfunction (SOD). Gastroenterology 108: A408

Corazziari E, Cieala M, Fortunee G et al 1994 Hepatoduodenal transit in cholecystectomized subjects: relationship with sphincter of Oddi function and diagnostic value. Digestive Diseases and Sciences 19: 1985–1993

Cuer JC, Abergel A, Dapoigny M et al 1995 The efficacy of glyceryl trinitrate in patients with sphincter of Oddi dysfunction. A prospective double-blind study. Gastroenterology 108: A412

Darweesh RMA, Dodds WJ, Hogan WJ et al 1988 Efficacy of quantitative hepatobiliary scintigraphy and fatty-meal sonography for evaluating patients with suspected partial common duct obstruction. Gastroenterology 94: 779–786

Darweesh RMA, Dodds WJ, Hogan WJ et al 1988 Fatty-meal sonography for evaluating patients with suspected partial common duct obstruction. American Journal of Radiology 151: 63–68

Dean RS, Geenen JE, Stewart ET et al 1991 Sphincter of Oddi manometry and ultrasound fatty-meal test in patients with suspected SO dyskinesia: a comparison of test results. Gastroenterology 100: A314

Dodds WJ 1990 Biliary tract motility and its relationship to clinical disorders. American Journal of Radiology 155: 247–258

Doran FSA 1967 The sites to which pain is referred from the common bile duct in man and its implication for the theory of referred pain. British Journal of Surgery 54: 599–606

Evans PR, Dowsett JF, Young-Tar B et al 1995 Abnormal sphincter of Oddi response to cholecystokinin in postcholecystectomy syndrome patients with irritable bowel syndrome: the irritable sphincter. Digestive Diseases and Sciences 40: 1149–1156

Gandolfi L, Corazziari E 1986 The international workshop on sphincter of Oddi manometry. Gastrointestinal Endoscopy 32: 46–49

Geenen JE, Hogan WJ, Dodds WJ et al 1980 Intraluminal pressure recording from the human sphincter of Oddi. Gastroenterology 78: 317–324

Geenen JE, Hogan WJ, Dodds WJ et al 1989 The efficacy of endoscopic sphincterotomy after cholecystectomy in patients with sphincter of Oddi dysfunction. New England Journal of Medicine 320: 82–87

Guelrud M 1993 Results of sphincter of Oddi manometry studies in healthy humans. Gastroenterology and Endoscopy Clinics of North America 3: 93–105

Guelrud M, Mendoza S, Rossiter G et al Effect of nifedipine on sphincter of Oddi motor function in humans. Studies in healthy volunteers and patients with biliary dyskinesia. Gastroenterology 92: 1418

Helm JF, Venu RP, Geenen JE et al 1988 Effects of morphine on the human sphincter of Oddi. Gut 29: 1402–1407

Hogan WJ, Geenen JE 1987 Dysmotility disturbances of the biliary tract; classification, diagnosis and treatment. Seminars in Liver Disease 7: 302–310

Hogan WJ, Geenen JE 1988 Biliary dyskinesia. Endoscopy 20: 179–183

Hogan WJ 1991 Sphincter of Oddi physiology and pathophysiology. Regulatory Peptide Letter III 2: 23–28

Jazrawi RP, Pazzi P, Letizia et al 1995 Postprandial gallbladder motor function: refilling and turnover of bile in health and in cholelithiasis. Gastroenterology 109: 582–591

Kaikaus RM, Jacob L, Geenen JE et al 1995 Long-term outcome of endoscopic sphincterotomy in patients with group II sphincter of Oddi dysfunction. Gastroenterology 108: A419

Lans JL, Parikh NP, Geenen JE 1991 Application of sphincter of Oddi manometry in routine clinical investigations. Endoscopy 23: 139–141

Magrini P, Badiali D, Bausano G et al 1988 Abdominal pain in response to rectal distension in patients with chronic constipation. Gastroenterology A277

National Institutes of Health Consensus Development Conference 1993 Statement on gallstones and laparoscopic cholecystectomy. American Journal of Surgery 165: 390–396

Padbury RTA, Furness JB, Baker RA, Toouli J, Messenger J 1993 Projections of nerve cells from the duodenum to the sphincter of Oddi and gallbladder of the Australian possum. Gastroenterology 104: 130–136

Pasricha PJ, Hylind LM, Sostre S et al 1993 Biliary-type pain in patients without gallstones: acalculous cholecystitis or sphincter of Oddi dysfunction? Gastroenterology 104: A375

Rolny P, Arleback A, Funch-Jensen P et al 1986 Paradoxical response of sphincter of Oddi to intravenous injection of cholecystokinin or ceruletide. Manometric findings and results of treatment in biliary dyskinesia. Gut 27: 1507–1511

Rolny P, Geenen JE, Hogan WJ et al 1991 Clinical features, manometric findings and endoscopic therapy results in group 1 patients with sphincter of Oddi dysfunction. Gastrointestinal Endoscopy 37: 252–253

Rolny P, Anderberg B, Ihse I et al 1990 Pancreatitis after sphincter of Oddi manometry. Gut 31: 821–824

Rolny P, Arleback A 1993 Effect of midazolam on sphincter of Oddi motility. Endoscopy 25: 381–383

Ruffolo TA, Sherman S, Lehman GA, Hawes RH 1994 Gallbladder ejection fraction and its relationship to sphincter of Oddi dysfunction. Digestive Diseases and Sciences 39: 289–292

Sherman S, Troiano FP, Hawes RH et al 1990 Sphincter of Oddi manometry: decreased risk of clinical pancreatitis with use of a modified aspirating catheter. Gastrointestinal Endoscopy 36: 462–466

Sherman S, Traiano FP, Hawes RH et al 1991 Frequency of abnormal sphincter of Oddi manometry compared with the clinical suspicion of sphincter of Oddi dysfunction. American Journal of Gastroenterology 86: 586–590

Sherman S, Hawes RH, Madura JA et al 1992 Comparison of intraoperative and endoscopic manometry of the sphincter of Oddi. Surgery Gynecology and Obstetrics 175: 410–418

Smithline A, Hawes R, Lehman G 1993 Sphincter of Oddi manometry: interobserver variability. Gastrointestinal Endoscopy 39: 486–491

Sostre S, Kalloo AN, Spiefls EJ et al 1992 A non-invasive test of sphincter of Oddi dysfunction in postcholecystectomy patients: the scintigraphic score. Journal of Nuclear Medicine 33: 1216–1222

Tanaka M, Ikeda S 1988 Sphincter of Oddi manometry: comparison of microtransducer and perfusion methods. Endoscopy 20: 184–188

Thune A, Saccone GTP, Scicchitano JP et al 1991a Distension of the gallbladder inhibits sphincter of Oddi motility in man. Gut 32: 690–693

Thune A, Scicchitano J, Roberts-Thomson I et al 1991b Reproducibility of endoscopic sphincter of Oddi manometry. Digestive Diseases and Sciences 36: 1401–1405

Toouli J, Hogan WJ, Geenen JE et al 1982a Action of cholecystokinin-octapeptide on sphincter of Oddi basal pressure and phasic wave activity in humans. Surgery 92: 497–503

Toouli J, Geenen JE, Hogan WJ et al 1982b Sphincter of Oddi motor activity: a comparison between patients with common bile duct stones and controls. Gastroenterology 82: 111–117

Torsoli A, Corazziari E, Habib FI et al 1986 Frequencies and cyclic pattern of the human sphincter of Oddi phasic activity. Gut 27: 363–369

Venu RP, Geenen JE, Hogan WJ et al 1992 Patients with biliary-type pain and a normal appearing gallbladder; where is the problem? Gastroenterology 102: A336

Westlake PJ, Hershfield NB, Kelly JK et al 1990 Chronic right upper quadrant pain without gallstones: does HIDA scan predict outcome after cholecystectomy? American Journal of Gastroenterology 85: 986–990

Yap L, Wycherley AG, Morpheh AD, Toouli J 1991 Acalculous biliary pain: cholecystectomy alleviates symptoms in patients with abnormal cholescintigraphy. Gastroenterology 101: 786–793

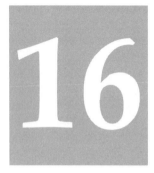

Biliary tract: clinical management

C Ainley

INTRODUCTION

There is an ever-increasing literature on functional abnormalities of the biliary tract and their relation to right upper quadrant pain. A number of tests of biliary motility are available to establish the diagnosis of dysmotility and treatment is by cholecystectomy for acalculous gall bladder disease and endoscopic sphincterotomy or surgical sphincteroplasty for sphincter of Oddi dysfunction.

However, for many practicing gastroenterologists there are a number of worrying anomalies and gaps leading to the suspicion that these are not definite clinical entities. First, several of the motility disturbances which have been described are shared with calculous disease and, with the recent recognition of the significance of biliary microcrystals, the distinction between calculous and acalculous biliary disease is becoming blurred. Second, is biliary dysmotility an isolated abnormality or part of a generalized motility problem and, more specifically, is there a relation between acalculous gall bladder disease and sphincter of Oddi dysfunction? Third, biliary manometry is the gold standard for making the diagnosis of sphincter of Oddi dysfunction and yet it is both unphysiological and practiced in only a few centers, particularly in Europe. What is happening to patients with sphincter of Oddi dysfunction treated elsewhere? Fourth, the information on the effects of smooth muscle relaxant drugs on the sphincter of Oddi is notable for its virtual absence. Fifth, both for acalculous gall bladder disease and sphincter of Oddi dysfunction, women predominate and there are few data on associated psychopathology, either as an etiological factor or influencing the effects of treatment.

THE SIZE OF THE PROBLEM

Approximately 30 000 cholecystectomies are carried out annually in the United Kingdom and the symptom threshold for surgery has probably fallen in the laparoscopic era such that the number of operations has increased (Lam et al 1996).

While a negative ultrasound scan of the liver and biliary system is an extremely common finding for patients with biliary pain, only rarely is biliary dyskinesia entertained as a cause for their symptoms. Thus, while cholecystokinin provocation testing and measurement of the gall bladder ejection fraction to detect acalculous gall bladder disease are relatively simple and non-invasive, neither has become established as part of routine clinical practice and yet cholecystectomy is the most frequent surgical operation performed. Unfortunately, there are no good data on the total number or proportion of cholecystectomies carried out for chronic acalculous gall bladder disease, but both figures are likely to be small. The position is similar for sphincter of Oddi dysfunction which may also occur with either a normal or diseased gall bladder in situ and potentially be the main cause of symptoms.

That up to 50% of patients continue to experience symptoms after cholecystectomy is well recognized (Stefanini et al 1974, Ros & Zambon 1987, Gilliland & Traverso 1990). The majority of patients with persisting symptoms experience functional dyspepsia, vague abdominal pain or altered bowel habit, but between 5% and 10% have recurrent biliary pain and persisting choledocholithiasis is usually only responsible for a minority of these cases. The results for laparoscopic cholecystectomy appear to be more satisfactory with 77–95% of patients reporting symptom relief (Peters et al 1991, Velpen et al 1993, McMahon et al 1995, Luman et al 1996), but the figures for persisting biliary pain are broadly similar. Thus annually in the UK, approximately 1500 new postcholecystectomy patients experience biliary pain for which sphincter of Oddi dysfunction may be the cause.

DO CALCULOUS AND ACALCULOUS BILIARY DISEASE DIFFER?

The frequent occurrence of biliary pain in the absence of gall stones has led to the proposition that gall bladder dysmotility may be responsible. Symptom precipitation (Lennard et al 1984, Sunderland & Carter 1988) and reduced gall bladder contractility assessed by cholecystography (Goldstein et al 1974, Rhodes et al 1988) following bolus IV cholecystokinin (CCK) have been proposed as tests of gall bladder dysmotility, but the results following cholecystectomy have been inconsistent – perhaps due to the subjectivity inherent in both techniques. In contrast, quantitative cholescintigraphy following CCK is objective and reproducible and studies have shown a reduced gall bladder ejection fraction to be associated with up to 95% symptom relief following chole-cystectomy and usually associated with histopathological changes in the resected gall bladder (Yap et al 1991, Misra et al 1991, Fink-Bennett et al 1991, Zech et al 1991, Reed et al 1993). In fact, overall the results far exceed gall stone disease! As a result, quantitative cholescintigraphy has become the gold standard for the diagnosis of chronic acalculous gall bladder disease even though a further study found only poor results after cholecystec-tomy (Westlake et al 1990).

It is surprising that acalculous chronic gall bladder disease has been considered separate from stone disease since both reduced motility and histopathological changes in the gall bladder wall are common to both. There is good evidence of impaired gall bladder emptying in patients with cholelithiasis (Fisher et al 1982, Forgacs et al 1984, Festi et al 1990), but cause and effect are not clear. In the prairie dog animal model of cholelithiasis, impaired gall bladder emptying occurs early and probably before cholest-erol crystal formation (Doty et al 1983, Chapman et al 1989). However, the story does not end with impaired motility as the primary abnormality since this in turn is influenced by bile litho-genicity (Lamorte 1993).

The distinction between calculous and acalculous gall bladder disease is based on ultrasound which, although accurate, may miss calculi. Thus 66% of patients with right upper quadrant pain diagnosed as having acute acalculous cholecystitis by ultrasound are subsequently shown to have stones by further imaging (Ekberg & Weiber 1991). Further, there is also the increasing recognition of the clinical importance of biliary microcrystals causing disease per se (Ros et al 1991) and leading on to gall stones (Editorial 1992). Microcrystals can only be detected by ultrasound as biliary sludge when present in large amounts in the gall bladder (Murray et al 1992) and while endoscopic ultra-sound is far more sensitive (Amouyal & Amouyal 1995), only a few centers can offer this technique. Evidence that microcrystals are associated with an abnormal gall bladder ejection fraction and chronic cholecystitis has been available for some time (Brugge et al 1986) and it is surprising that the studies proposing the diagnosis of acalculous biliary pain made by abnormal chole-scintigraphy (Yap et al 1991, Misra et al 1991, Fink-Bennett et al 1991, Zech et al 1991, Reed et al 1993) have not considered the potential importance of biliary microlithiasis. In addition to symptom relief after cholecystectomy, these authors cite the high frequency of histological chronic cholecystitis in the excised gall bladders as further evidence that gall bladder dysmotility without stones is a definite clinical entity. However, no mention is made of how dysmotility causes pathological changes in the gall bladder wall in spite of the most likely link being via microlithiasis formation.

For acute acalculous cholecystitis, the importance of biliary microlithiasis as biliary sludge in clinical conditions associated with reduced gall bladder motility is established (Editorial 1992) and it can be reasonably argued that the same may be true of chronic acalculous gall bladder disease and that it is part of the spectrum of calculus biliary disease. Perhaps this is an academic point since both are treated by cholecystectomy, but this is not always successful and it would be interesting to determine whether the presence of microcrystals is a reliable prognostic factor in surgery for acalculous gall bladder disease.

In contrast with the gall bladder, sphincter of Oddi dysfunction does not appear to be an important factor in choledocholithiasis (Yuasa et al 1994), although there is an association with microlithiasis in patients with a normal gall bladder in situ (Shiben et al 1996).

IS BILIARY DYSMOTILITY AN ISOLATED ABNORMALITY?

Most of acalculous gall bladder disease and sphincter of Oddi dysfunction have been carried out in isolation, but sphincter of Oddi dysfunction has been linked with esophageal (Johnson et al 1986), gastric (Botoman et al 1992) and small intestinal dysmotility (Soffer & Johlin 1994). The investigations are often complex and hence this restriction is understandable, but comparative information concerning motility or functional problems elsewhere in the gut would be useful. The usual description is of a cohort of patients with biliary pain in whom gall stones have been excluded by appropriate investigation. Only a proportion of patients are shown to have evidence of biliary dysmotility and they are then treated by either cholecystectomy or sphincterotomy as appropriate and followed up. The fate of the patients without biliary dysmotility is variable and they are either excluded from further analysis, treated 'medically' or have continuing pain of varying severity. In only a few of these patients is alternative organic disease diagnosed and hence their symptoms are functional even though clinically it is impossible to differentiate them from patients with biliary dyskinesia.

Although not studied systematically, there is a body of evidence linking biliary dysmotility and functional abdominal symptoms. In common with irritable bowel syndrome, there is a marked predominance of women with sphincter of Oddi dysfunction in all series of patients. Gall bladder motility is abnormal in a proportion of patients with irritable bowel syndrome (Kellow et al 1987, Kamath et al 1991) and functional symptoms (predominantly flatulent dyspepsia) are common following cholecystectomy (Ros & Zambon 1987). Balloon distension of the right side of the colon (Swarbrick et al 1980) or small intestine (Moriarty & Dawson 1982) causes right upper quadrant pain in 10–15% of patients with irritable bowel syndrome. Soffer & Johlin (1994) showed abnormal duodenojejunal manometry in patients with sphincter of Oddi dysfunction affecting both the biliary and pancreatic sphincters who failed to respond to combined biliary sphincterotomy and pancreatic septotomy. Further, most of these patients showed a paradoxical response to cholecystokinin during manometry. In a series of 42 patients Evans et al (1995) also showed a paradoxical response to cholecystokinin to be more common in patients with both sphincter of Oddi dysfunction and irritable bowel syndrome (33%) compared to patients with sphincter of Oddi dysfunction alone (67%) but they did not go on to report the results of sphincterotomy.

That functional abnormalities of the sphincter of Oddi are associated with functional abnormalities elsewhere in the GI tract is not surprising. However, there is little information on the relevance of concomitant functional abnormalities to either symptoms or to the response to sphincterotomy which is often suboptimal. Further reports are therefore required but these will be difficult to perform and interpret because of the number of variables which potentially will need to be studied including: daily versus intermittent biliary pain, associated irritable bowel syndrome or other functional problems; psychological factors; Geenen–Hogan types I, II and III; manometric abnormalities including the response to cholecystokinin; small intestinal manometry; response to sphincterotomy.

In health, gall bladder motility and the sphincter of Oddi function as a unit under dual neural and hormonal control such that gall bladder contraction is accompanied by sphincter relaxation and vice versa. Therefore, there could well be an association with both being abnormal. While cases have been described, there is no definite link (Ruffolo et al 1991).

BILIARY MANOMETRY AS THE GOLD STANDARD FOR SPHINCTER OF ODDI DYSFUNCTION

Most reviews of the subject include the statement that biliary manometry is the gold standard for the diagnosis of sphincter of Oddi dysfunction and then list the advantages and disadvantages of the technique. The position is in fact more complex since it is biliary manometry which has done most to establish sphincter of Oddi dysfunction as a clinical entity. The Wisconsin group have been at the forefront and their two main contributions have been the Geenen–Hogan classification of sphincter of Oddi dysfunction and the only prospective double-blind prospective trial of the efficacy of endoscopic sphincterotomy in patients with group II dysfunction (Geenen et al 1989).

In addition to the standard criticisms of biliary manometry (unphysiological, short term, technically difficult and pancreatitis), there are other difficulties. For obvious reasons, the total number of normal controls in the world literature is small and probably not in three figures. Of the various manometric parameters (basal pressure, contraction wave frequency, pressure and propagation and response to cholecystokinin), only a basal sphincter pressure greater than 40 mmHg and possibly a paradoxical response to cholecystokinin (Rolny et al 1986) appear to be of any relevance to symptoms.

While most series report a beneficial clinical effect of endoscopic sphincterotomy in patients with an elevated basal sphincter pressure, there are frequent treatment failures (Aronchik et al 1984, Neoptolemos et al 1988, Geenen et al 1989, Sherman et al 1991a, Soffer & Johlin 1994). There are also reports of little clinical benefit from sphincterotomy (Roberts-Thomson & Toouli 1985, Thatcher et al 1987). Even in the Wisconsin prospective double-blind study, sphincterotomy was not 100% effective in patients with an elevated basal sphincter pressure and there was a 40% improvement at 4 years in the other patient groups, i.e. raised pressure with sham sphincterotomy and normal pressure whether or not sphincterotomy had been carried out (Geenen et al 1989). The authors termed these 'placebo responders' and by implication their symptoms were not organic, which casts doubt on sphincter of Oddi dysfunction as a discrete entity if clinically it presents with symptoms that cannot be differentiated from those with a functional etiology.

The availability of biliary manometry shows considerable variation. Even in the USA, only the large centers offer a service and in Europe it is limited to a small number of interested groups such that in the United Kingdom there is only one reliable established unit. There are therefore obvious problems comparing patients in different series but this patchy distribution begs the question of how patients with possible sphincter of Oddi dysfunction are managed without biliary manometry. Indeed, it could be argued from the limited availability that most gastrointestinal centers rarely miss such a facility. Patients with group I sphincter of Oddi dysfunction do not pose a problem since the clinical evidence for sphincter stenosis or dysfunction is adequate for endoscopic sphincterotomy to be carried out without resorting to biliary manometry. In fact, it is a problem for the validity of biliary manometry as a technique that the basal pressure is only elevated in 65–86% of patients with group I dysfunction (Rolny et al 1991, Sherman et al 1991a). The difficulty arises with patients having group II or III dysfunction. Other approaches including quantitative hepatobiliary scanning and clinical assessment are less reliable than biliary manometry and if sphincter of Oddi dysfunction were a common problem, there would be a significant number of patients either subjected to unnecessary sphincterotomy or with continuing biliary pain due to undiagnosed sphincter dysfunction.

In practice, the number of such patients is small and they are managed on an ad hoc basis with sphincterotomy if there is a reasonable clinical suspicion of sphincter of Oddi dysfunction, e.g. bile duct dilation or abnormal liver blood tests, corresponding to Geenen–Hogan group II in which there is a 50% prevalence of sphincter of Oddi dysfunction (Sherman et al 1991a). In the absence of any objective evidence of dysfunction (group III), most patients are managed with smooth muscle relaxant drug therapy since only a minority (13–28%) have abnormal manometry (Sherman et al 1991a). However, such a *laissez-faire* approach may no longer be acceptable in the United Kingdom due to rising patient expectation and also to medicolegal issues relating to the increased risk of pancreatitis associated both with biliary manometry itself (Albert et al 1991) and sphincterotomy for sphincter of Oddi dysfunction, especially group III patients in whom the bile duct is of normal caliber (Sherman et al 1991b). This increased risk of pancreatitis complicating ERCP in patients with sphincter of Oddi dysfunction is a consistent finding and adds to the evidence that the syndrome is a clinical entity.

While biliary manometry is currently the gold standard for the diagnosis of sphincter of Oddi dysfunction, of the many problems associated with the technique, the fact that it does not reliably diagnose those patients who will benefit from sphincterotomy, and from sphincterotomy alone, is likely to prevent its widespread use in the United Kingdom. Measured at ERCP, biliary manometry is neither physiological nor long term and in common with small intestinal manometry (Kellow et al 1990), prolonged recording is probably required to provide more useful data. Prolonged biliary manometry poses considerable problems, but techniques have been developed (Tanaka et al 1983).

DRUGS AND THE SPHINCTER OF ODDI

The neural and hormonal control of the sphincter of Oddi have been studied in detail with nitric oxide-mediated inhibition being the final common path for sphincter relaxation (Baker et al 1983). In contrast, there is little information on the effect of smooth muscle relaxant drugs which could clearly be useful in sphincter of Oddi dysfunction, not only in the context of a therapeutic trial to assess possible benefit from sphincterotomy but also as definitive treatment. Glyceryl trinitrate relaxes the sphincter (Staritz et al 1985) and similar changes have been claimed for long-acting nitrates (Nowakowska-Dulawa et al 1990). Similarly, butyl scopolamine is an effective sphincter relaxant (Brandstatter et al 1996). Although nifedipine and other calcium antagonists have been proposed as drug treatment for sphincter of Oddi dysfunction (Viceconte & Micheletti 1995), there are no data on their effects on sphincter pressure. At first sight, it is surprising that there have been no trials of spasmolytic drug treatment for sphincter of Oddi dysfunction, but these drugs would also affect smooth muscle elsewhere in the GI tract which would render such investigations difficult both to conduct and to interpret.

Nonetheless, the lack of information on drug treatment for sphincter of Oddi dysfunction, with or without concomitant irritable bowel syndrome, is an additional factor detracting from acceptance of the syndrome as a clinical entity. The generalized effects of systemic drug treatment are not relevant with the injection of botulinum toxin into the sphincter, but a preliminary report suggested no benefit (Pasricha et al 1994). In relation to the numerous reports of the effects of sphincterotomy for sphincter of Oddi dysfunction, there is a dearth of information on drug treatment which needs to be rectified.

PSYCHOLOGICAL ASPECTS

There is considerable indirect evidence that psychological factors are relevant to biliary dyskinesia and pain. Both for acalculous gall bladder disease (Yap et al 1991, Misra et al 1991) and sphincter of Oddi dysfunction (Geenen et al 1989, Soffer & Johlin 1994, Evans et al 1995) women are far more frequently affected than men. As stated above, gall bladder motility is abnormal in irritable bowel syndrome (Kellow et al 1987, Kamath et al 1991), and approximately 33% of patients with sphincter of Oddi dysfunction also have irritable bowel syndrome (Evans et al 1995). Unfortunately, there is little direct evidence other than a single abstract showing an increased incidence of anxiety, depression and somatoform disorders in patients, predominantly women, with sphincter of Oddi dysfunction (Troiano et al 1990).

CONCLUSION

While biliary dysmotility has been shown to exist as either a reduced gall bladder ejection fraction or sphincter of Oddi dysfunction, the association with biliary pain and its relief by either cholecystectomy or endoscopic sphincterotomy is not clearcut in a large proportion of patients. There are problems with the techniques in use and a lack of information about other concomitant functional disease, psychological aspects and drug treatment. It is to be hoped that future research will correct these deficiencies so that the frequency and importance of biliary dyskinesia can be more clearly defined.

REFERENCES

Albert MB, Steinberg WM, Irani SK 1988 Severe acute pancreatitis complicating sphincter of Oddi manometry. Gastrointestinal Endoscopy 34: 342–345
Amouyal G, Amouyal P 1995 Endoscopic ultrasound in gallbladder stones. Gastroscopy and Endoscopy Clinics of North America 5: 825–830
Aronchick CA, Long WB, Soloway RD 1984 Endoscopic biliary manometry and a modified morphine prostigmine test as predictors of clinical response to sphincterotomy in biliary dyskinesia. Gastrointestinal Endoscopy 30: 140
Baker RA, Saccone GTP, Brookes SLH, Toouli J 1993 Nitric oxide mediates nonadrenergic noncholinergic neural relaxation in the Australian possum. Gastroenterology 105: 1746–1753
Botoman VA, Kozarek RA, Novell LA et al 1992 Gastroparesis in patients with unexplained biliary colic and suspected sphincter of Oddi dysfunction. Gastroenterology 102: 303
Brandstatter G, Schinzel S, Wurzer H 1996 Influence of spasmolytic analgesics on motility of sphincter of Oddi. Digestive Diseases and Sciences 41: 1814–1818
Brugge WR, Brand DL, Atkins HL et al 1986 Gallbladder dyskinesia in chronic acalculous cholecystitis. Digestive Diseases and Sciences 31: 461–467
Chapman WC, Peterkin GA, Lamorte WW et al 1989 Alterations in biliary motility correlate with increased gallbladder prostaglandin synthesis in early cholelithiasis in prairie dog. Digestive Diseases and Sciences 34: 1420–1424
Doty JE, Pitt HA, Kuchenbecker SL, DenBesten L 1983 Impaired gallbladder

emptying before gallstone formation in the prairie dog. Gastroenterology 85: 168–174

Editorial 1992. Biliary sludge: more than a curiosity. Lancet 339:1087

Ekberg O, Weiber S 1991. The clinical importance of a thick walled, tender gallbladder without stones on ultrasonography. Clinical Radiology 44: 38–41

Evans PR, Dowsett JF, Bak Y-T et al 1995 Abnormal sphincter of Oddi response to cholecystokinin in postcholecystectomy syndrome patients with irritable bowel syndrome. Digestive Diseases and Sciences 40: 1149–1156

Festi D, Frabboni R, Bazzoli F et al 1990 Gallbladder motility in cholesterol gallstone disease. Effect of ursodeoxycholic acid administration and gallstone dissolution. Gastroenterology 99; 1779–1785

Fink-Bennett D, DeRidder P, Kolozsi WZ et al 1991 Cholecystokinin cholescintigraphy: detection of abnormal gallbladder motor function in patients with chronic acalculous gallbladder disease. Journal of Nuclear Medicine 32: 1695–1699

Fisher RS, Stelzer F, Rock E, Malmud LS 1982 Abnormal gallbladder emptying in patients with gallstones. Digestive Diseases and Sciences 27: 1019–1024

Forgacs IC, Maisey MN, Murphy GM, Dowling RH 1984. Influence of gallstones and ursodeoxycholic acid therapy on gallbladder emptying. Gastroenterology 87: 299–307

Geenen JE, Hogan WJ, Dodds WJ et al 1989 The efficacy of endoscopic sphincterotomy after cholecystectomy in patients with sphincter of Oddi dysfunction. New England Journal of Medicine 320: 82–87

Gilliland TM, Traverso LW 1990 Modern standards for comparison of cholecystectomy with alternative treatments for symptomatic cholithiasis with emphasis on long term relief of symptoms. Surgery, Gynecology and Obstetrics 170: 39–44

Goldstein R, Grunt R, Margulies M 1974 Cholecystokinin cholecystography in the differential diagnosis of acalculous gallbladder disease. Digestive Diseases and Sciences 19: 835–849

Johnson DA, Cattau EL Jr, Winters C Jr 1986 Biliary dyskinesia with associated high amplitude esophageal peristaltic contractions. American Journal of Gastroenterology 81: 254–256

Kamath PS, Gaisano HY, Phillips SF et al 1991 Abnormal gallbladder motility in irritable bowel syndrome: evidence for target-organ defect. American Journal of Physiology 260: G815–819

Kellow JE, Miller LJ, Phillips SF et al 1987 Altered sensitivity of the gallbladder to cholecystokinin octapeptide in irritable bowel syndrome. American Journal of Physiology 253: G650–655

Kellow JE, Gill RC, Wingate DL 1990 Prolonged ambulant recordings of small bowel motility demonstrate abnormalities in the irritable bowel syndrome. Gastroenterology 98: 1208–1218

Lam CM, Murray FE, Cuschieri A 1996 Increased cholecystectomy rate after the introduction of laparoscopic cholecystectomy in Scotland. Gut 38: 282–284

Lamorte WW 1993 Biliary motility and abnormalities associated with cholesterol cholelithiasis. Current Opinion in Gastroenterology 9: 810–816

Lennard TWJ, Farndon JR, Taylor RMR 1984 Acalculous biliary pain: diagnosis and selection for cholecystectomy using the cholecystokinin test for pain reproduction. British Journal of Surgery 71: 368–370

Luman W, Adams WH, Nixon SN et al 1996 Incidence of persisting symptoms after laparoscopic cholecystectomy: a prospective study. Gut 39: 863–866

McMahon AJ, Ross S, Baxter JN et al 1995 Symptomatic outcome 1 year after laparoscopic and minilaparotomy cholecystectomy: a randomised trial. British Journal of Surgery 82: 1378–1382

Misra DC, Blossom GB, Fink-Bennett D, Glover JL 1991 Results of surgical therapy for biliary dyskinesia. Archives of Surgery 126: 957–960

Moriarty KJ, Dawson AM 1982 Functional abdominal pain: further evidence that whole gut is affected. British Medical Journal 284: 1670–1672

Murray FE, Stinchcombe SJ, Hawkey CJ 1992 Development of biliary sludge in patients on intensive care unit: results of a prospective ultrasonographic study. Gut 33: 1123–1125

Neoptolemos JP, Bailey IS, Carr-Locke DL 1988 Sphincter of Oddi dysfunction: results of treatment by endoscopic sphincterotomy. British Journal of Surgery 75: 454–459

Nowakowska-Dulawa E, Nowak A, Kaczor R 1990 Effects of isosorbide dinitrate and Hymecromone on the motor activity of the sphincter of Oddi in man. World Congress of Gastroenterology, Sydney, 1990, p 160

Pasricha PJ, Miskovsky EP, Kalloo AN 1994 Intrasphincteric injection of botulinum toxin for suspected sphincter of Oddi dysfunction. Gut 35: 1319–1321

Peters JH, Ellison C, Innes JE 1991 Safety and efficacy of laparoscopic cholecystectomy. A prospective analysis of 100 initial patients. Annals of Surgery 213: 3–12

Reed DN, Fernandez M, Hicks PD 1993 Kinevac-assisted cholescintigraphy as an accurate predictor of chronic acalculous gallbladder disease and the likelihood of symptoms relief with cholecystectomy. American Surgeon 59: 273–277

Rhodes M, Lennard TWJ, Farndon JR, Taylor RMR 1988 Cholecystokinin (CCK) provocation test: long term follow-up after cholecystectomy. British Journal of Surgery 75: 951–953

Roberts-Thomson IC, Toouli J 1985 Is endoscopic sphincterotomy for disabling biliary type pain after cholecystectomy effective? Gastrointestinal Endoscopy 31: 370–375

Rolny P, Geenen JE, Hogan WJ et al 1991 Clinical features, manometric findings and endoscopic therapy in group I patients with sphincter of Oddi dysfunction. Gastrointestinal Endoscopy 37: 252–253

Rolny P, Arleback A, Funch-Jensen P et al 1986 Paradoxical response of sphincter of Oddi to intravenous injection of cholecystokinin or ceruletide. Manometric findings and results of treatment in biliary dyskinesia. Gut 27: 1507–1511

Ros E, Zambon D 1987 Postcholecystectomy symptoms. A prospective study of gallstone patients before and two years after surgery. Gut 28: 1500–1508

Ros E, Navarro S, Bru C et al 1991 Occult microlithiasis in 'idiopathic' acute pancreatitis. Prevention of relapses by cholecystectomy or ursodeoxycholic acid therapy. Gastroenterology 101: 1701–1709

Ruffolo TA, Sherman S, Silverman WB, Lehman GA 1991 The gallbladder ejection fraction and its relationship to sphincter of Oddi dysfunction. Gastrointestinal Endoscopy 37: 256

Sherman S, Ruffolo TA, Hawes RH, Lehman GA 1991b Complications of endoscopic sphincterotomy: a prospective series with emphasis on the increased risk associated with sphincter of Oddi dysfunction and nondilated bile ducts. Gastroenterology 101: 1068–1075

Sherman S, Troiano FP, Hawes RH et al 1991a Frequency of abnormal sphincter of Oddi manometry after cholecystectomy in patients with sphincter of Oddi dysfunction. American Journal of Gastroenterology 86: 586–590

Shiben T, Thomas A, Brodmerkel RM Jr et al 1996 Calcium bilirubinate crystals are an indicator of sphincter of Oddi dysfunction in patients with gallbladder in situ and biliary type pain. Gastroenterology 106: A3559

Soffer EE, Johlin FC 1994 Intestinal dysmotility in patients with sphincter of Oddi dysfunction. Digestive Diseases and Sciences 39: 1942–1946

Staritz M, Poralla T, Ewe K, Meyer zum Buschenfelde K-H 1985 Effect of glyceryl trinitrate on the sphincter of Oddi motility and baseline pressure. Gut 26: 194–197

Stefanini P, Carboni M, Patrassi N et al 1974 Factors influencing the long term results of cholecystectomy. Surgery, Gynecology and Obstetrics 139: 734–738

Sunderland GT, Carter DC 1988 Clinical application of the cholecystokinin provocation test. British Journal of Surgery 75: 444–449

Swarbrick ET, Hegarty JE, Bat L et al 1980 Site of pain from the irritable bowel syndrome. Lancet ii: 443–446

Tanaka M, Ikeda S, Nakayama F 1983 Continuous measurement of common bile duct pressure with an indwelling microtransducer introduced by duodenoscopy: a new diagnostic aid for postcholecystectomy dyskinesia: a preliminary report. Gastrointestinal Endoscopy 29: 83–88

Thatcher BS, Sivak MV, Tedesco FJ et al 1987 Endoscopic sphincterotomy for suspected dysfunction of the sphincter of Oddi. Gastrointestinal Endoscopy 33: 91–95

Troiano F, O'Connor, Sherman S 1990 Psychological aspects of sphincter of Oddi dysfunction patients. American Journal of Gastroenterology 85: 1261A

Velpen GCV, Shimi SM, Cuschieri A 1993 Outcome after cholecystectomy for symptomatic gallstone disease and effect of surgical of surgical access: laparoscopic open approach. Gut 34: 1448–1451

Viceconte G, Micheletti A 1995 Endoscopic manometry for the sphincter of Oddi: its usefulness for the diagnosis and treatment of benign apaillary stenosis. Scandinavian Journal of Gastroenterology 30: 797–803

Yap L, Wycherly AG, Morphett AD, Toouli J 1991 Acalculous biliary pain: cholecystectomy alleviates symptoms in patients with abnormal cholescintigraphy. Gastroenterology 101: 786–793

Yuasa N, Nimura Y, Yasiu A et al 1994 Sphincter of Oddi motility in patients with bile duct stones: a comparative study using percutaneous transhepatic manometry. Digestive Diseases and Sciences 39: 289–292

Westlake PJ, Hershfield NB, Kelly JK et al 1990 Chronic right upper quadrant pain without gallstones: does Hida scan predict outcome after cholecystectomy? American Journal of Gastroenterology 85: 986–990

Zech ER, Simmons LB, Kendrick RR et al 1991 Cholecystokinin enhanced hepatobiliary excretion with ejection fraction calculation as an indicator of disease of the gallbladder. Surgery, Gynecology and Obstetrics 172: 21–24

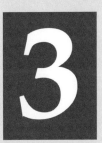

Functional disorders in context

Irritable bowel

H Spiro

I think of the 'irritable bowel' (IB) as no disease at all, but rather as one of many entirely human responses to economic, social, emotional and even spiritual malaise, a hard-wired reaction to stress. I take IB to be churned up in some people when their energies and emotions are channeled into other than the usual directions: 'The sorrow that has no vent in tears makes other organs weep' provides my guide.

For physicians, consideration of IB seems comparable to their assessment of pain. Too many doctors think of pain as sensations rattling along the c-fibers; they would do better sometimes to think of pain, especially chronic pain, in its more metaphorical guise of punishment or guilt. 'What have you done that you should be tormented in this way?' is a question with little currency in our secular age but, however transmuted, it still gets helpful answers.

Unfortunately, few modern physicians will agree, so accustomed are they to seeing disease and measuring it. Over the past 25 years many processes have been turned into diseases; the homely 'irritable bowel', no more important an affliction than gray hair, has matured into 'functional bowel disease' (FBD) and is now accounted an important – and fundable – economic problem. Yet when I ask an audience of physicians how often they themselves have taken time off because of gastrointestinal complaints like irritable bowel or dyspepsia, no one stands up. I take that to mean that the work days lost because of FBD are taken off more because of the job than because of the gut. In the philosophical world what has happened to IB is known as *reification*, where an idea becomes a thing. That is accounted a mistake.

That change has come about for several reasons. The first and most important is the increasing reliance of physicians on the eye for diagnosis. By 'eye', I mean all the visions of our new instruments which have enhanced what we doctors can see and measure; visual displays have become so breathtaking that the eye – seeing – has almost entirely replaced the ear – hearing. As far as physicians are concerned, it has become essential for their diagnoses. Cardiologists may hang a stethoscope about the neck, but to scrutinize diseases they look to wave patterns and scans rather than to the ear, to listen for a 'presystolic rumble', for example; gastroenterologists search out peptic ulcer on endoscopy and the coils of video film rather than deducing it from what the patient says. By greatly expanding our medical vision, modern technology has helped to convert a number of once unoffending everyday processes into 'things' that we can see and name, and dread. Sour stomach and dyspepsia once meant nervous indigestion or maybe an 'ulcer', but now ulcer has become 'peptic ulcer disease' and needs to be 'ruled out' and erased with antibiotics.

A second reason for reification comes in the frenzy for nosology or classification, fueled in the past by 'third-party payers' and now by managed care, whose accountants find it easier to pay for a specific 'entity' than for a symptom: this has turned esophageal reflux, once only the very common 'heartburn', into the more sonorous and dreaded 'gastroesophageal reflux disease', haunted by Barrett's mucosa and the specter of cancer. Modern doctors believe mainly in what they can see, while third-party payers pay only for what can be named and numbered.

A third reason is more peripheral to the considerations of this volume, but no less important. Modern Americans are unwilling to bear pain of any variety and therapeutic triumphalism has made most of our fellow citizens feel that doctors can take away the pain of existence with anodynes and diagnostic tests.

And so tomes like this explore functional bowel disease, even if, as many of the preceding chapters will suggest, it is not easy to mark the exact boundaries of that 'disease'. Is diarrhea from the stress of examinations in medical school quite the same as the diarrhea of depression or disappointment? Does functional bowel disease have specific qualities that can be enumerated and assessed or is FBD simply a *gestalt*, that is, a pattern which cannot be derived from enumeration of its components. I take IB and FBD to be concepts with fuzzy borders, unlikely subjects for enumeration or conclaves of experts in pleasant watering holes. Excitement, not disdain, makes burglars defecate in the rooms of the houses they have despoiled, just as soldiers during the First World War had diarrhea on 'going over the top'. There are countless other examples which seem more like natural responses to stress than symptoms of functional bowel disease. What about the teacher 'burned out' on the job or the pipe-fitter worried about losing his livelihood? Do they have FBD that requires colonoscopy, motility studies and more?

As a gastroenterologist who does no procedures, I see many patients who have complaints that have defied a host of usually 'invasive' diagnostic procedures. I find some comfort in dividing their symptoms into the *pathophysiologic*, with a clear relation to normal gut physiology, or *symbolic*, what used to be called 'hysterical' because they are unsophisticatedly *non*-physiologic. I try to ascertain whether abdominal pain bears any relation to gut function, that is, whether it is worsened or relieved by moving the bowels, whether eating brings on the pain or makes it better, and so forth. But when I talk with patients who can tell me only of their 'pain', I begin to suspect that pain will make no appearance in any of the usual abdominal scans or endoscopic scrutinies. I recall Elaine Scarry's advice that 'To hear about pain is to be in doubt, to have pain is to know', but then I begin to explore the mystical, symbolic socioeconomic origin of that pain on my very first encounter with the patient. That is not always easy and here I will be content simply with reminding the practitioner that diarrhea sometimes may prove only diarrhea, but that sometimes it turns out to be sorrow or despair or grief.

Having foraged in the fields of functional complaints for many years, less and less often rejoicing in the discovery of an organic disease as the number of gastroenterologists in Connecticut has grown from five to over 200, I have found in certain aphorisms great support. One holds that neither character nor bowel habits change very much over a lifetime, without some specific new stimulus. The boy or girl who cheats on examinations in high school may well smooth out curves in the laboratory; the young man or woman who makes friends with a cripple in a wheelchair will go the proverbial 'extra mile' as a doctor in a medical extremity. Thus the man or woman who boasts a bowel movement every morning after breakfast will continue the same matutinal evacuation at 60, unless cancer or depression has supervened. New-onset diarrhea calls for a sigmoidoscopy, to be sure, but much patient–doctor conversation should precede the ordering of gastrin or VIP assays or even of computerized scans for FBD.

Simple but strict criteria hold for what I still prefer to call irritable bowel. Whatever the complaints, whether diarrhea or constipation, they must have begun by adolescence; my long-time prejudice, affirmed by modern observations, holds that women are more likely to have constipation where men are more likely to have diarrhea. So convinced am I of this that when a young woman complains of diarrhea, I am as inclined to look for a specific cause as when I see a young man with constipation. In the typical IB pattern as I generalize it, with age, constipation is followed by abdominal pain made worse by failure to empty the bowel and relieved by so doing. I do not expect the diarrhea of IB to occur at night nor to lead to accidents; it will wax and wane depending on life events.

Lactose intolerance becomes common around adolescence and many other processes can simulate IB. By and large, however, if symptoms are gradual in onset and characteristic, I carry out no diagnostic studies in the young before testing their response to treatment. That may seem overly cavalier but failure to recognize ulcerative proctitis, which could account for an irritable bowel picture, in someone who responds to mild measures brings no trouble for no one is harmed. In persons (I do not consider them patients) with diarrhea, I routinely rule out lactose intolerance; diagnosis enough for me is relief from avoiding milk products or worsening complaints after drinking milk.

More important, however, having an irritable bowel does not protect people from developing other disorders and so I am always wary about another problem, like a colon cancer coming on over the years and I warn these persons about that.

I quarrel with those who think first of 'functional bowel disease' when they hear about new colonic disturbances from the man or woman of 45 or 50. I cannot make that diagnosis when colonic dysfunction comes on in mid-life. Character and bowel habits, let me repeat, do not change throughout life. The diagnosis of FBD goes out the window until after a thorough diagnostic work-up. That is all those persons may have, but only after thorough testing can I come to that conclusion. I continue to reserve the diagnosis of 'irritable bowel' for persons with the lifelong patterns already described, partly because I can help them and partly because I believe that middle-age 'FBD' has a different origin from that which begins in adolescence.

The symptomatic management of such people comes from optimism born of experience. The constipated are asked to follow the following ritual:

1. Drink half a glass of hot water mixed with half a glass of orange juice on an empty stomach on awakening.
2. Eat three servings (three cups) of stewed or cooked fruit and three cups of stewed or cooked vegetables each day.
3. Drink 12 glasses of water each day.
4. Eat or drink anything else that you want.

People with diarrhea are instructed to omit fruits and vegetables from the diet for 2–3 weeks and to take some Metamucil or similar substance, to firm up the stool. Sometimes, they need to take a tablet or two of Lomotil or Imodium after the first diarrheal movement in the morning; most patients with diarrhea or FBD usually respond, but some need more pills. After that, I lay out a long-term plan not dissimilar from that described elsewhere in this book.

Only when patients are not quickly relieved do I go on to diagnostic studies quite similar to those laid out elsewhere. Others have argued for the reassurance of early diagnosis, but my unenumerated impression is that the reassurance of a firm opinion and the sacrament of a written program suffice, along with the appropriate dietary modifications.

This is not the place to discuss the management of patients with functional bowel disease which does *not* fulfill the criteria for life-long colonic responses, the patients with 'agonizing' abdominal pain 'all over' without any elicitable precipitants. They fall into a category of 'psychogenic' pain and are more likely to be helped by exploration of life events and by serotonin reuptake inhibitors. Incidentally, for such gastrointestinal complaints the old standby of Elavil is still as effective as any of the newer agents, thanks in part to its antimuscarinic effects. My son and daughter, both psychiatrists, reassure me that even though Elavil is now 30 years old, it remains ideal for this intention.

I must close this brief discussion with a tip of the hat to alternative medicine practitioners who have reminded us in the mainstream about the patient as a person. While it seems unlikely that alternative practitioners follow their prescribed rituals to the letter, any more than we mainstream practitioners, still their emphasis on taking the time for a *complete* history seems important. Catharsis, the purging of emotions by weeping or by talking, brings relief. The words of the doctor or the words of the patient have as much to do with relief as the program that we prescribe. Catharsis does more than any cathartics!

Index